S0-AQJ-974

Study Guide for

Memmler's

Structure and Function
of the Human Body

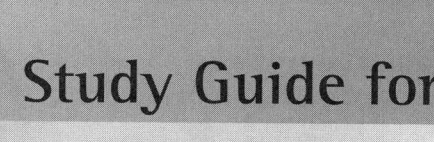
Study Guide for

Memmler's
Structure and Function
of the Human Body

Eighth Edition

Barbara Janson Cohen, BA, MA
Delaware County Community College
Media, Pennslyvania

Kerry L. Hull, BSc, PhD
Associate Professor
Department of Biology
Bishop's University
Lennoxville, Quebec
Canada

Jason Taylor, BSc, MSc
Instructor, Red River College
Winnepeg, Canada
Consulting Editor

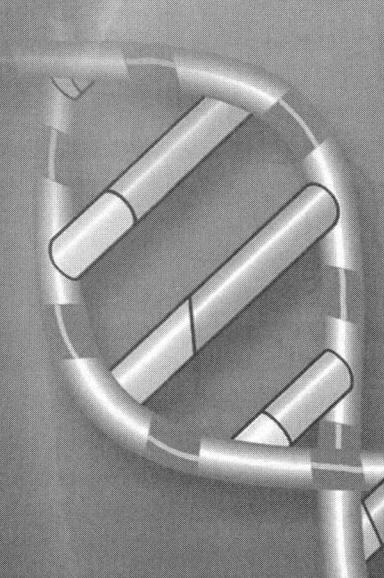

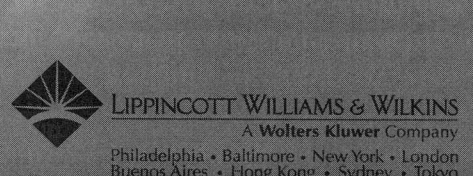
LIPPINCOTT WILLIAMS & WILKINS
A **Wolters Kluwer** Company

Philadelphia • Baltimore • New York • London
Buenos Aires • Hong Kong • Sydney • Tokyo

Editor: *John Goucher*
Managing Editor: *Molly M. Ward*
Marketing Manager: *Hilary Henderson*
Project Editor: *Kevin Johnson*
Designer: *Armen Kojoyian*
Artwork: *Dragonfly Media Group*
Cover Illustration and Cover Design: *Armen Kojoyian*
Typesetter: *Maryland Composition*
Printer: *Victor Graphics*

Copyright © 2005 Lippincott Williams & Wilkins

351 West Camden Street
Baltimore, Maryland 21201-2436 USA

530 Walnut Street
Philadelphia, Pennsylvania 19106

All rights reserved. This book is protected by copyright. No part of this book may be reproduced in any form or by any means, including photocopying, or utilized by any information storage and retrieval system without written permission from the copyright owner.

Printed in the United States of America

ISBN 0-7817-5185-3

The publishers have made every effort to trace the copyright holders for borrowed material. If they have inadvertently overlooked any, they will be pleased to make the necessary arrangements at the first opportunity.

To purchase additional copies of this book, call our customer service department at **(800) 638-3030** or fax orders to **(301) 824-7390**. For other book services, including chapter reprints and large quantity sales, ask for the Special Sales department.

For all other calls originating outside of the United States, please call **(301) 714-2324**.

Visit *Lippincott Williams & Wilkins* on the Internet: **http://www.lww.com**. Lippincott Williams & Wilkins customer service representatives are available from 8:30 am to 6:00 pm, EST, Monday through Friday, for telephone access.

05 06 07 08
1 2 3 4 5 6 7 8 9 10

The *Study Guide for Memmler's Structure and Function of the Human Body*, eighth edition, assists the beginning student to learn basic information required in the health occupations. Although it will be more effective when used in conjunction with the eighth edition of *Structure and Function of the Human Body*, the Study Guide may also be used to supplement other textbooks on basic anatomy and physiology.

The questions in this edition reflect revisions and updating of the text. The labeling and coloring exercises are taken from the all-new illustrations designed for the book. The "Practical Applications" section of each chapter uses clinical situations to test understanding of a subject. Comparing the normal with the abnormal helps a student to gain some understanding of disease prevention and health maintenance.

The exercises are planned to help in student learning, not merely to test knowledge. A certain amount of repetition has been purposely incorporated as a means of reinforcement. Matching questions require the student to write out complete answers, giving practice in spelling as well as recognition of terms. Other question formats include multiple choice, completion, true–false, and short essays. The true–false questions must be corrected if they are false. The essay answers provided are examples of suitable responses, but other presentations of the material are acceptable.

All answers to the Study Guide questions are in the Instructor's Manual that accompanies the text.

Learning about the Human Body

You already have some ideas about the human body that will influence how you learn the information in this textbook. Many of your theories are correct, and this Study Guide, created to accompany the eighth edition of Memmler's *Structure and Function of the Human Body*, will simply add detail and complexity to these ideas. Other theories, however, may be too simplistic. It can be difficult to replace these ingrained beliefs with more accurate information. For instance, many students think that the lungs actively inflate and deflate as we breathe, but it is the diaphragm and the rib-cage muscles that accomplish all of the work. Learning physiology or any other subject therefore involves:

1. **Construction**: Adding to and enhancing your previous store of ideas.
2. **Reconstruction**: Replacing misconceptions (prior views and ideas) with scientifically sound principles.
3. **Self-monitoring**. Construction and reconstruction require that you also monitor your personal understanding of a particular topic and consciously formulate links between what you are learning and what you have previously learned. Rote learning is not an effective way to learn anatomy and physiology (or almost anything else, for that matter). **Metacognition** is monitoring your own understanding. Metacognition is very effective if it takes the form of self-questioning during the lectures. Try to ask yourself questions during lectures such as "What is the prof trying to show here?" "What do these numbers really mean?" or "How does this stuff relate to the stuff we covered yesterday?" Self-questioning will help you create links between concepts. In other words, try to be an **active learner** during the lectures. Familiarity with the material is not enough; you will have to internalize it and apply it to succeed. You can greatly enhance your ability to be an active learner by reading the appropriate sections of the textbook before the lecture.

Each field in biology has its own language. This language is not designed to make your life difficult; the terms often represent complex concepts. Rote memorization of definitions will not help you learn. Indeed, because biological terms often have different meanings in everyday conversation, you probably hold some definitions that are misleading and must be revised. For example, you may say that someone has a "good metabolism" if they can eat enormous meals and stay slender. However, the term "metabolism" actually refers to all of the chemical reactions that occur in the body, including those that build muscle and fat. We learn a new language not by reading about it but by using it. The Study Guide you hold in your hands employs a number of learning techniques in every chapter to help you become comfortable with the language of anatomy and physiology.

"Addressing the Learning Outcomes"

This section will help you master the material both verbally and visually. The first activity, writing out answers to the learning outcomes, will provide you with a good overview of the important concepts in the chapter. The labeling and coloring atlas will be especially useful for mastering anatomy. You can use the atlas in two ways. First, follow the instructions to label and color (when appropriate) each exercise, using your textbook if necessary. You will use the same color to write the name of the structure and to color it. Colored pencils work best, but you may have to outline in black names written in light colors. Coloring exercises are fun, and have been shown to enhance learning.

"Making the Connections": Learning through Concept Maps

This learning activity uses concept mapping to master definitions and concepts. You can think of concept mapping as creating a web of information. Individual terms have a tendency to get lost, but a web of terms is more easily maintained in memory. You can make a concept map by following these steps:

1. Select the concepts to map (6–10 is a good number). Try to use a mixture of nouns, verbs, and processes.
2. If one exists, place the most general, important, or over-riding concept at the top or in the center and arrange the other terms around it. Organize the terms so that closely related terms are close together.
3. Draw arrows between concepts that are related. Write a sentence to connect the two concepts that begins with the term at the beginning of the arrow and ends with the term at the end of the arrow.

For instance, consider a simple concept map composed of three terms: *student learning*, *professors*, and *textbooks*. Write the three terms at the three corners of a triangle, separated from each other by 3–4 inches. Next is the difficult part: devising connecting phrases that explain the relationship between any two terms. What is the essence of the relationship between student learning and professors? An arrow could be drawn from *professors* to *student learning*, with the connecting phrase "***can explain difficult concepts to facilitate***". The relationship would be "*Professors **can explain difficult concepts to facilitate** student learning.*" Draw arrows between all other term pairs (*student learning* and *textbooks*, *textbooks* and *professors*) and try to come up with connecting phrases. Make sure that the phrase is read in the direction of the arrow.

There are two concept mapping exercises for most chapters. The first exercise consists of filling in boxes and, in the later maps, connecting phrases. The guided concept maps for Chapters 1 through 7 ask you to think of the appropriate term for each box. The guided concept maps for Chapters 8 through 25 are more traditional concept maps. Pairs of terms are linked together by a connecting phrase. The phrase is read in the direction of the arrow. For instance, an arrow leading from "*genes*" to "*chromosomes*" could result in the phrase "*Genes **are found on pieces of DNA called** chromosomes.*" The second optional exercise provides a suggested list of terms to use to construct your own map. This second exercise is a powerful learning tool, because you will identify your own links between concepts. **The act of creating a concept map is an effective way to understand terms and concepts.**

"Testing Your Knowledge"

These questions should be completed after you have read the textbook and completed the other learning activities in the study guide. Try to answer as many questions as possible without referring to your notes or the text. As in the end-of-chapter questions, there are three different levels of questions. Type I questions (Building Understanding) test simple recall: how well have you learned the material? Type II questions (Understanding Concepts) examine your ability to integrate and apply the information in simple practical situations. Type III questions (Conceptual Thinking) are the most challenging. They ask you to apply your knowledge to new situations and concepts. There is often more than one right answer to Conceptual Thinking questions. The answers to all questions are available from your instructor.

Learning from the World Around You

The best way to learn anatomy and physiology is to immerse yourself in the subject. Tell your friends and family what you are learning. Discover more about recent health advances from television, newspapers, and magazines. Our knowledge about the human body is constantly changing. The work you will do using the Study Guide can serve as a basis for life-long learning about the structure and function of the human body.

Contents

Study Guide for

Memmler's

Structure and Function

of the Human Body

unit **I**

The Body as a Whole

chapter 1

Organization of the Human Body

Overview

Anatomy is the study of body structure, whereas **physiology** is the study of how the body functions.

Living things are organized from simple to complex levels. The simplest living form is the **cell**, the basic unit of life. Specialized cells are grouped into **tissues**, which, in turn, are combined to form **organs**; these organs form systems, which work together to maintain the body.

The systems include the integumentary system, the body's covering; the skeletal system, the framework of the body; the muscular system, which moves the bones; the nervous system, the central control system that includes the organs of special sense; the endocrine system, which produces the regulatory hormones; the circulatory system, consisting of the heart, blood vessels, and lymphatic vessels that transport vital substances; the respiratory system, which adds oxygen to the blood and removes carbon dioxide; the digestive system, which converts raw food materials into products usable by cells; the urinary system, which removes wastes and excess water; and the reproductive system, by which new individuals of the species are produced.

All the cellular reactions that sustain life comprise **metabolism**, which can be divided into **catabolism** and **anabolism**. In catabolism, complex substances are broken down into simpler molecules. When the nutrients from food are broken down by catabolism, energy is released. This energy is stored in the compound **ATP** (adenosine triphosphate) for use by the cells. In anabolism, simple compounds are built into substances needed for cell activities.

All the systems work together to maintain a state of balance or **homeostasis**. The main mechanism for maintaining homeostasis is **negative feedback**, by which the state of the body is the signal to keep conditions within set limits.

The human body is composed of large amounts of fluid, the amount and composition of which must be constantly regulated. The **extracellular fluid** consists of the fluid that surrounds the cells as well as the fluid circulated in blood and lymph. The fluid within cells is the **intracellular fluid**.

Study of the body requires knowledge of directional terms to locate parts and to relate various parts to each other. Several planes of division represent different directions in which cuts can be made through the body. Separation of the body into areas and regions, together with the use of the special terminology for directions and locations, makes it possible to describe an area within the human body with great accuracy.

The large internal spaces of the body are cavities in which various organs are located. The **dorsal cavity** is subdivided into the **cranial cavity** and the **spinal cavity (canal)**. The **ventral cavity** is subdivided into the **thoracic** and **abdominopelvic cavities**. Imaginary lines are used to divide the abdomen into regions for study and diagnosis.

The metric system is used for all scientific measurements. This system is easy to use because it is based on multiples of 10.

Learning the Language: Word Anatomy

Complete the following table by writing the correct word part or meaning in the space provided. For each word part, write a term that contains the word part.

Word Part	Meaning	Example
1. -tomy	_____	_____
2. -stasis	_____	_____
3. _____	nature, physical	_____
4. homeo-	_____	_____
5. _____	apart, away from	_____
6. _____	down	_____
7. _____	upward	_____

Addressing the Learning Outcomes

I. Writing Exercise

The learning outcomes for Chapter 1 are listed below. These outcomes provide an overview of the major topics covered in this chapter. On a separate piece of paper, try to write out an answer to each outcome. All of the answers can be found in the pages of the textbook. Learning Outcomes 2, 9, 10, 11, and 12 are also addressed in the Coloring Atlas.

1. Define the terms *anatomy* and *physiology*.
2. Describe the organization of the body from chemicals to the whole organism.
3. List 11 body systems and give the general function of each.
4. Define *metabolism* and name the two phases of metabolism.
5. Briefly explain the role of ATP in the body.
6. Differentiate between extracellular and intracellular fluids.
7. Define and give examples of homeostasis.
8. Compare negative feedback and positive feedback.
9. List and define the main directional terms for the body.

10. List and define the three planes of division of the body.
11. Name the subdivisions of the dorsal and ventral cavities.
12. Name and locate subdivisions of the abdomen.
13. Name the basic units of length, weight, and volume in the metric system.
14. Define the metric prefixes *kilo-, centi-, milli-,* and *micro-.*
15. Show how word parts are used to build words related to the body's organization.

II. Labeling and Coloring Atlas

EXERCISE 1-1: Levels of Organization (text Fig. 1-1)

INSTRUCTIONS

1. Write the name or names of each labeled part on the numbered lines in different colors.
2. Color the different structures on the diagram with the corresponding color. For instance, if you wrote "cell" in blue, color the cell blue.

1. _____

2. _____

3. _____

4. _____

5. _____

6. _____

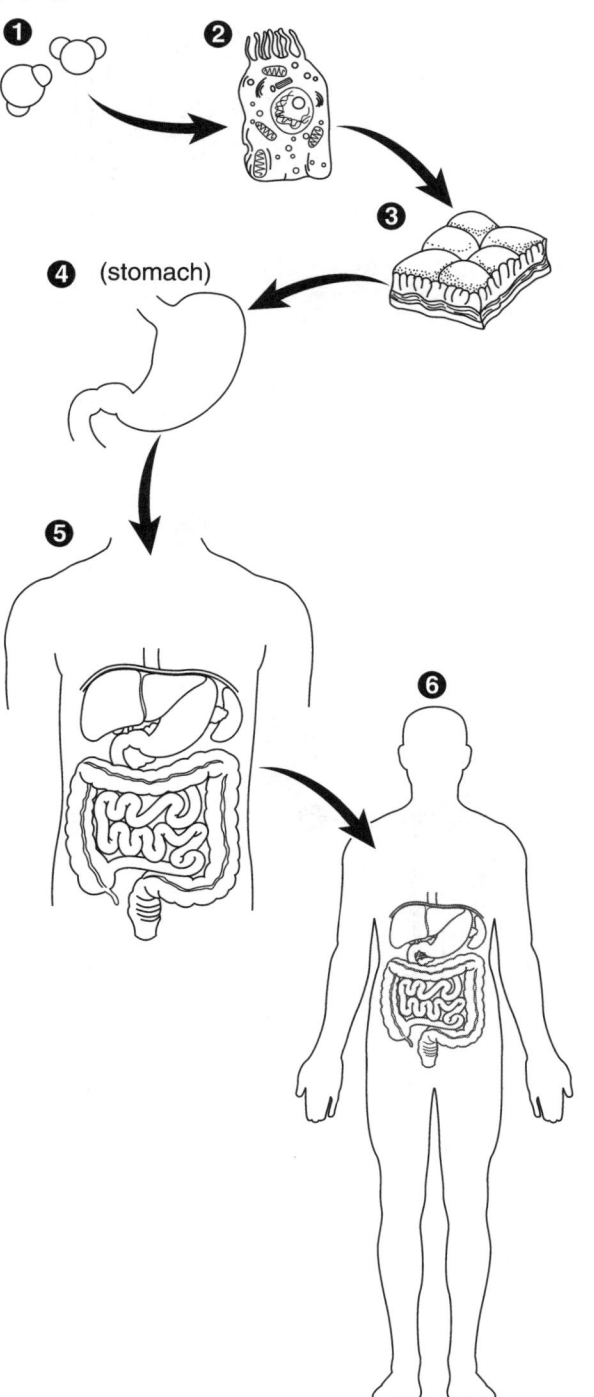

❹ (stomach)

Exercise 1-2: Directional Terms (text Fig. 1-7)

Instructions

1. Write the name of each directional term on the numbered lines in different colors.
2. Color the arrow corresponding to each directional term with appropriate color.

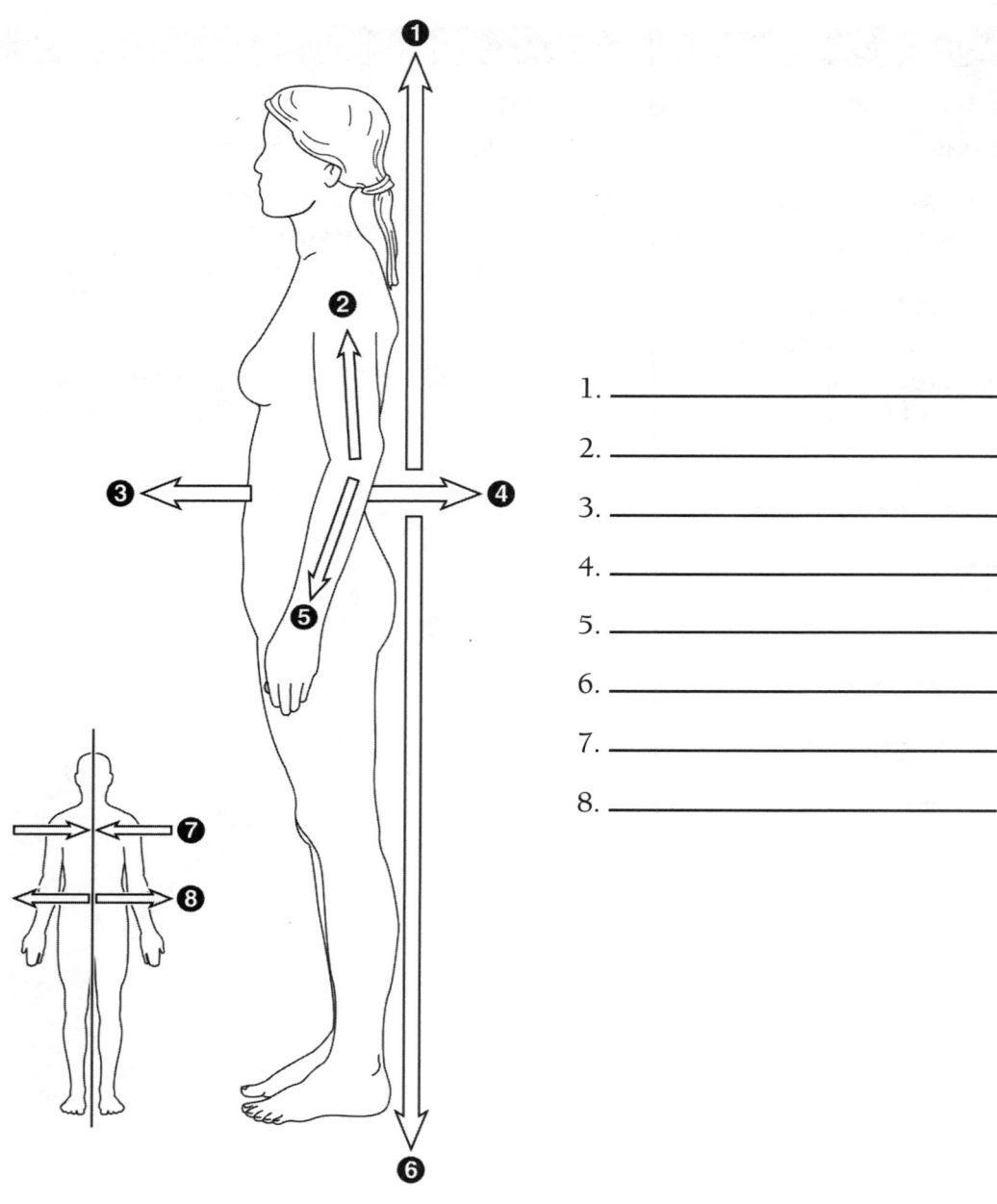

1. _____

2. _____

3. _____

4. _____

5. _____

6. _____

7. _____

8. _____

EXERCISE 1-3: Planes of Division (text Fig. 1-8)

INSTRUCTIONS

1. Write the names of the three planes of division on the correct numbered lines in different colors.
2. Color each plane in the illustration with its corresponding color.

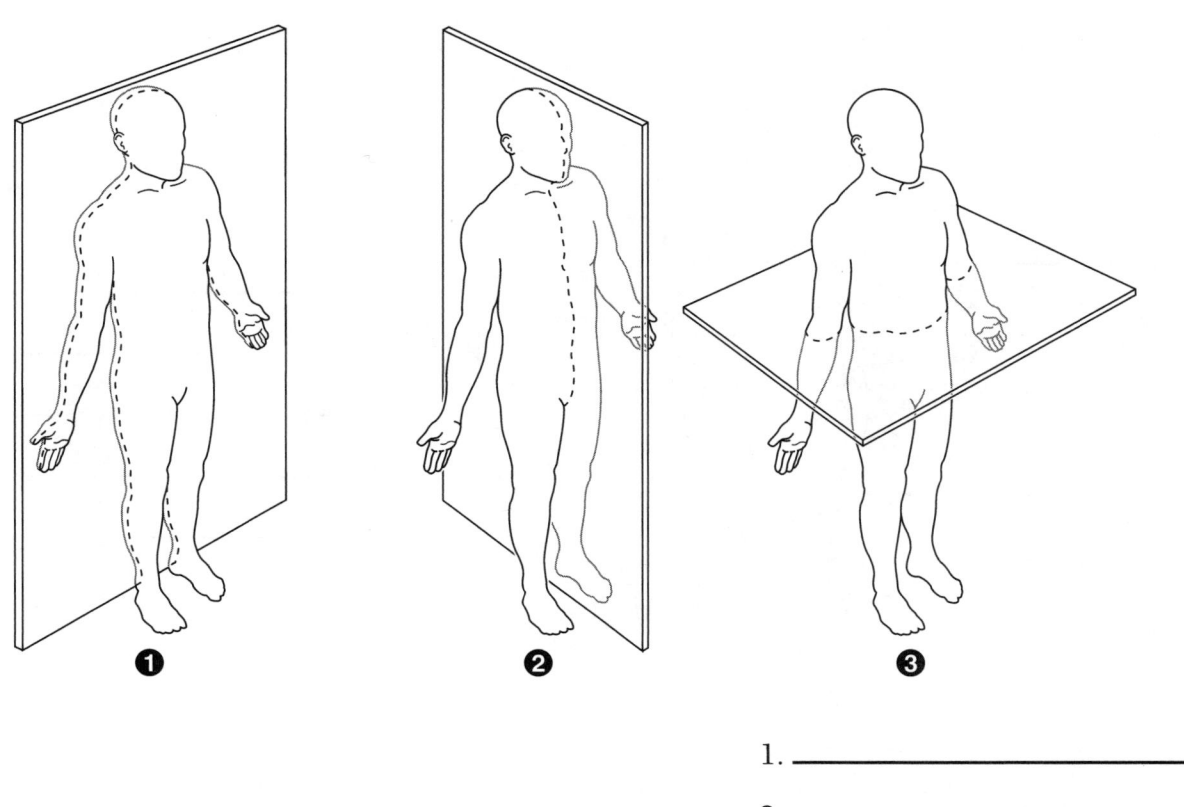

1. _____

2. _____

3. _____

Exercise 1-4: Lateral View of Body Cavities (text Fig. 1-11)

Instructions

1. Write the names of the different body cavities and other structures in the appropriate spaces in different colors. Try to choose related colors for the dorsal cavity subdivisions and for the ventral cavity subdivisions.
2. Color each part with the corresponding color.

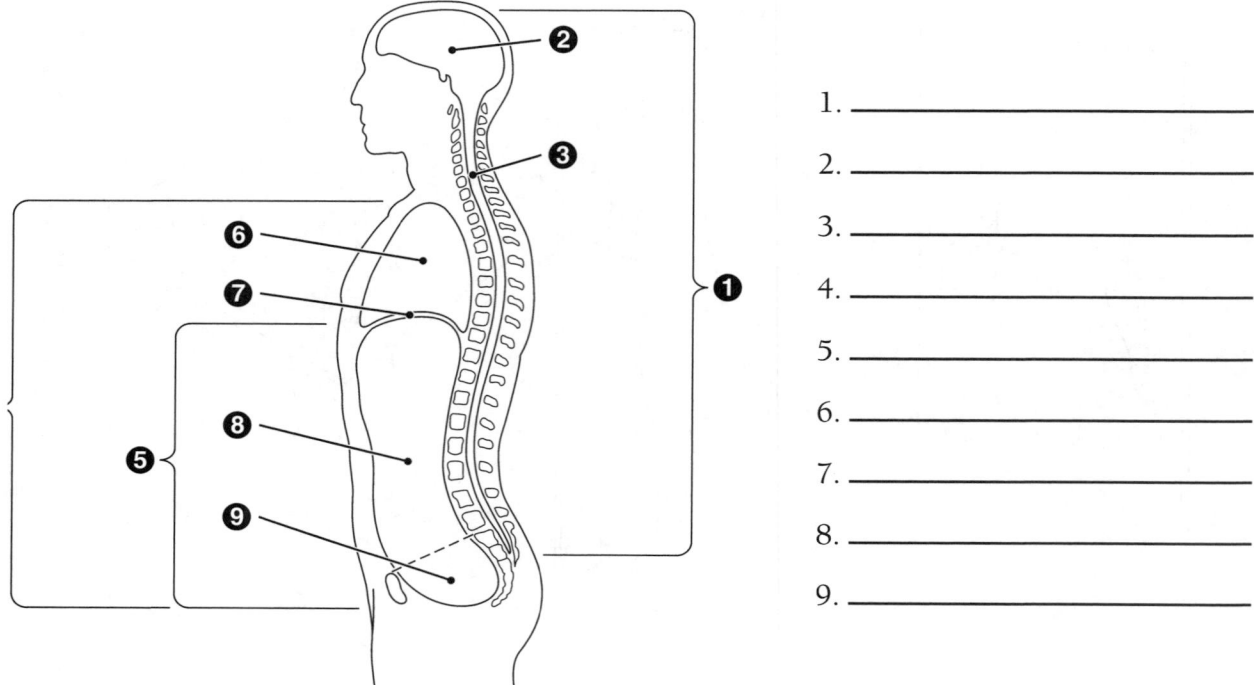

1. _____

2. _____

3. _____

4. _____

5. _____

6. _____

7. _____

8. _____

9. _____

EXERCISE 1-5: Regions of the Abdomen (text Fig. 1-13)

INSTRUCTIONS

1. Write the names of the nine regions of the abdomen on the appropriate numbered lines in different colors.
2. Color the corresponding region with the appropriate color.

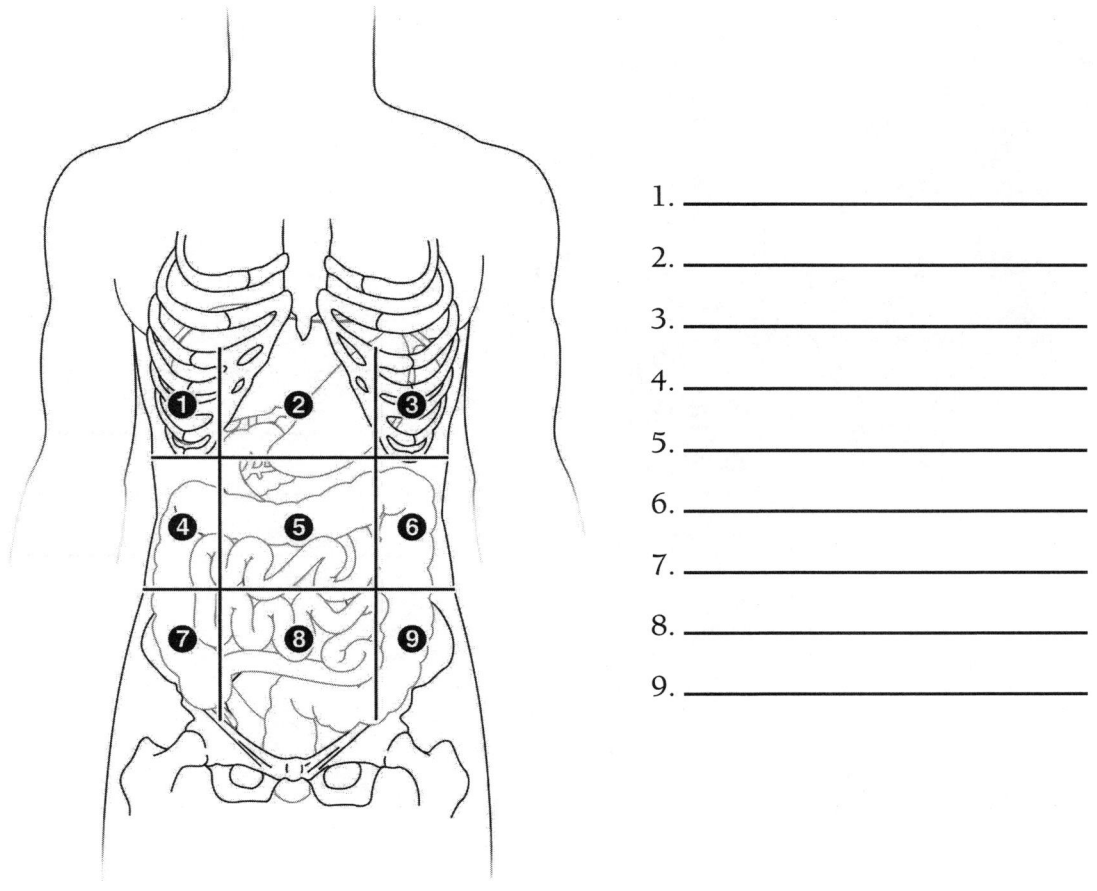

1. _____
2. _____
3. _____
4. _____
5. _____
6. _____
7. _____
8. _____
9. _____

EXERCISE 1-6: Quadrants of the Abdomen (text Fig. 1-14)

INSTRUCTIONS

1. Write the names of the four quadrants of the abdomen on the appropriate numbered lines in different colors.
2. Color the corresponding quadrant in the appropriate color.

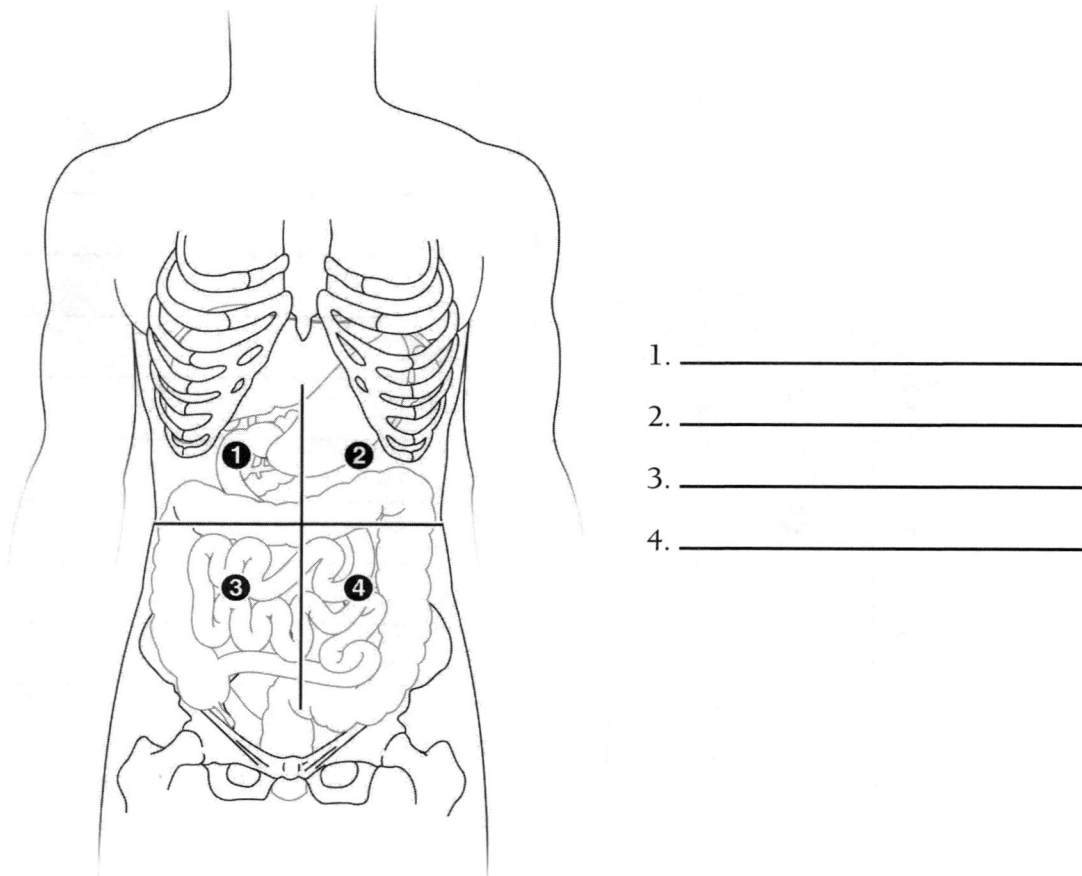

1. _____

2. _____

3. _____

4. _____

Making the Connections

The following concept map deals with the body's cavities and their divisions. Complete the concept map by filling in the blanks with the appropriate word or term for the cavity, division, subdivision, or region.

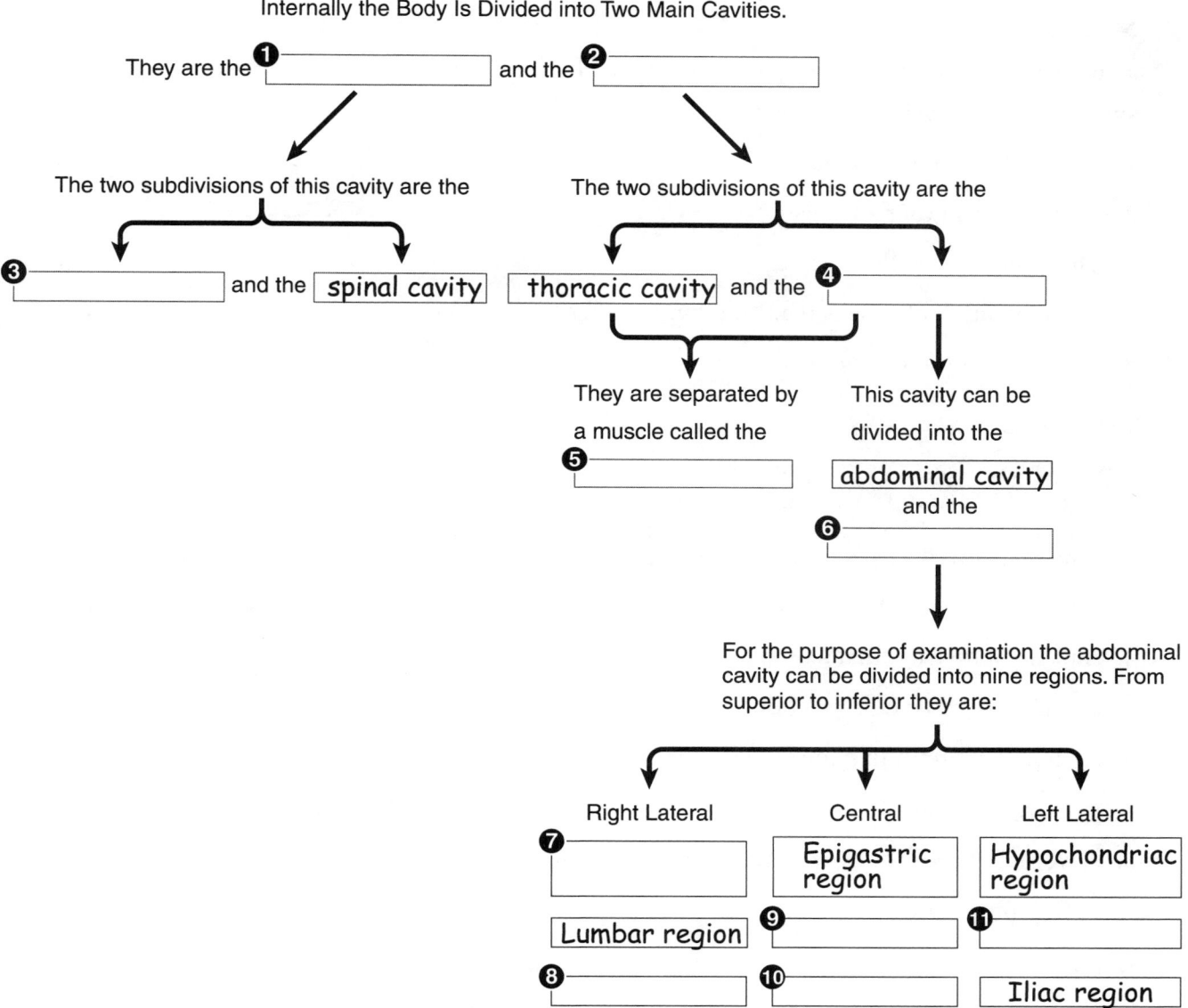

Internally the Body Is Divided into Two Main Cavities.

They are the **❶** _____ and the **❷** _____

The two subdivisions of this cavity are the   The two subdivisions of this cavity are the

❸ _____ and the   spinal cavity   thoracic cavity   and the   **❹** _____

They are separated by   This cavity can be
a muscle called the   divided into the

❺ _____   abdominal cavity
                                   and the
                              ❻ _____

For the purpose of examination the abdominal cavity can be divided into nine regions. From superior to inferior they are:

Right Lateral	Central	Left Lateral
❼ _____	Epigastric region	Hypochondriac region
Lumbar region	**❾** _____	**⓫** _____
❽ _____	**❿** _____	Iliac region

Testing Your Knowledge
Building Understanding

I. Matching Exercises

Matching only within each group, write the answers in the spaces provided.

➤ **Group A**

anatomy   tissue   organ   cell

system   physiology   chemical

1. The study of body function   _____

2. A specialized group of cells   _____

3. The basic unit of life   _____

4. A combination of tissues that function together   _____

5. The study of body structure   _____

➤ **Group B**

posterior   anterior   medial

caudal   lateral   horizontal   distal

1. A term that indicates a location toward the front   _____

2. A term that means farther from the origin of a part   _____

3. A plane of division that also is described
   as a transverse or cross-section   _____

4. A directional term that means away from the midline
   (toward the side)   _____

5. A word that means nearer to the sacral (lowermost) region
   of the spinal cord   _____

➤ **Group C**

hypochondriac   thoracic   sagittal   epigastric

frontal   transverse   hypogastric

1. A plane of division that is also called the coronal plane   _____

2. A plane that divides the body into superior and inferior parts   _____

3. Term describing the lateral regions of the abdomen
   just below the ribs   _____

4. A term that describes the uppermost (chest) portion of the
   ventral body cavity   _____

5. A plane that divides the body into left and right parts _____

6. The abdominal region below the umbilical region _____

➤ **Group D**

nervous sytem   integumentary system   cardiovascular system

endocrine system   lymphatic system   digestive system   urinary system

1. The system that processes sensory information _____

2. The system that delivers nutrients to body tissues _____

3. The system that breaks down and absorbs food _____

4. The system that includes the fingernails _____

5. The system that includes the bladder _____

II. Multiple Choice

Select the best answer and write the letter of your choice in the blank.

1. The energy currency of the cell is: 1. _____
   a. PTA
   b. ATP
   c. steroids
   d. proteins
2. The diaphragm separates: 2. _____
   a. the cranial and the spinal cavities
   b. the dorsal and ventral cavities
   c. the thoracic and abdominal cavities
   d. the abdominal and pelvic cavities
3. The breakdown of complex molecules into more simple ones is called: 3. _____
   a. anabolism
   b. synthesis
   c. negative feedback
   d. catabolism
4. Fluids located outside the cells are described as: 4. _____
   a. extracellular
   b. intracellular
   c. superior
   d. extraneous
5. The heart and the blood vessels compose the: 5. _____
   a. circulatory system
   b. nervous system
   c. integumentary system
   d. digestive system
6. The navel is found in the: 6. _____
   a. lumbar region
   b. umbilical region
   c. iliac region
   d. hypogastric region

7. The study of normal body function is called: 7. _____
   a. physiology
   b. homeology
   c. anatomy
   d. chemistry
8. A penny-shaped slice of a banana is probably which type of section?   8. _____
   a. longitudinal section
   b. sagittal section
   c. cross-section
   d. coronal section

III. Completion Exercise

Write the word or phrase that correctly completes each sentence.

➤ Group A: General Terminology

1. In the anatomical position, the body is upright and palms

   are facing   _____

2. Fluid inside cells is called   _____

3. Catabolism can generate energy in the form of   _____

4. Negative feedback is a mechanism for maintaining an internal

   state of balance known as   _____

5. The sum of all catabolic and anabolic reactions in the body

   is called   _____

6. The process of childbirth is an example of a type of feedback

   called   _____

➤ Group B: Body Cavities, Directional Terms, and Planes of Division

1. The term that means nearer to the head is   _____

2. The space enclosing the brain and spinal cord forms a

   continuous cavity called the   _____

3. The abdomen may be divided into four regions, each of

   which is called a(n)   _____

4. The cavity that houses the bladder is the   _____

5. The plane that divides the body into anterior and posterior

   parts is the   _____

6. The ventral body cavity that contains the stomach, most of

   the intestine, the liver, and the spleen is the   _____

7. The abdomen may be subdivided into nine regions,

   including three along the midline. The region closest to the

   sternum (breastbone) is the   _____

8. The space between the lungs is called the   _____

9. The diaphragm separates the abdominopelvic cavity from the   _____

➤ **Group C: The Metric System**
Write the word that correctly completes each sentence.

1. The number of milligrams in a gram is   _____

2. The number of centimeters in an inch is   _____

3. The number of millimeters in a centimeter is   _____

4. Using the metric system, your height would probably

   be calculated in   _____

5. A liter is a slightly greater volume than a   _____

Understanding Concepts

I. True or False

For each question, write "T" for true or "F" for false in the blank to the left of each number. If a statement is false, correct it by replacing the underlined term and write the correct statement in the blanks below the question.

_____ 1. Proteins are broken down into their component parts by the process of <u>anabolism</u>.

_____

_____ 2. Your mouth is <u>inferior</u> to your nose.

_____

_____ 3. The brain is <u>caudal</u> to the spine.

_____

_____ 4. Your umbilicus is <u>lateral</u> to the left lumbar region.

_____

_____ 5. The right iliac region is found in the <u>right lower quadrant</u>.

_____

II. Practical Applications

Study each discussion. Then write the appropriate word or phrase in the space provided.

➤ **Group A: Directional Terms**

1. The gallbladder is located just above the colon. The directional term that describes the position of the gallbladder with regard to the colon is _____

2. The kidneys are closer to the sides of the body than is the stomach. The directional term that describes the kidneys with regard to the stomach is _____

3. The entrance to the stomach is nearest the point of origin or beginning of the stomach, so this part is said to be _____

4. The knee is located closer to the hip than is the ankle. The term that describes the position of the ankle with regard to the knee is _____

5. The ears are closer to the back of the head than is the nose. The term that describes the position of the ears with regard to the nose is _____

6. The stomach is below the esophagus; it may be described as _____

7. The head of the pancreas is nearer the midsagittal plane than is its tail portion, so the head part is more _____

➤ **Group B: Body Cavities and the Metric System**

Study the following cases and answer the questions based on the nine divisions of the abdomen and your knowledge of the metric system.

1. Mr. A bruised his ribs in a dirt buggy accident. He experienced tenderness in the upper left side of his abdomen. In which of the nine abdominal regions are the injured ribs located? _____

2. Ms. D had a history of gallstones. The operation to remove these stones involved the upper right part of the abdominal cavity. Which abdominal division is this? _____

3. After her operation, Ms. D was able to bring her stones home in a jar. She was told that her stones weighed 0.025 kilograms in total. How many milligrams do her stones weigh? _____

4. Ms. C is 8 weeks pregnant. Her uterus is still confined to the most inferior division of the abdomen. This region is called the _____

5. Ms. C is experiencing heartburn as a result of her pregnancy. The discomfort is found just below the breastbone, in the _____

6. After the birth of her child, Ms. C opted for a tubal ligation. The doctor threaded a fiberoptic device through a small incision in her navel as part of the surgery. Ms. C will now have a very small incision in which portion of the abdomen? _____

7. Ms. C's incision was 2 millimeters in length. What is the length of her incision in centimeters? _____

➤ Group C: Body Systems

The triage nurse in the emergency room was showing a group of students how she assessed patients with disorders in different body systems. Study each situation, and answer the following questions based on your knowledge of the 11 body systems.

1. One person was describing dizziness and blurred vision. Vision is controlled by the _____

2. One person had been injured in a snowboarding accident, spraining his wrist joint. The wrist joint is part of the _____

3. A woman had attempted a particularly onerous yoga pose and felt a sharp pain in her left thigh. Now she is limping. The nurse suspected a tear to structures belonging to the _____

4. An extremely tall individual entered the clinic, reporting a headache. The nurse suspected that he had excess production of a particular hormone. The specialized glands that synthesize hormones comprise the _____

5. A middle-aged woman was brought in with loss of ability to move the right side of her body. The nurse felt that a blood clot in a blood vessel of the brain was producing the symptoms. Blood vessels are part of the _____

6. A man reporting pain in the abdomen and vomiting blood was brought in by his family. A problem was suspected in the system responsible for taking in food and converting it to usable products. This system is the _____

7. Each client was assessed for changes in the color of the outer covering of the body. The outer covering is called the skin, which is part of the _____

8. A young woman was experiencing pain in her pelvic region. The doctor suspected a problem with her ovaries. The ovaries are part of the _____

9. An older man was experiencing difficulty with urination. The production of urine is the function of the _____

III. Short Essays

1. Compare and contrast the terms **anabolism** and **catabolism**. List one similarity and one difference.

   _____

   _____

   _____

   _____

2. Which type of feedback, negative or positive, is used to maintain homeostasis? Defend your answer, referring to the definition of homeostasis.

   _____

   _____

   _____

   _____

3. Explain why specialized terms are needed to indicate different positions and directions within the body. Provide a concrete example.

_____

_____

_____

_____

Conceptual Thinking

1. Consider the role of negative feedback in the ability of a thermostat to keep your house at the same temperature. What would happen on a hot day if your thermostat worked according to the principles of positive feedback?

_____

_____

_____

2. Consider the role of positive feedback in childbirth. Is childbirth a good example of homeostasis? Would the baby be delivered if stretching of the uterine muscles inhibited oxytocin secretion?

_____

_____

_____

3. A change at the chemical level can have an effect on the whole body. That is, a change in a chemical affects a cell, which alters the functioning of a tissue, which disrupts an organ, which disrupts a system, which results in body dysfunction. Illustrate this concept by rewriting the following description in your own words using the different levels of organization: chemical, cell, tissue, organ, system, and body (hint: blood is a tissue). Which of the bolded terms applies to each level of organization? Which level of organization is not explicitly stated?

Mr. S. experiences pain throughout his **body**. The movement of **blood** through his vessels is impaired. His **blood cells** are misshapen. A chemical found in red blood cells called **hemoglobin** is abnormal.

_____

_____

_____

_____

_____

Expanding Your Horizons

As a student of anatomy and physiology, you have joined a community of scholars stretching back into pre-history. The history of biological thought is a fascinating one, full of murder and intrigue. We think that scientific knowledge is entirely objective. However, as the books below will show, theories of anatomy and physiology depend on societal factors such as economic class, religion, and gender issues.

Resource List

Serafini A. The Epic History of Biology. Cambridge, MA: Perseus; 1993.
Magner LN. A History of the Life Sciences. New York: Dekker; 1993.
Asimov I. A Short History of Biology. Westport, CT: Greenwood; 1980.

chapter 2

Chemistry, Matter, and Life

Overview

Chemistry is the physical science that deals with the composition of matter. To appreciate the importance of chemistry in the field of health, it is necessary to know about elements, atoms, molecules, compounds, and mixtures. An **element** is a substance consisting of just one type of atom. Although exceedingly small particles, atoms possess a definite structure. The **nucleus** contains **protons** and **neutrons**, and the element's **atomic number** indicates the number of protons in its nucleus. The **electrons** surround the nucleus where they are arranged in specific orbits called **energy levels**.

Union of two or more atoms produces a **molecule**; the atoms in the molecule may be alike (as in the oxygen molecule) or different (sodium chloride, for example). In the latter case, the substance is called a **compound**. A combination of compounds, each of which retains its separate properties, is a **mixture**. Mixtures include solutions, such as salt water, and suspensions. In the body, chemical compounds are constantly being formed, altered, broken down, and recombined into other substances.

Water is a vital substance composed of hydrogen and oxygen. It makes up more than half of the body and is needed as a solvent and a transport medium. Hydrogen, oxygen, carbon, and nitrogen are the elements that constitute approximately 96% of living matter, whereas calcium, sodium, potassium, phosphorus, sulfur, chlorine, and magnesium account for most of the remaining 4%.

When atoms combine with each other to form compounds they are held together by chemical bonds. Bonds that form as the result of the attraction between oppositely charged ions are called **ionic bonds**. Bonds that form when two atoms share electrons between them are called **covalent bonds**.

Inorganic compounds include acids, bases, or salts. **Acids** are compounds that can donate hydrogen ions (H^+) when in solution. **Bases** usually contain the hydroxide ion (OH^-) and can accept hydrogen ions. The **pH scale** is used to indicate the strength of an acid or base. **Salts** are formed when an acid reacts with a base.

Isotopes (forms of elements) that give off radiation are said to be **radioactive**. Because they can penetrate tissues and can be followed in the body, they are useful in diagnosis. Radioactive substances also have the ability to destroy tissues and can be used in the treatment of many types of cancer.

Proteins, carbohydrates, and lipids are the organic compounds characteristic of living organisms. **Enzymes**, an important group of proteins, function as catalysts in metabolism.

Learning the Language: Word Anatomy

Complete the following table by writing the correct word part or meaning in the space provided. For each word part, write a term that contains the word part.

Word Part	Meaning	Example
1. _____	to fear	_____
2. _____	to like	_____
3. glyc/o-	_____	_____
4. _____	different	_____
5. hydr/o-	_____	_____
6. hom/o-	_____	_____
7. _____	many	_____
8. aqu/e-	_____	_____
9. sacchar/o-	_____	_____
10. _____	together	_____

Addressing the Learning Outcomes

I. Writing Exercise

The learning outcomes for Chapter 2 are listed below. These learning outcomes provide an overview of the major topics covered in this chapter. On a separate piece of paper, try to write out an answer to each learning outcome. All of the answers can be found in the pages of the textbook. Learning Outcomes 2, 13, and 14 are also addressed in the Coloring Atlas.

1. Define an element.
2. Describe the structure of an atom.
3. Differentiate between molecules and compounds.
4. Explain why water is so important to the body.
5. Define *mixture*; list the three types of mixtures and give two examples of each.
6. Differentiate between ionic and covalent bonds.
7. Define an electrolyte.
8. Define the terms *acid, base,* and *salt*.
9. Explain how the numbers on the pH scale relate to acidity and basicity (alkalinity).
10. Define *buffer* and explain why buffers are important in the body.
11. Define *radioactivity* and cite several examples of how radioactive substances are used in medicine.

12. List three characteristics of organic compounds.
13. Name the three main types of organic compounds and the building blocks of each.
14. Define *enzyme*; describe how enzymes work.
15. Show how word parts are used to build words related to chemistry, matter, and life.

II. Labeling and Coloring Atlas

EXERCISE 2-1: Parts of the Atom, Molecule of Water (text Figs. 2-1 and 2-2)

INSTRUCTIONS

1. Write the names of the types of atoms in this figure (1 hydrogen and 2 oxygen) on the appropriate lines in two different light colors.
2. LIGHTLY color the hydrogen and oxygen atoms in the figure with the corresponding color.
3. Write the names of the parts of the atom (electron, proton, neutron) on the appropriate lines in different, darker colors.
4. Color the electrons, protons, and neutrons on the figure in the appropriate colors. You should find 10 electrons, 10 protons, and 8 neutrons in total.

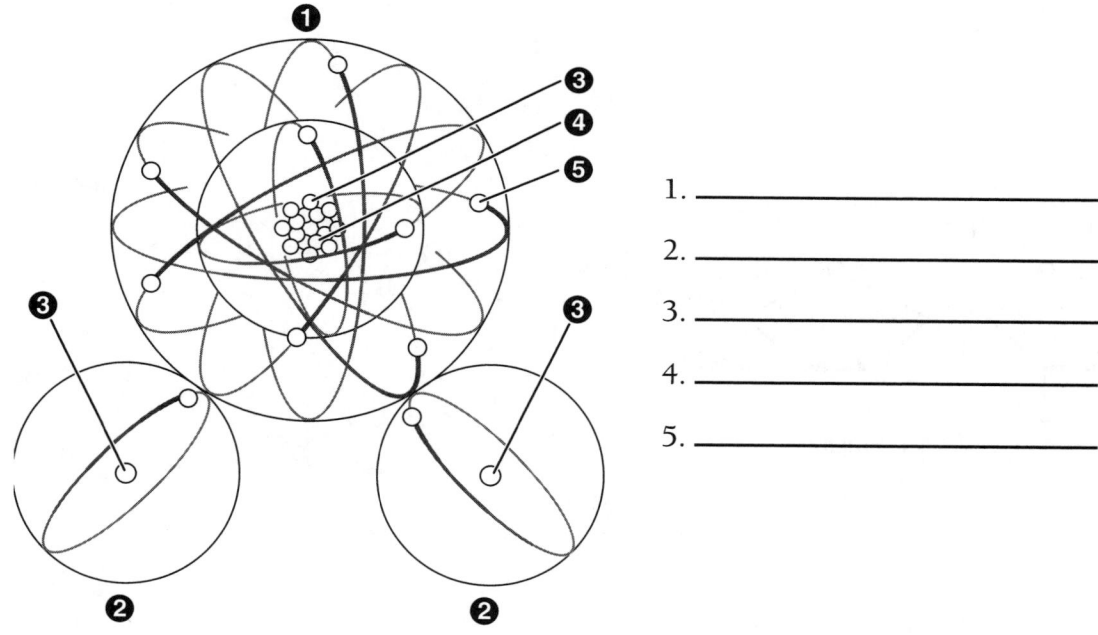

1. _____

2. _____

3. _____

4. _____

5. _____

EXERCISE 2-2: Carbohydrates (text Fig. 2-7)

INSTRUCTIONS

1. Write the terms *monosaccharide*, *disaccharide*, and *polysaccharide* in the appropriate numbered boxes 1 to 3.
2. Write the terms *glucose*, *sucrose*, and *glycogen* in the appropriate numbered boxes 4 to 6 in different colors.
3. Color the glucose, sucrose, and glycogen molecules with the appropriate colors. To simplify your diagram, only use the glucose color to shade the glucose molecule in the monosaccharide.

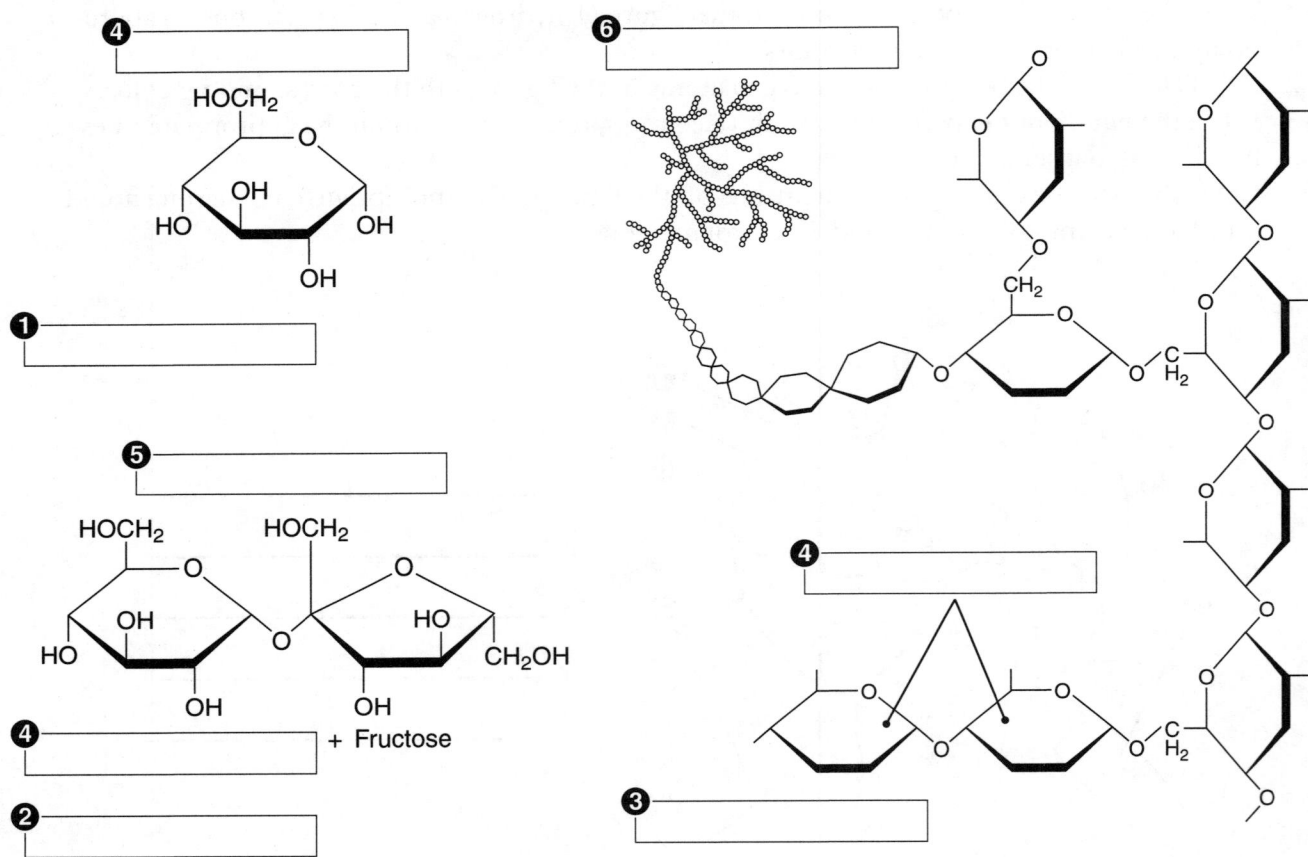

+ Fructose

EXERCISE 2-3: Lipids (text Fig. 2-8)

INSTRUCTIONS

1. Write the terms *glycerol* and *fatty acids* on the appropriate lines in two different colors.
2. Find the boxes surrounding these two components on the diagram, and color them lightly in the appropriate colors.
3. Write the terms *triglyceride* and *cholesterol* in the boxes under the appropriate diagrams.

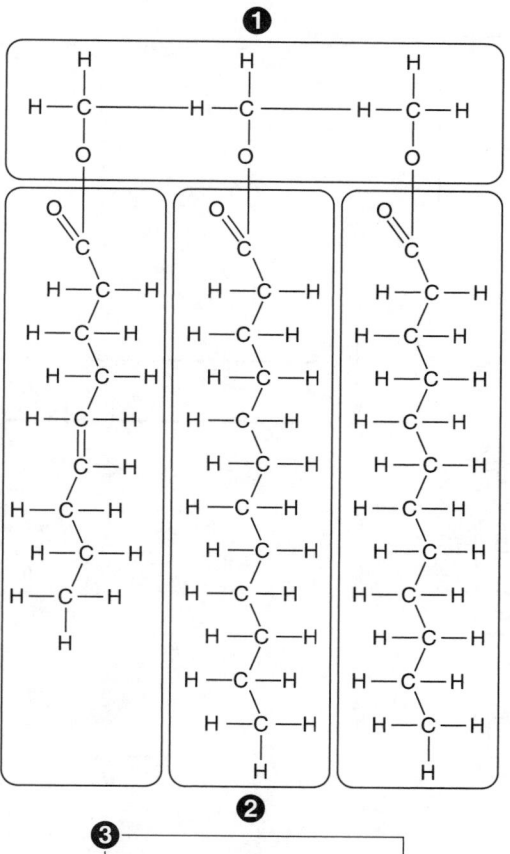

1. _____

2. _____

EXERCISE 2-4: Proteins (text Fig. 2-9)

INSTRUCTIONS

1. Write the terms *amino group* and *acid group* on the appropriate lines in different colors.
2. Find the shapes surrounding these two components on the diagram, and color them lightly in the appropriate colors.
3. Place the following terms in the appropriate numbered boxes: amino acid, coiled, pleated, folded.

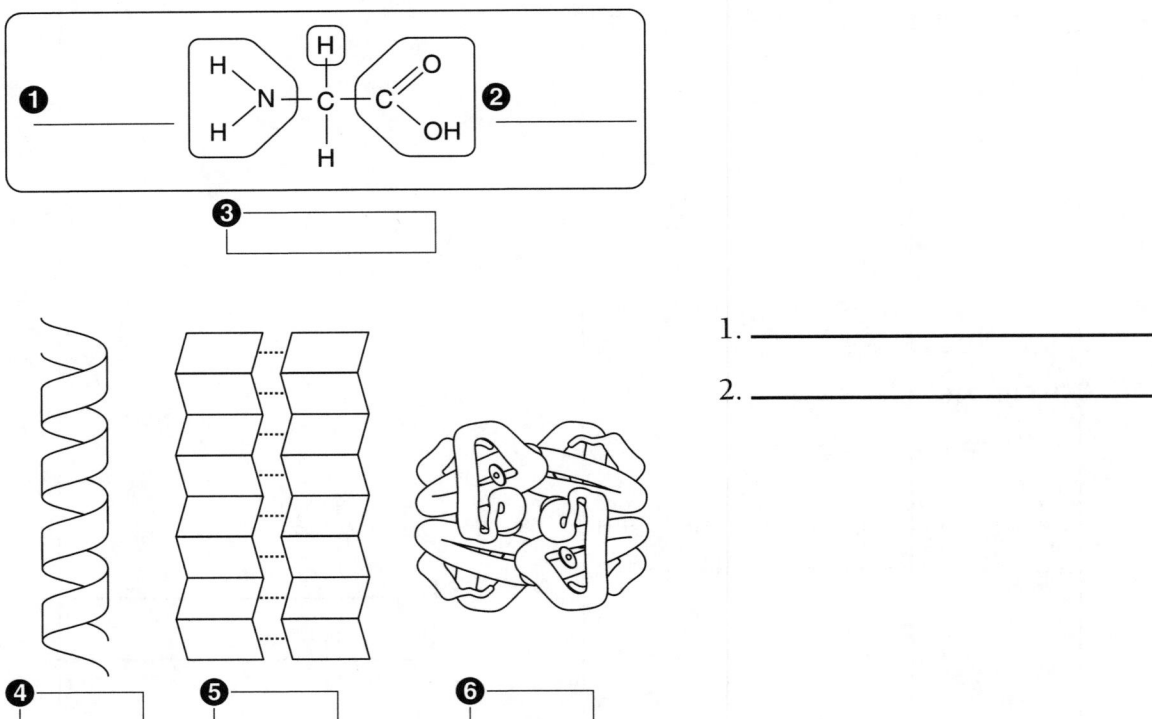

1. —————————————

2. —————————————

EXERCISE 2-5: Enzyme Action (text Fig. 2-10)

INSTRUCTIONS

1. Write the terms *substrate 1, substrate 2,* and *enzyme* on the appropriate numbered lines in different colors (red and blue are recommended for the substrates).
2. Color the structures on the diagram with the appropriate color.
3. What color will result from the combination of your two substrate colors? Write "product" in this color on the appropriate line, and then color the product.

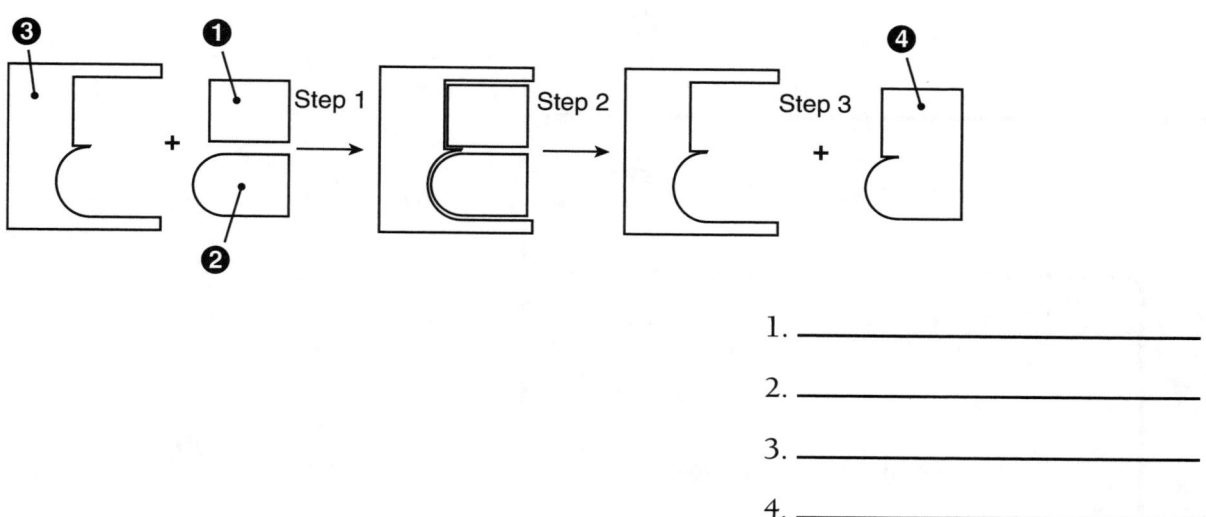

1. _____

2. _____

3. _____

4. _____

Making the Connections

The following concept map deals with the components of matter. Complete the concept map by filling in the blanks with the appropriate word or term.

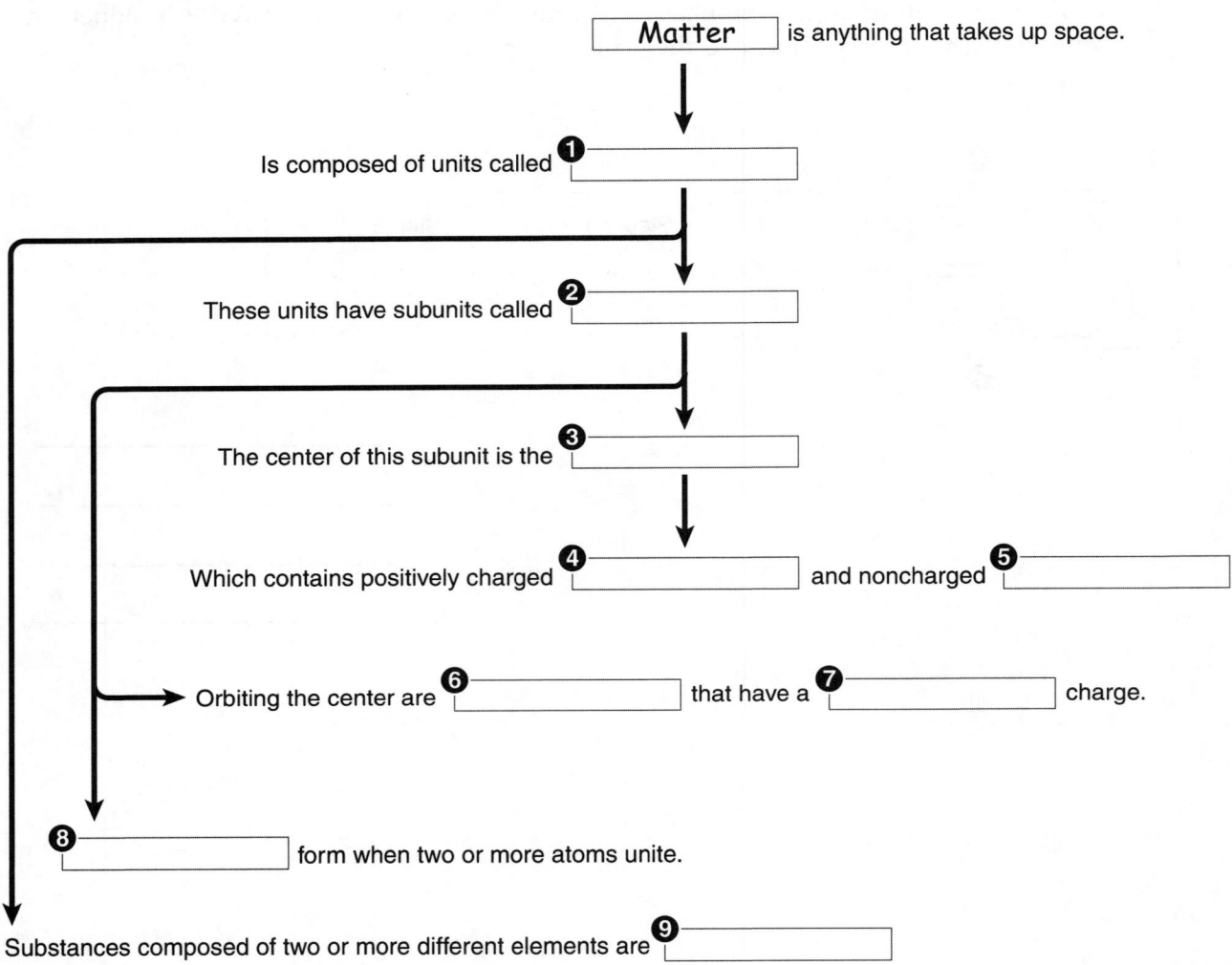

Optional Exercise: Construct your own concept map using the following terms: amino acid, protein, monosaccharide, enzyme, polysaccharide, glycogen, glucose, lipid, triglyceride.

Testing Your Knowledge
Building Understanding

I. Matching Exercises

Matching only within each group, write the answers in the spaces provided.

➤ Group A

nucleus	proton	element	electrons
neutrons	atom	isotopes	ions

1. A positively charged particle inside the atomic nucleus _____

2. The smallest complete unit of matter _____

3. Two forms of an element with unequal numbers of neutrons _____

4. A substance composed of one type of atom _____

5. The part of the atom containing protons and neutrons _____

6. A negatively charged particle outside the atomic nucleus _____

➤ Group B

solution	molecule	suspension	solute
compounds	mixture	colloid	

1. A substance that is dissolved in another substance _____

2. A mixture in which substances will settle out unless the mixture is shaken _____

3. The unit formed by the union of two or more atoms _____

4. Substances that result from the union of two or more different atoms _____

5. Cytoplasm and blood plasma are examples of this type of mixture _____

➤ Group C

cations	ionic	acid
electrolytes	anions	pH buffer

1. Negatively charged ions _____

2. A substance that donates a hydrogen ion to another substance _____

3. Compounds that form ions when in solution _____

4. Positively charged ions _____

5. A measure of the acidity of a solution _____

6. A substance that helps to maintain a stable hydrogen ion

   concentration in a solution _____

➤ **Group D**

| protein | amino acid | phospholipid | carbohydrate |
| monosaccharide | steroid | disaccharide | |

1. Two simple sugars linked together _____

2. A building block of proteins _____

3. A lipid containing a ring of carbon atoms _____

4. A lipid that contains phosphorus in addition to carbon,

   hydrogen, and oxygen _____

5. A category of organic compounds that includes simple sugars

   and starches _____

II. Multiple Choice

Select the best answer and write the letter of your choice in the blank.

1. The element that is the basis for organic chemistry is: 1._____
   - a. nitrogen
   - b. carbon
   - c. oxygen
   - d. hydrogen
2. The smallest particle of an element that has all the properties of that
   element is a(n): 2._____
   - a. proton
   - b. neutron
   - c. electron
   - d. atom
3. If an electron is added to an atom it becomes a charged particle, also
   known as a(n): 3._____
   - a. proton
   - b. anion
   - c. cation
   - d. electrolyte
4. Electrons are arranged around the nucleus in specific orbits called: 4._____
   - a. energy levels
   - b. ellipses
   - c. pathways
   - d. isotopes

5. A pH of seven is said to be: 5. _____
    a. basic
    b. neutral
    c. acidic
    d. radioactive

6. Building block for sugars are: 6. _____
    a. amino acids
    b. free fatty acids
    c. glycerol molecules
    d. monosaccharides

7. Covalent bonds are: 7. _____
    a. formed between two ions
    b. polar or nonpolar
    c. never used in organic molecules
    d. usually very unstable

8. Salt completely dissolved in water is an example of a: 8. _____
    a. colloid
    b. suspension
    c. aqueous solution
    d. isotope

9. A fat can also be called a(n):   9. _____
    a. polysaccharide
    b. lipid
    c. inorganic molecule
    d. isotope

III. Completion Exercise

Write the word or phrase that correctly completes each sentence.

1. The most abundant element by mass in the human body is _____

2. An isotope that disintegrates, giving off rays of atomic particles, is said to be _____

3. The number of electrons lost or gained by an atom in a chemical reaction is called its _____

4. Water can dissolve many different things. For this reason it is called the _____

5. Sugar water is a mixture in which one substance is dissolved in another and remains evenly distributed. This type of mixture is a(n) _____

6. A mixture that is not a solution but does not separate because the particles in the mixture are so small is a(n) _____

7. Metabolic reactions require organic catalysts called _____

8. Many essential body activities depend on certain compounds that form ions when in solution. Such compouds are called _____

9. The name given to a chemical system that prevents changes in hydrogen ion concentration is _____

10. The study of the composition and properties of matter is called _____

Understanding Concepts

I. True or False

For each question, write "T" for true or "F" for false in the blank to the left of each number. If a statement is false, correct it by replacing the underlined term and write the correct statement in the blanks below the question.

_____ 1. Sodium chloride (NaCl) is an example of an element.

_____

_____ 2. If a neutral atom has 12 protons, it will have 11 electrons.

_____

_____ 3. An atom with an atomic number of 15 will have 15 protons.

_____

_____ 4. Butter dissolves poorly in water. Butter is thus an example of a hydrophobic substance.

_____

_____ 5. When table salt is dissolved in water, the sodium ion donates one electron to the chloride ion. The chloride ion has 17 protons, so it will have 17 electrons.

_____

_____ 6. You put some soil in water and shake well. After 10 minutes, you note that some of the dirt has settled to the bottom of the jar. With respect to the dirt at the bottom of the jar, your mixture is a colloid.

_____

_____ 7. A pH of 10.0 is basic.

_____

_____ 8. Carbon dioxide is composed of two oxygen atoms and one carbon atom bonded by the sharing of electrons. The shared electrons are usually closer to the oxygens than to the carbon. Carbon dioxide is formed by ionic bonds.

_____

_____ 9. Maltose, a <u>disaccharide</u>, is composed of two glucose molecules.

_____

_____ 10. Hemoglobin, a protein, is composed of long chains of <u>phospholipids</u>.

_____

II. Practical Applications

Study each discussion. Then write the appropriate word or phrase in the space provided. The following medical tests are based on principles of chemistry and physics.

1. Young Ms. M was experiencing intense thirst and was urinating more than usual. Her doctor suspected that she might have diabetes mellitus. This diagnosis was confirmed by the finding of glucose in her urine and high glucose levels in her blood. Glucose and other sugars belong to a group of organic compounds classified as _____ .

2. Young Mr. L was brought to the clinic because he had experienced two convulsions during the night. The doctor suspected that he might have epilepsy. He obtained a graphic record of his brain-wave activity to aid in this diagnosis. This brain wave record is called a(n) _____ .

3. Ms. F just ran a 50-kilometer ultramarathon in the Sahara desert. She was brought into the clinic with symptoms of decreased function of many systems. Her history revealed poor fluid intake for several weeks. Her symptoms were caused by a shortage of the most abundant compound in the body, which is _____ .

4. Mr. Q has been experiencing diarrhea, intestinal gas, and bloating whenever he drinks milk. Deficiency in an enzyme called lactase, which digests the sugar in milk, was diagnosed. Enzymes, like all proteins, are composed of building blocks called _____ .

5. Mr. V came to the clinic reporting severe headaches. The doctor ordered a PET scan that measures the use of a monosaccharide by the brain. This monosaccharide, which can be assembled into a glycogen molecule in body tissues, is called _____ .

6. Daredevil Mr. L was riding his skateboard on a high wall when he fell. He had pain and swelling in his right wrist. His examination included a procedure in which rays penetrate body tissues to produce an image on a photographic plate. The rays used for this purpose are called _____ .

7. Ms. F was given an intravenous solution, containing sodium, potassium, and chloride ions. These elements come from salts that separate into ions in solution and are referred to as _____ .

III. Short Essays

1. Describe the structure of a protein. Make sure you include the following terms in your answer: pleated sheet, helix, protein, amino acid.

_____

_____

_____

_____

_____

2. What is the difference between a solvent and a solute? Name the solvent and the solute in salt water.

_____

_____

_____

3. What is the difference between inorganic and organic chemistry?

_____

_____

_____

4. Why is the shape of an enzyme important in its function?

_____

_____

_____

5. Compare and contrast solutions and suspensions. Name one similarity and one difference.

_____

_____

_____

Conceptual Thinking

1. Using the periodic table of the elements in Appendix 3, answer the following questions:
   a. How many protons does silicon (Si) have? _____
   b. How many electrons does copper (Cu) have? _____
   c. Phosphorus (P) exists as many isotopes. One isotope is called P^{32}, based on its atomic weight. The atomic weight can be calculated by adding up the number of protons and the number of neutrons. How many neutrons does P^{32} have? _____
   d. How many electrons does the magnesium ion Mg^{2+} have? (The 2+ indicates that the magnesium atom has lost two electrons). _____

2. There is much more variety in proteins than in carbohydrates. Explain why.

_____

_____

_____

Expanding Your Horizons

You may have read the term "antioxidant" in newspaper articles or on the Web. But what is an antioxidant, and why do we want them? An understanding of atomic structure is required to answer this question. Radiation or chemical reactions can cause molecules to pick up or lose an electron, resulting in an unpaired electron. Molecules with unpaired electrons are called **free radicals**. For instance, an oxygen molecule can gain an electron, resulting in superoxide (O_2^-), and a hydroxyl ion (OH^-) can lose an electron, resulting in a neutral OH_2 free radical. Unpaired electrons are very unstable; thus, free radicals steal electrons from other substances, converting them into free radicals. This chain reaction disrupts normal cell metabolism and can result in cancer. Antioxidants, including vitamin C, give up electrons without converting into free radicals, thereby stopping the chain reaction. The two references listed below will tell you more about free radicals and how antioxidants may fight the aging process and protect against Parkinson disease.

Resource List

Brown K. A Radical Proposal. Scientific American Presents 2000;11:38–43.
Youdim MB, Riederer P. Understanding Parkinson's Disease. Sci Am 1997;276:52–59.

chapter 3

Cells and Their Functions

Overview

The **cell** is the basic unit of life; all life activities result from the activities of cells. The study of cells began with the invention of the light microscope and has continued with the development of electron microscopes. Cell functions are performed by specialized structures within the cell called **organelles**. These include the nucleus, ribosomes, mitochondria, Golgi apparatus, endoplasmic reticulum (ER), lysosomes, peroxisomes, and centrioles. Two specialized organelles, cilia and flagella, function in cell locomotion and the movement of materials across the surface of cells.

An important cell function is the manufacture of proteins, including enzymes (organic catalysts). Protein manufacture is performed by the ribosomes in the cytoplasm according to information coded in the deoxyribonucleic acid (DNA) of the nucleus. Specialized molecules of RNA called messenger RNA play a key role in the process by carrying copies of the information in DNA to the ribosomes. DNA also is involved in the process of cell division or mitosis. Before cell division can occur, the DNA must double itself so each daughter cell produced by mitosis will have exactly the same kind and amount of DNA as the parent cell.

The **plasma (cell) membrane** is important in regulating what enters and leaves the cell. Some substances can pass through the membrane by **diffusion**, which is simply the movement of molecules from an area where they are in higher concentration to an area where they are in lower concentration. The diffusion of water through the cell membrane is termed **osmosis**. Because water can diffuse very easily across the membrane, cells must be kept in solutions that have the same concentrations as the cell fluid. If the cell is placed in a solution of higher concentration (a **hypertonic solution**), it will shrink; in a solution of lower concentration (a **hypotonic solution**), it will swell and may burst. The cell membrane can also selectively move substances into or out of the cell by **active transport**, a process that requires energy (ATP) and transporters. Large particles and droplets of fluid are taken in by the processes of **phagocytosis** and **pinocytosis**.

Learning the Language: Word Anatomy

Complete the following table by writing the correct word part or meaning in the space provided. For each word part, write a term that contains the word part.

Word Part	Meaning	Example
1. phag/o-	_____	_____
2. _____	to drink	_____
3 –some	_____	_____
4. lys/o-	_____	_____
5. _____	cell	_____
6. _____	above, over, excessive	_____
7. hem/o-	_____	_____
8. _____	same, equal	_____
9. hypo-	_____	_____
10. _____	in, within	_____

Addressing the Learning Outcomes

I. Writing Exercise

The learning outcomes for Chapter 3 are listed below. These learning outcomes provide an overview of the major topics covered in this chapter. On a separate piece of paper, try to write out an answer to each learning outcome. All of the answers can be found in the pages of the textbook. Learning Outcomes 2, 3, 4, 7, and 9 are also addressed in the Coloring Atlas, and Learning Outcome 10 is addressed in the Word Anatomy exercise above.

1. List three types of microscopes used to study cells.
2. Describe the function and composition of the plasma membrane.
3. Describe the cytoplasm of the cell, including the name and function of the main organelles.
4. Describe the composition, location, and function of DNA in the cell.
5. Compare the function of three types of RNA in the cells.
6. Explain briefly how cells make proteins.
7. Name and briefly describe the stages in mitosis.
8. Define eight methods by which substances enter and leave cells.
9. Explain what will happen if cells are placed in solutions with concentrations the same as or different from those of the cell fluids.
10. Show how word parts are used to build words related to cells and their functions.

II. Labeling and Coloring Atlas

Exercise 3-1: Typical Animal Cell Showing the Main Organelles (text Fig. 3-2)

Instructions

1. Write the name of each labeled part on the numbered lines in different colors. Make sure you use light colors for structures 1 and 7.
2. Color the different structures on the diagram with the corresponding color.

*Note: It is impossible to distinguish between parts 12 and 15 based on this diagram.

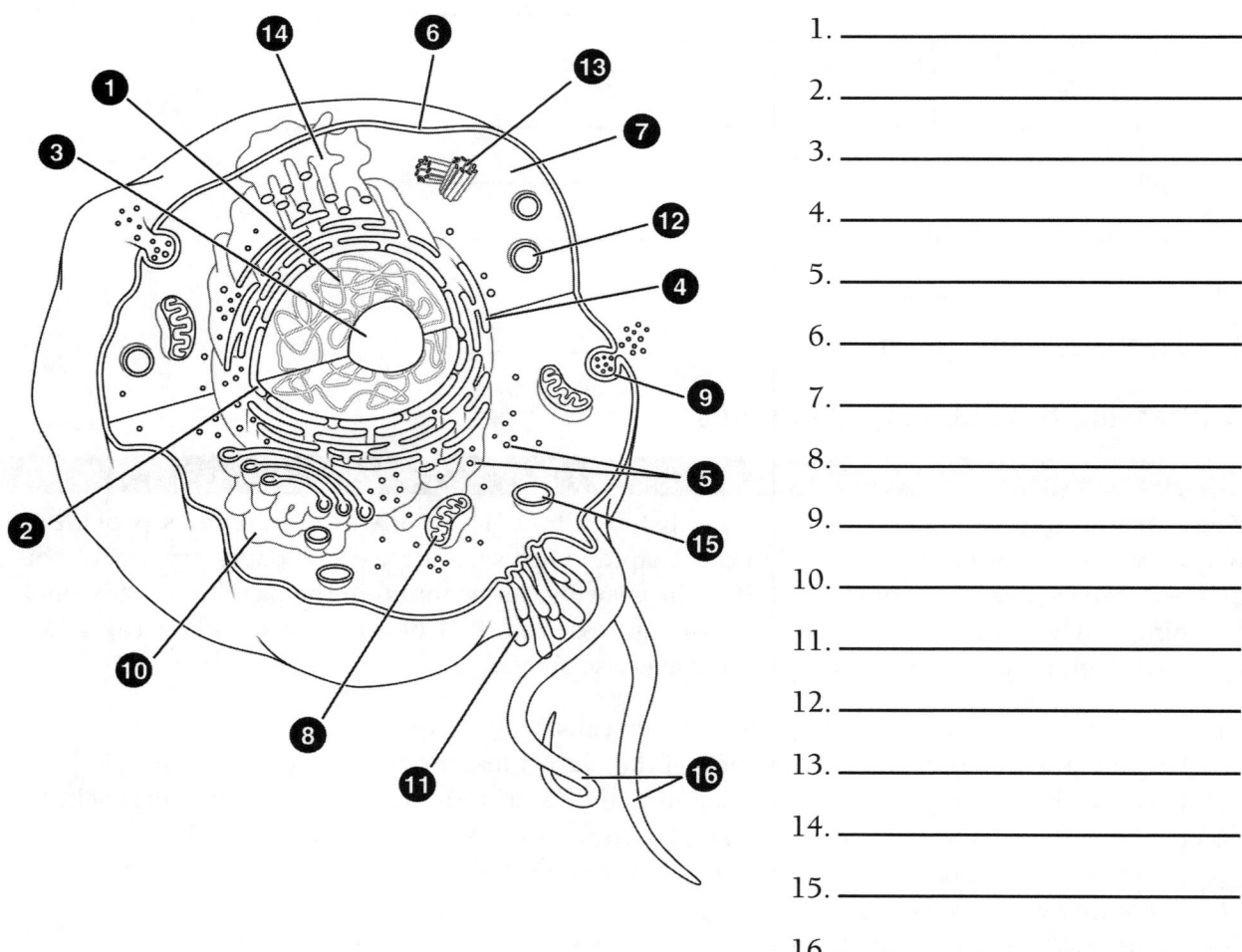

1. _____
2. _____
3. _____
4. _____
5. _____
6. _____
7. _____
8. _____
9. _____
10. _____
11. _____
12. _____
13. _____
14. _____
15. _____
16. _____

EXERCISE 3-2: Structure of the Plasma Membrane (text Fig. 3-3)

INSTRUCTIONS

1. Write the name of each labeled membrane component on the numbered lines in different colors. Choose a light color for component number 3.
2. Color the different structures on the diagram with the corresponding color (except for structures 6–8). Color ALL of components 1 and 3 through 5, not just those indicated by the leader lines. For instance, component 1 is found in three locations.

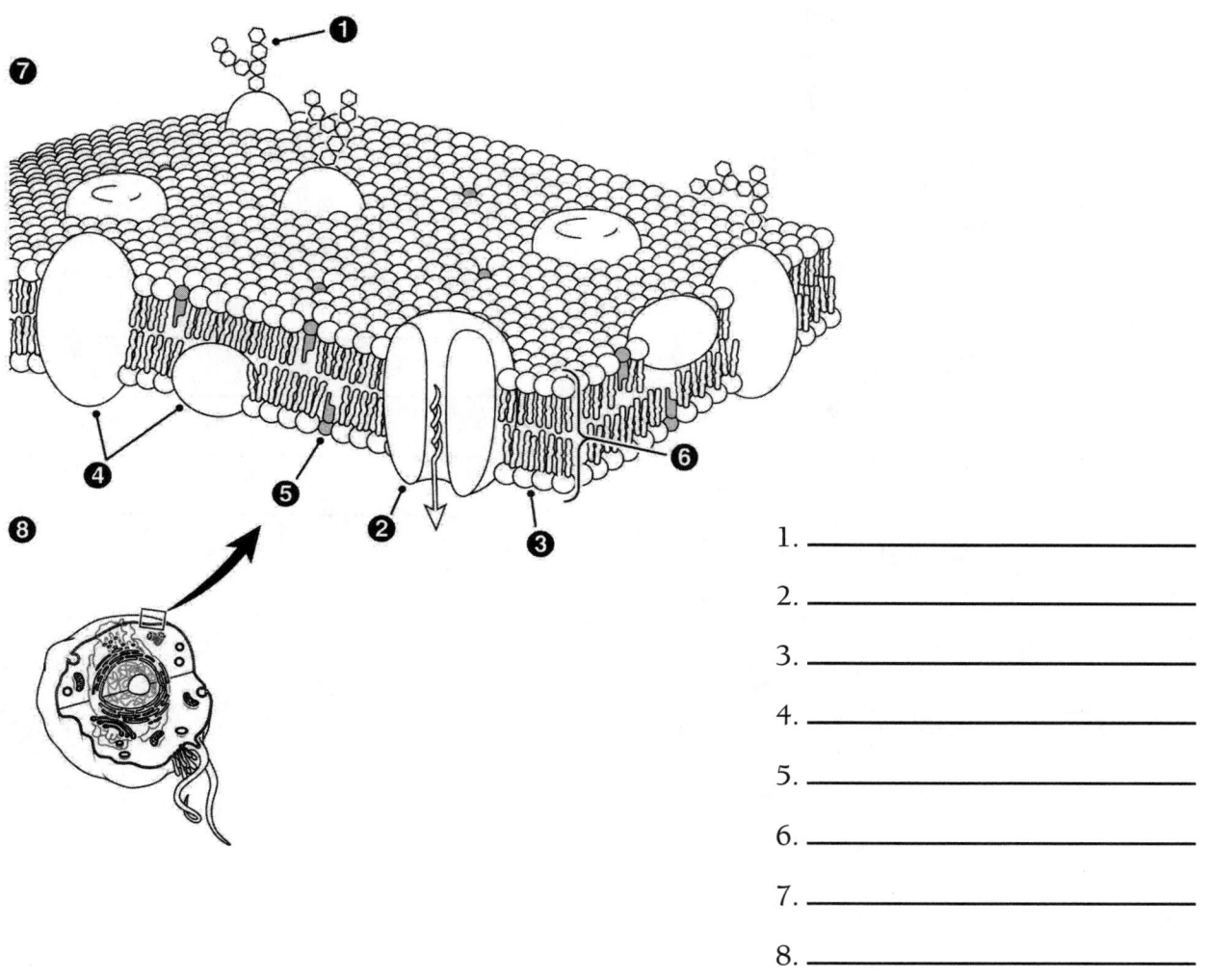

1. _____

2. _____

3. _____

4. _____

5. _____

6. _____

7. _____

8. _____

EXERCISE 3-3: Basic Structure of a DNA Molecule (text Fig. 3-6)

INSTRUCTIONS

1. Write the name of each part of the DNA molecule on the numbered lines in contrasting colors.
2. Color the different parts on the diagram with the corresponding color. Try to color each part everywhere it occurs in the DNA molecule.

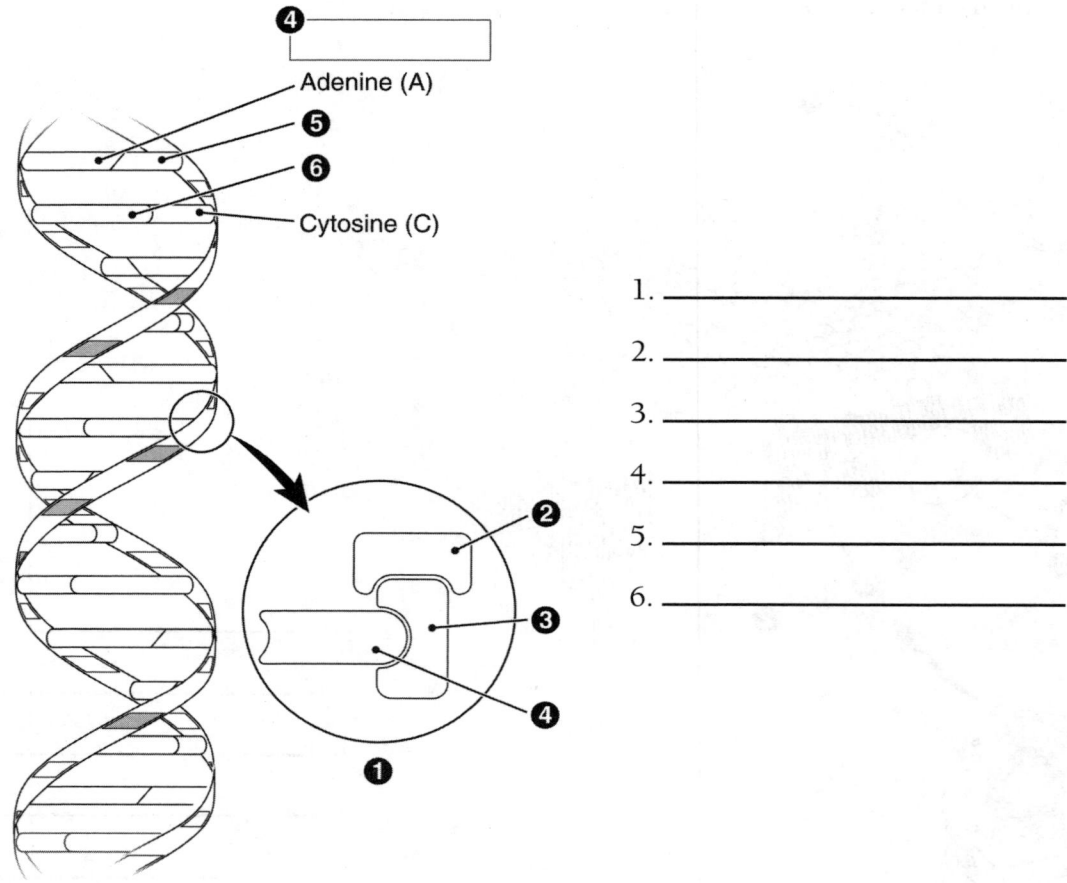

Adenine (A)

Cytosine (C)

1. _____

2. _____

3. _____

4. _____

5. _____

6. _____

EXERCISE 3-4: Stages of Mitosis (text Fig. 3-9)

INSTRUCTIONS

Identify interphase and the indicated stages of mitosis. Find the DNA in each stage and color it.

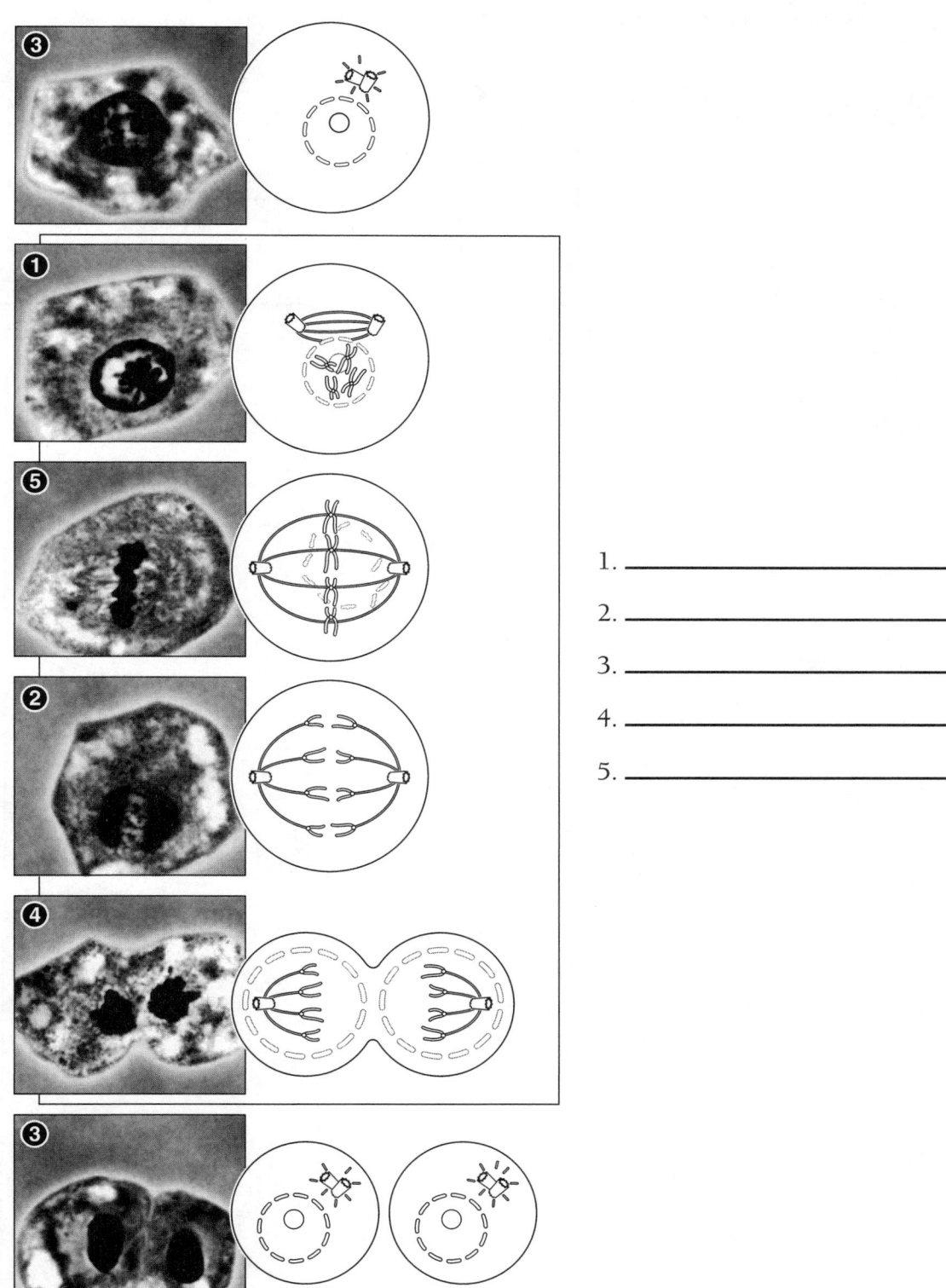

1. _____

2. _____

3. _____

4. _____

5. _____

EXERCISE 3-5: Osmosis (text Fig. 3-18)

INSTRUCTIONS

Label each of the following solutions using the appropriate term that indicates the concentration of solute in the solution relative to the concentration of solute in the cell.

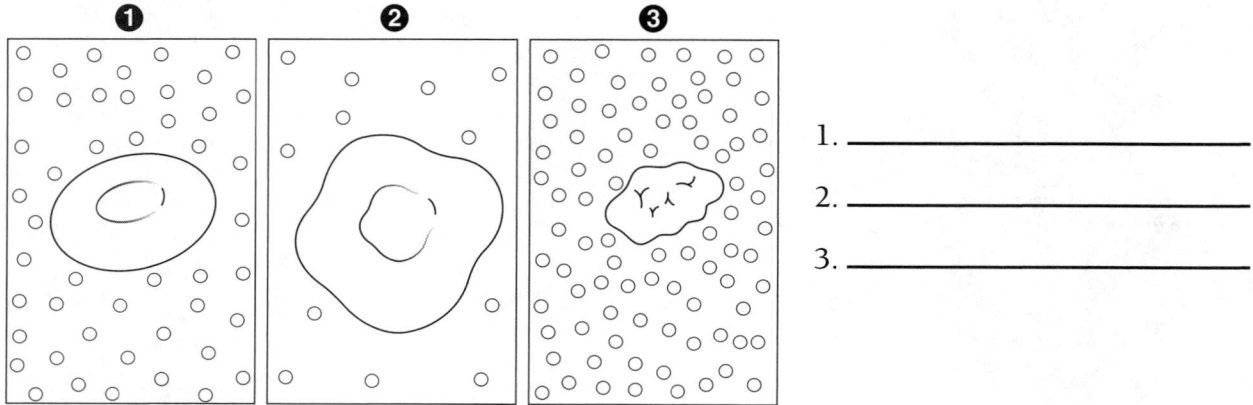

1. _____

2. _____

3. _____

EXERCISE 3-6: Membrane Proteins (text Table 3-2)

INSTRUCTIONS

1. Write the appropriate membrane protein function in boxes 1 to 6 in different colors.
2. Color the protein in each diagram the appropriate color.

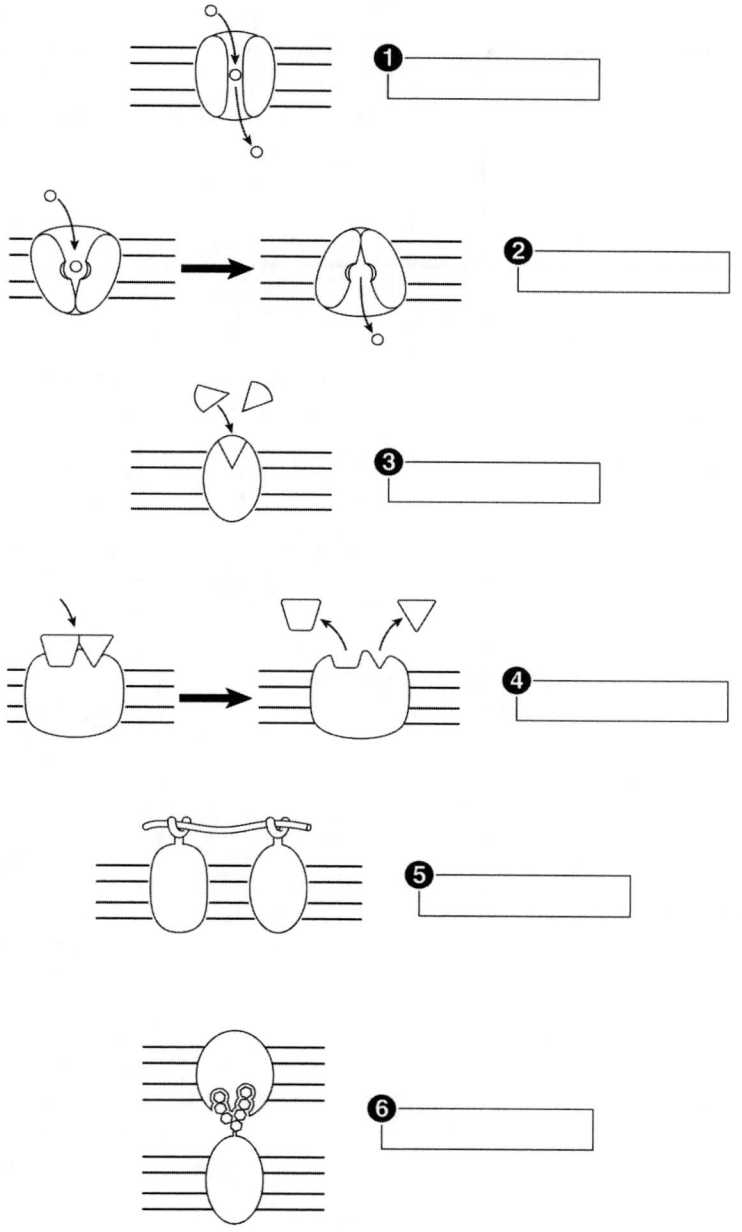

Making the Connections

The following concept map deals with the movement of materials through the plasma membrane. Complete the concept map by filling in the appropriate word or phrase that describes the indicated process.

1. Processes that move small quantities of material through the plasma membrane include…

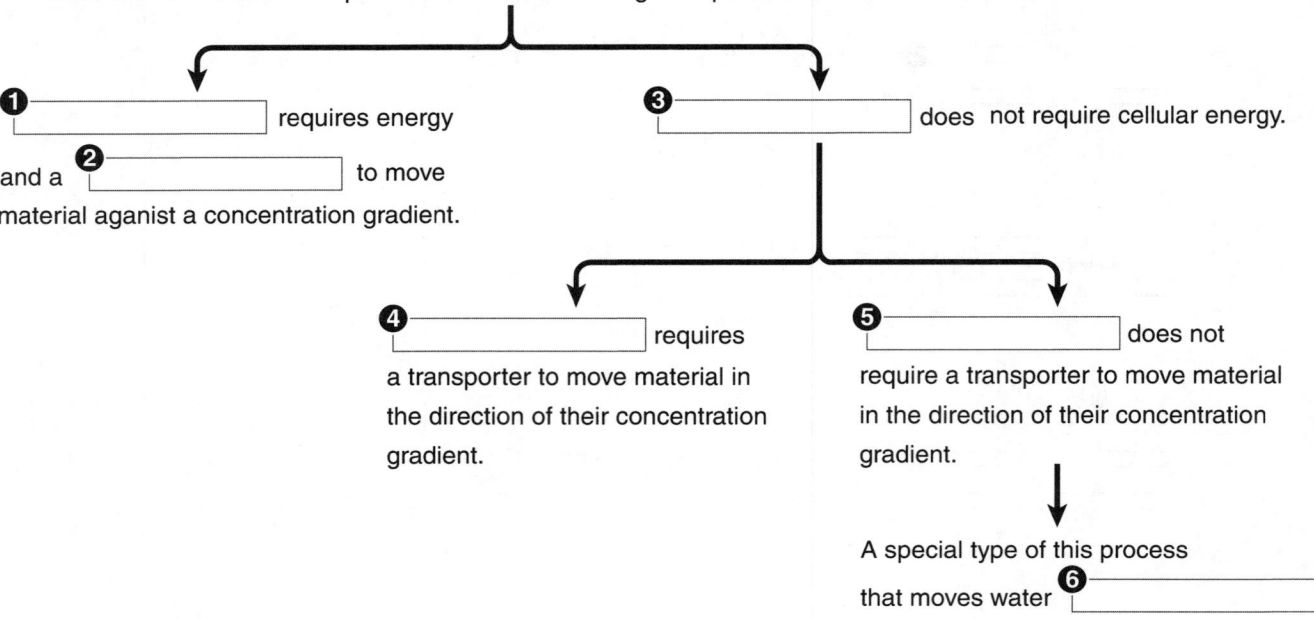

2. Processes that move large quantities of material through the plasma membrane include…

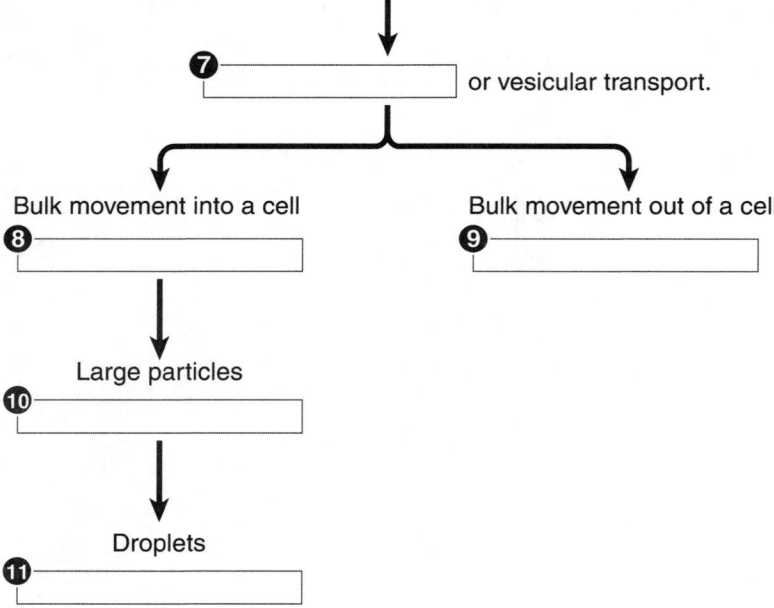

Optional Exercise: Make your own concept map, based on the components of the cell. Choose your own terms to incorporate into your map, or use the following list: nucleus, mitochondria, cell membrane, protein, RNA, DNA, ATP, vesicle, ribosome, endoplasmic reticulum.

Testing Your Knowledge
Building Understanding

I. Matching Exercises

Matching only within each group, write the answers in the spaces provided.

➤ Group A: Transport Processes

| endocytosis | active transport | diffusion | osmosis | facilitated diffusion |
| filtration | isotonic | hypotonic | hypertonic | |

1. The process that uses a carrier to move materials across the plasma membrane against the concentration gradient using ATP _____

2. The use of hydrostatic force to move fluids through a membrane _____

3. The process that uses a carrier to move materials across the plasma membrane in the direction of the concentration gradient _____

4. A special form of diffusion that applies only to water _____

5. The spread of molecules throughout an area _____

6. The process by which a cell takes in large particles _____

7. Term for a solution with a salt concentration equal to 0.9% _____

8. Term for a solution that is more concentrated than the fluid within the cell _____

➤ Group B: Structure of the Cell

| lysosome | nucleolus | cilia | ribosome |
| mitochondrion | nucleus | Golgi apparatus | vesicle |

1. A structure that assembles ribosomes _____

2. A structure that assembles amino acids into proteins _____

3. A set of membranes involved in packaging proteins for export _____

4. A small sac-like structure used to transport substances within the cell _____

5. A membraneous organelle that generates ATP _____

6. A small sac-like structure that degrades waste products _____

7. The site of DNA storage _____

➤ Group C: Protein Synthesis

DNA	nucleotide	transcription	translation
ribosomal RNA (rRNA)	transfer RNA (tRNA)	messenger RNA (mRNA)	

1. The process by which an mRNA is synthesized from the DNA   _____

2. A building block of DNA and RNA   _____

3. An important component of ribosomes   _____

4. The structure that carries amino acids to the ribosome   _____

5. The nucleic acid that carries information from the nucleus to the ribosomes   _____

➤ Group D: General Terminology

telophase	phospholipid	cholesterol	mitosis
anaphase	metaphase	prophase	interphase

1. The chromosomes become visible during this phase   _____

2. A substance that strengthens the plasma membrane   _____

3. The substance that makes up the bulk of the plasma membrane   _____

4. The phase of mitosis when chromosomes are aligned in the middle of the cell   _____

5. DNA synthesis occurs during this phase   _____

6. The chromosomes are being pulled apart in this phase   _____

II. Multiple Choice

Select the best answer and write the letter of your choice in the blank.

1. Which of the following organelles consists of a series of membranes studded with ribosomes?   1. _____
   a. mitochondrion
   b. rough endoplasmic reticulum
   c. smooth endoplasmic reticulum
   d. Golgi apparatus

2. A natural part of growth and remodeling involves the process of programmed cell death known as: 2. _____
   a. mitosis
   b. mutation
   c. apoptosis
   d. phagocytosis

3. Which of the following are required for active transport?   3. _____
   a. vesicles and cilia
   b. transporters and ATP
   c. osmotic pressure and centrioles
   d. osmosis and lysosomes

4. The stage of mitosis during which the DNA condenses into visible chromosomes is called: 4. _____
   a. metaphase
   b. anaphase
   c. prophase
   d. telophase

5. Large proteins can be secreted from the cell using the process of: 5. _____
   a. pinocytosis
   b. osmosis
   c. endocytosis
   d. exocytosis

6. Which of the following substances is NOT a constituent of the plasma membrane?   6. _____
   a. DNA
   b. proteins
   c. carbohydrates
   d. phospholipids

7. Which of the following tools has the greatest magnification?   7. _____
   a. scanning electron microscope
   b. transmission electron microscope
   c. light microscope
   d. magnifying glass

8. A membrane protein that permits the passage of specific substances is called a(n):   8. _____
   a. channel
   b. receptor
   c. linker
   d. enzyme

III. Completion Exercise

Write the word or phrase that correctly completes each sentence.

1. The type of light microscope in use today is the   _____

2. The plasma membrane contains two kinds of lipids: cholesterol and   _____

3. In some cells the plasma membrane is folded outward into multiple small projections called   _____

4. The four bases found in DNA are A, C, G, and   _____

5. The four bases found in RNA are A, C, G, and   _____

6. The assembly of amino acids into proteins is called   _____

7. When a red blood cell draws in water and bursts, it is said
   to undergo   _____

8. The chromosomes duplicate during the period between
   mitoses, which is called   _____

9. A cell has four chromosomes before entering the process of
   mitosis. After mitosis, the number of chromosomes in each
   daughter cell will be   _____

10. Transporters are used for the processes of active transport and   _____

11. Droplets of water and dissolved substances are brought ino
    the cell by the process of   _____

12. The number of daughter cells formed when a cell undergoes
    mitosis is   _____

13. Bacteria are brought into the cell by the process of   _____

Understanding Concepts

I. True or False

For each question, write "T" for true or "F" for false in the blank to the left of each number. If a statement is false, correct it by replacing the underlined term and write the correct statement in the blanks below the question.

_____ 1. The nucleotide sequence "ACCUG" would be found in DNA.

    _____

_____ 2. A living cell (with a tonicity equivalent to 0.9% NaCl) is placed in a solution containing
          2% NaCl. This solution is hypertonic.

    _____

_____ 3. Glucose is moving into a cell, down its concentration gradient, using a carrier protein.
          Glucose is traveling by active transport.

    _____

_____ 4. A toxin has entered a cell. The cell is no longer capable of generating ATP. The most
          likely explanation for this effect is that the toxin has destroyed the mitochondria.

    _____

_____ 5. The best microscope to view a ribosome would be a scanning electron microscope.

    _____

_____ 6. It is impossible to count individual chromosomes during interphase.

    _____

II. Practical Applications

Study each discussion. Then write the appropriate word or phrase in the space provided. The following are observations you might make while working for the summer in a hospital laboratory.

1. A sample of breast tissue that was thought to be cancerous arrived at the pathology laboratory. Breast cells that produce milk synthesize large amounts of protein. The small RNA-containing bodies that synthesize proteins are called _____

2. The tissue was in a liquid called normal saline so that the cells would neither shrink nor swell. Normal saline contains 0.9% salt, and is thus considered to be _____

3. The pathologist (Dr. C) sliced the tissue very thinly and placed it on a microscope slide, but he was unable to see anything. Unfortunately, he had forgotten to add a dye to the tissue. These special dyes are called _____

4. Dr. C went back to his bench to get the necessary dye. He noticed that there were many impurities floating in the dye, and he decided to screen them out. He separated the solid particles from the liquid by forcing the liquid through a membrane, a process called _____

5. Dr. C was clumsy and accidentally spilled the dye into a sink full of dishes. The water in the sink rapidly turned pink. The dye molecules had moved through the water by the process of _____

6. Dr. C made up some new dye and treated the tissue. Finally, the tissue was ready for examination. Which type of microscope uses light to view stained tissues? _____

7. The pathologist looked at the tissue and noticed that the nuclei of many cells were in the process of dividing. This division process is called _____

8. Some cells were in the stage of cell division called prophase. The DNA was condensed into structures called _____

III. Short Essays

1. Compare and contrast active transport and facilitated diffusion. List at least 1 similarity and at least 1 difference.

   _____

   _____

   _____

2. You are in the hospital for a minor operation, and the technician is hooking you up to an IV. He knows you are a nursing student and jokingly asks if you would like a hypertonic, hypotonic, or isotonic solution to be placed in your IV. Which solution would you pick? Explain your answer.

   _____

   _____

   _____

3. Compare the transmission electron microscope with the scanning electron microscope. List 1 similarity and 1 difference.

   _____

   _____

   _____

Conceptual Thinking

1. Compare the structure of a cell to a factory or a city. Try to find cell structures that accomplish all of the different functions of the city or a factory.

   _____

   _____

   _____

   _____

   _____

2. Your great-aunt M is 96 years old and loves to hear about what you are learning in class. She recently attended an Elderhostel camp, where people were talking about this "new-fangled" notion called DNA.

   a. She asks you to explain why DNA is so important. Explain the role of DNA in protein synthesis, using clear uncomplicated language. You must define any term that your great-aunt might not know. You can use an analogy if you like.

_____

_____

_____

_____

_____

   b. Next, your great-aunt wonders how the proteins get out of the cell. Explain the pathway a protein takes from the ribosome to the blood. You can use an illustration if you like.

_____

_____

_____

_____

_____

3. You are a xenobiologist studying an alien cell isolated on Mars. Surprisingly, you notice that the cell contains some of the same substances as our cells. You quantify the concentration of these substances and determine that the cell contains 10% glucose and 0.3% calcium. The cell is placed in a solution containing 20% glucose and 0.1% calcium. The plasma membrane of this cell is is very different from ours. It is permeable to glucose but not to calcium. That is, only glucose can cross the plasma membrane without using transporters. Use this information to answer the following questions:

   a. Will glucose move into the cell or out of the cell? Which transport mechanism will be involved?

_____

_____

   b. Carrier proteins are present in the membrane that can transport calcium. If calcium moves down its concentration gradient, will calcium move into the cell or out of the cell? Which transport mechanism will be involved?

_____

_____

    c. You place the cell in a new solution to study the process of osmosis. You know that sodium does not move across the alien cell membrane. You also know that the concentration of the intracellular fluid is equivalent to 1% sodium. The new solution contains 2% sodium.

        (i) Is the 2% sodium solution hypertonic, isotonic, or hypotonic?

       _____

        (ii) Will water flow into the cell or out of the cell? _____

       (iii) What will be the effect of the water movement on the cell?

       _____

Expanding Your Horizons

Trees can be dated by counting the rings. Is it possible to tell the age of a cell? The answer is a qualified "yes." It is usually possible to estimate the number of divisions a cell has undergone. The DNA region at the end of chromosomes (the telomere) shortens every time a cell undergoes mitosis. Older cells thus have shorter telomeres. When telomeres become very short, the cell stops dividing or dies. Abnormally short telomeres result in premature aging of skin and other tissues. Some cells have a special enzyme (telomerase) that restores the telomeres, making the cells essentially immortal. Perhaps this enzyme can be inserted into human heart and skin cells—a true fountain of youth. You can read about telomeres and their importance in cell aging and cancer in the following article.

Resource List

Strauss E. Counting the Lives of a Cell. Sci Am Presents 2000;11:50–55.

chapter 4

Tissues, Glands, and Membranes

Overview

The cell is the basic unit of life. Individual cells are grouped according to function into **tissues**. The four main groups of tissues include **epithelial tissue**, which forms glands, covers surfaces, and lines cavities; **connective tissue**, which gives support and form to the body; **muscle tissue**, which produces movement; and **nervous tissue**, which conducts nerve impulses.

Glands produce substances used by other cells and tissues. **Exocrine glands** produce secretions that are released through ducts to nearby parts of the body. **Endocrine glands** produce hormones that are carried by the blood to all parts of the body.

The simplest combination of tissues is a **membrane**. Membranes serve several purposes, a few of which are mentioned here. They may serve as dividing partitions, may line hollow organs and cavities, and may anchor various organs. Membranes that have epithelial cells on the surface are referred to as **epithelial membranes**. Two types of epithelial membranes are **serous membranes**, which line body cavities and cover the internal organs, and **mucous membranes**, which line passageways leading to the outside.

Connective tissue membranes cover or enclose organs, providing protection and support. These membranes include the fascia around muscles, the meninges around the brain and spinal cord, and the tissues around the heart, bones, and cartilage.

The study of tissues—**histology**—requires much memorization. In particular, you may be challenged to learn the different types of epithelial and connective tissue, as well as the classification scheme of epithelial and connective membranes. Learning the structure of these different tissues and membranes will help you understand the amazing properties of the body—how we can jump from great heights, swim without becoming waterlogged, and fold our ears over without breaking them.

Learning the Language: Word Anatomy

Complete the following table by writing the correct word part or meaning in the space provided. For each word part, write a term that contains the word part.

Word Part	Meaning	Example
1. _____	cartilage	_____
2. _____	on, upon	_____
3. oste/o-	_____	_____
4. _____	heart	_____
5. osse/o-	_____	_____
6. blast-	_____	_____
7. peri-	_____	_____
8. _____	muscle	_____
9. _____	false	_____
10. hist/o-	_____	_____
11. neur/o-	_____	_____
12. _____	side, rib	_____

Addressing the Learning Outcomes

I. Writing Exercise

The learning outcomes for Chapter 4 are listed below. These learning outcomes provide an overview of the major topics covered in this chapter. On a separate piece of paper, try to write out an answer to each learning outcome. All of the answers can be found in the pages of the textbook. Learning Outcomes 1–3 are also addressed in the Coloring Atlas, and Learning Outcome 6 is addressed in the Word Anatomy exercise above.

1. Name the four main groups of tissues and give the location and general characteristics of each.
2. Describe the difference between exocrine and endocrine glands and give examples of each.
3. Give examples of liquid, soft, fibrous, and hard connective tissues.
4. Describe three types of epithelial membranes.
5. List several types of connective tissue membranes.
6. Show how word parts are used to build words related to tissues, glands, and membranes.

II. Labeling and Coloring Atlas

EXERCISE 4-1: Three Types of Epithelium (text Fig. 4-1)

INSTRUCTIONS

Label each of the following types of epithelium.

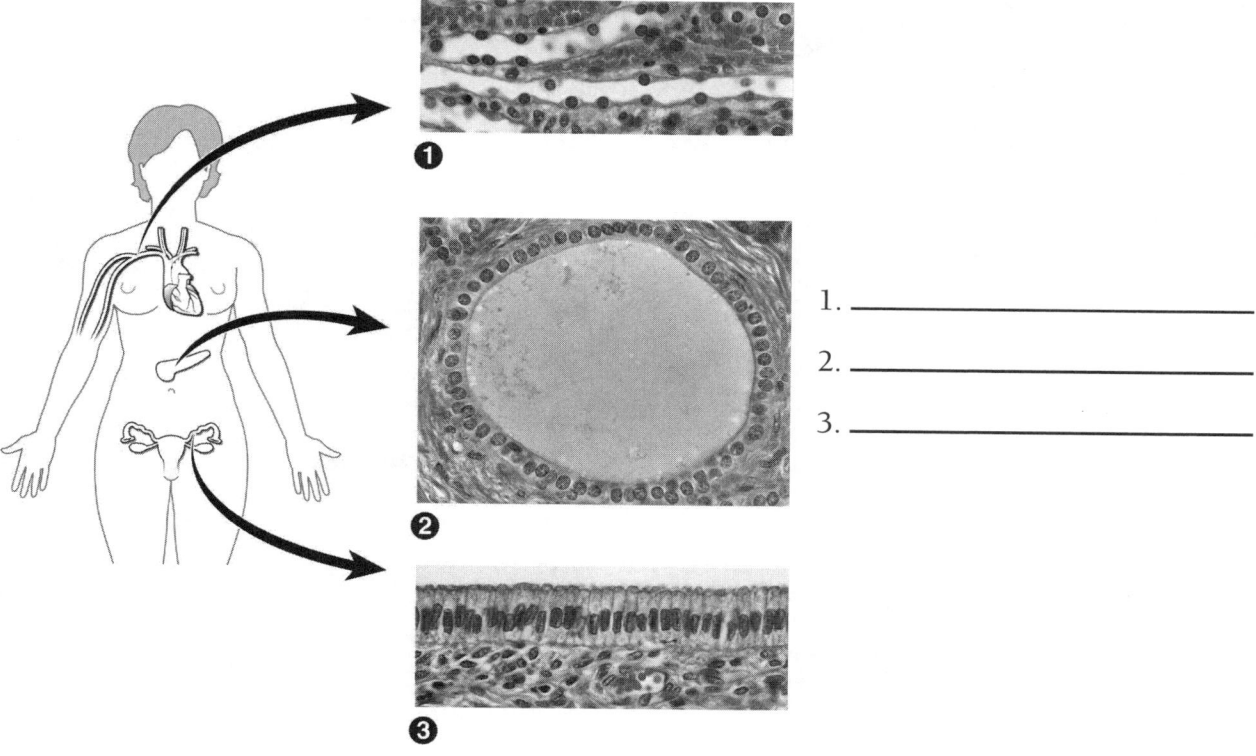

1. _____

2. _____

3. _____

EXERCISE 4-2: Connective Tissue (text Figs. 4-5 and 4-6)

INSTRUCTIONS

Write the names of the six types of connective tissue in the appropriate blanks in six different colors. Color some of the **cells** of each tissue type with the corresponding color.

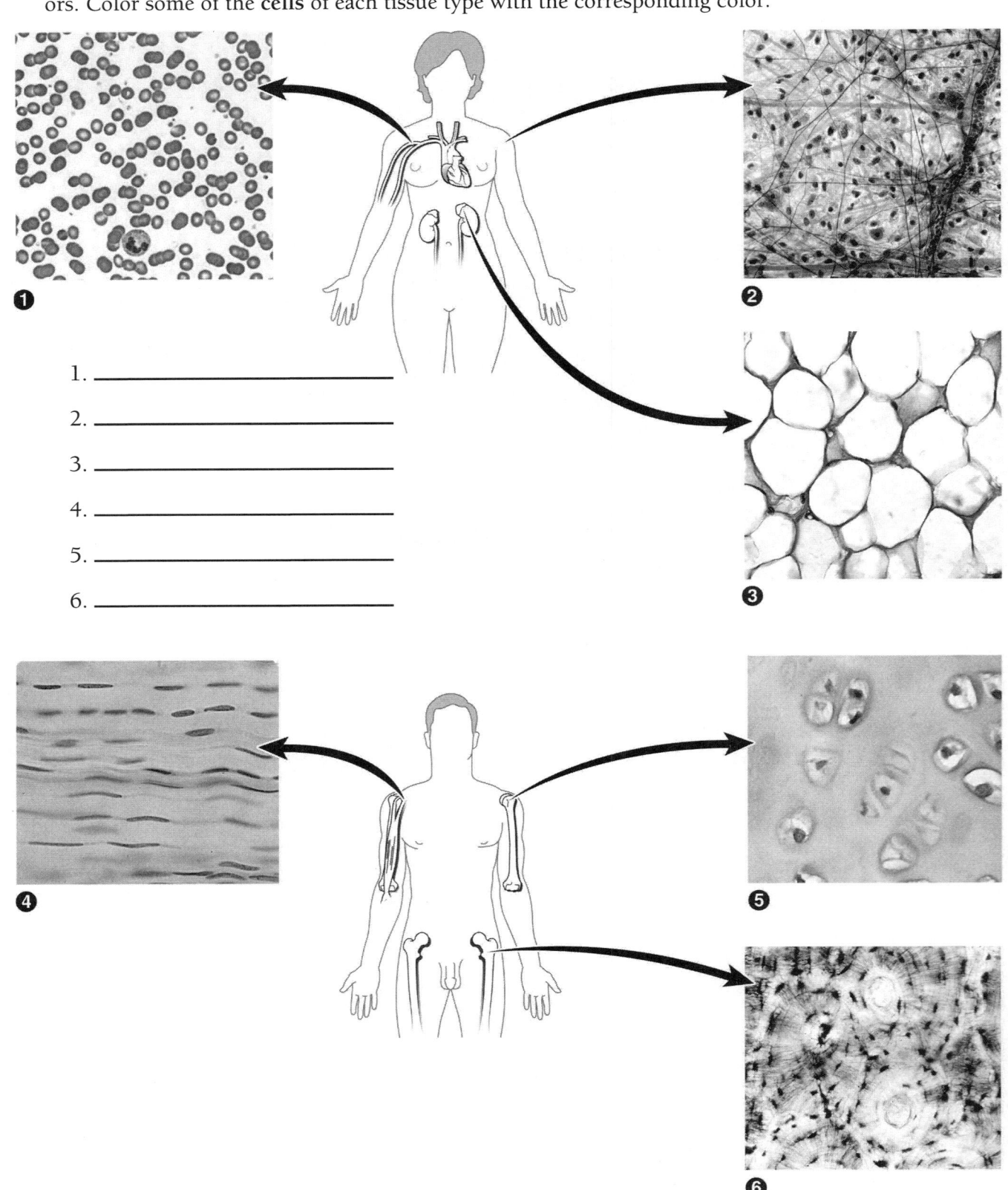

1. _____

2. _____

3. _____

4. _____

5. _____

6. _____

EXERCISE 4-3: Muscle Tissue (text Fig. 4-7)

INSTRUCTIONS

Write the names of the three types of muscle tissue in the appropriate blanks in different colors. Color some of the muscle cells the appropriate color. Look for the nuclei, and color them a different color.

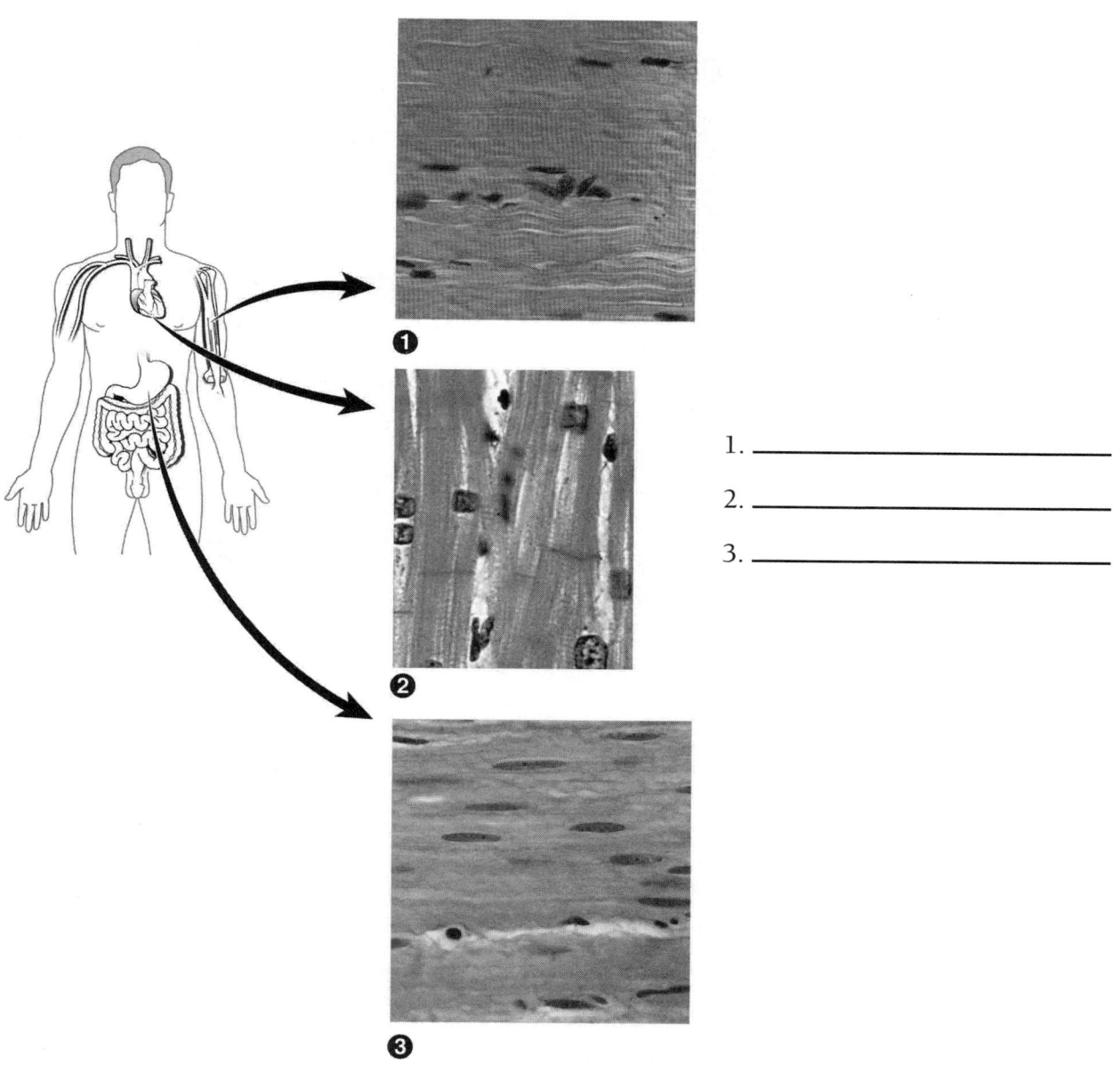

1. _____

2. _____

3. _____

Exercise 4-4: Nervous Tissue (text Fig. 4-8)

Instructions

1. Write the names of each tissue (indicating the plane of the section where appropriate) in boxes 7–9.
2. Label the neural structures and tissues (parts 1–6) using different colors. When possible, color each structure or tissue with the appropriate color.

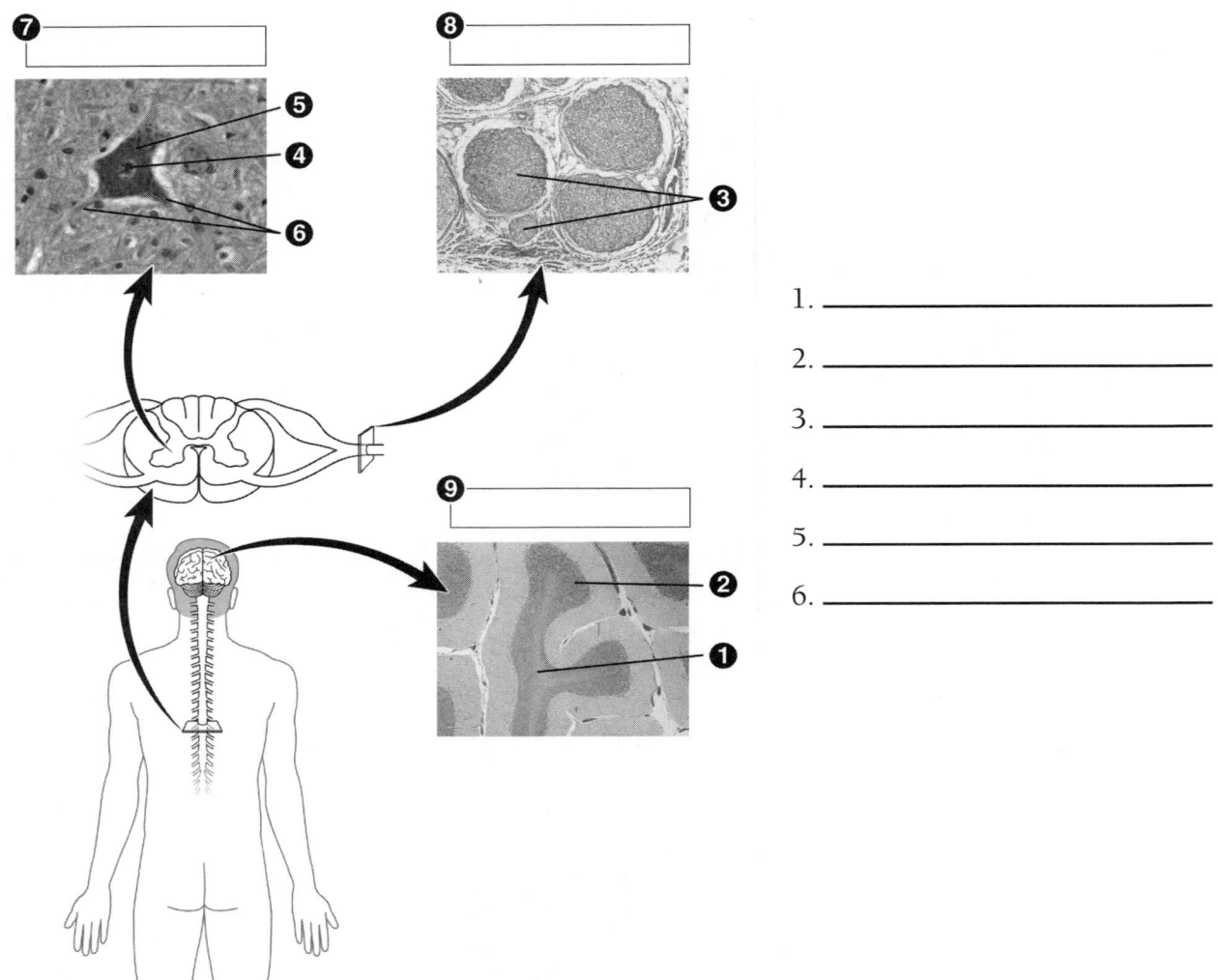

1. _____
2. _____
3. _____
4. _____
5. _____
6. _____

Making the Connections

The following concept map deals with the classification of tissues. Complete the concept map by filling in the appropriate word or phrase that classifies or describes the tissue.

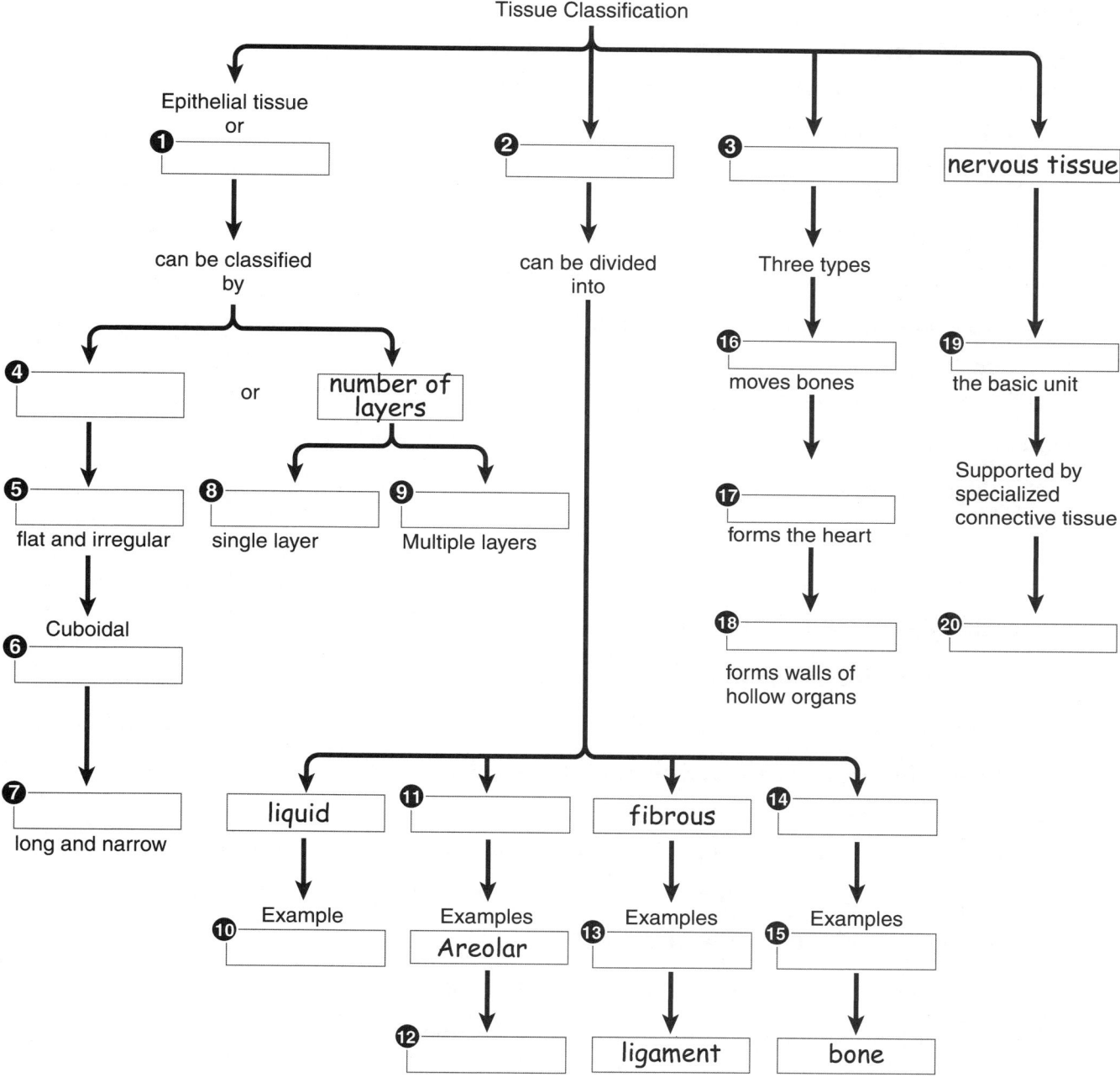

Optional Exercise: Assemble your own concept map summarizing the classification of membranes. Use the following terms: membrane, epithelial tissue membrane, connective tissue membrane, serous, mucous, cutaneous, peritoneum, pleurae, serous pericardium, parietal layer, visceral layer, meninges, fascia, deep, superficial, fibrous pericardium, periosteum, perichondrium. You could also provide some examples of the different membranes, as shown in the concept map provided above.

Testing Your Knowledge
Building Understanding

I. Matching Exercises

Matching only within each group, write the answers in the spaces provided.

➤ **Group A**

tissue   membrane   adipose   squamous

stratified   transitional   columnar

1. A group of cells similar in structure and function _____

2. A term that describes flat, irregular epithelial cells _____

4. A term that means *in layers* _____

5. Any thin sheet of tissue that separates two or more structures _____

6. Term that describes long and narrow epithelial cells _____

➤ **Group B**

bone   myocardium   voluntary muscle   axon

neuron   fat   smooth muscle   neuroglia

1. The thigh muscle is an example of _____

2. Tissue that forms when cartilage gradually becomes

   impregnated with calcium salts _____

3. The thick, muscular layer of the heart wall _____

4. Visceral muscle is also known as _____

5. A cell that carries nerve impulses is called a(n) _____

6. Nerve impulses are carried away from the cell body by the _____

➤ **Group C**

mesothelium   serous membrane   cutaneous membrane   parietal layer

visceral layer   synovial membrane   superficial fascia   deep fascia

1. The sheet of tissue that underlies the skin _____

2. A tough membrane composed entirely of connective tissue that

   serves to anchor and support an organ or to cover a muscle _____

3. The pleurae are an example of this type of membrane _____

4. The portion of a serous membrane attached to an organ _____

5. The connective tissue membrane that lines joint cavities _____

6. A tissue found in serous membranes _____

7. The portion of a serous membrane attached to the body wall _____

➤ Group D

ligament   tendon   collagen   chondrocyte

capsule   fibrocartilage   hyaline cartilage   elastic cartilage

1. A cord of connective tissue that connects a muscle to a bone _____

2. A tough membranous connective tissue that encloses an organ _____

3. The cartilage found between the bones of the spine _____

4. A fiber found in most connective tissues _____

5. A cell that synthesizes cartilage _____

6. A strong, gristly cartilage that makes up the trachea _____

➤ Group E

exocrine   endocrine   periosteum   peritoneum

epithelium   mucous membrane   perichondrium

1. A term that describes glands that secrete through ducts _____

2. A layer of fibrous connective tissue around a bone _____

3. A type of tissue found in membranes and glands _____

4. A term that describes glands that secrete into the blood _____

5. The membrane that covers cartilage _____

6. A membrane that lines spaces open to the outside of the body _____

II. Multiple Choice

Select the best answer and write the letter of your choice in the blank.

1. Which of the following is a type of connective tissue?   1. _____
   a. transitional
   b. squamous
   c. cuboidal
   d. areolar
2. The phrase stratified cuboidal epithelium describes: 2. _____
   a. flat, irregular, epithelial cells in a single layer
   b. square epithelial cells in many layers
   c. long, narrow, epithelial cells in a single layer
   d. flat, irregular, epithelial cells in many layers
3. The only type of muscle that is under voluntary control is: 3. _____
   a. smooth muscle
   b. skeletal muscle
   c. cardiac muscle
   d. visceral muscle

4. The proper scientific name for a nerve cell is: 4. _____
   a. neuroglia
   b. nevus
   c. neuron
   d. axon

5. Mucus is secreted from: 5. _____
   a. endocrine glands
   b. goblet cells
   c. areolar tissue
   d. tendons

6. Cartilage is produced by: 6. _____
   a. chondrocytes
   b. fibroblasts
   c. osteoblasts
   d. osteocytes

7. Adipose tissue stores: 7. _____
   a. mucus
   b. water
   c. protein
   d. fat

8. The tough connective tissue membrane that covers most parts of all
   bones is the: 8. _____
   a. perichondrium
   b. periosteum
   c. fascia
   d. ligament

III. Completion Exercise

Write the word or phrase that correctly completes each sentence.

1. The secretion that traps dust and other inhaled foreign

   particles is _____

2. Cells that form bone are called _____

3. The cartilage found at the end of long bones is called _____

4. The axons of some neurons have an insulating coating called _____

5. The study of tissues is called _____

6. The epithelial membrane that lines the walls of the abdominal

   cavity is called the _____

7. A mucous membrane can also be called the _____

8. A lubricant that reduces friction between the ends of bones is

   produced by the _____

9. The microscopic, hairlike projections found in the cells lining

most of the respiratory tract are called _____

Understanding Concepts

I. True or False

For each question, write "T" for true or "F" for false in the blank to the left of each number. If a statement is false, correct it by replacing the underlined term and write the correct statement in the blanks below the question.

_____ 1. The mouth is lined by a type of epithelial membrane called a <u>serous</u> membrane.

_____

_____ 2. The heart is an example of <u>skeletal muscle</u>.

_____

_____ 3. The strip of tissue connecting the kneecap to the thigh muscle is an example of a <u>tendon</u>.

_____

_____ 4. Inflammation of the large abdominal serous membrane is <u>pleuritis</u>.

_____

_____ 5. The <u>visceral</u> layer of a serous membrane is in contact with the stomach.

_____

_____ 6. You have identified a new gland in the neck. This gland is connected to the mouth by a duct. Your new gland is an example of an <u>exocrine</u> gland.

_____

II. Practical Applications

You are working as a sports therapist for a wrestling team. At a particularly brutal competition, you are asked to evaluate a number of injuries.

1. Mr. K experienced a crushing injury to the lower leg

   yesterday in a sumo wrestling match when his opponent

   fell on him. Initially, he had little pain. Now, he reports

   numbness and pain in the foot and leg. This type of injury is

   made worse by the tight, fibrous covering of the muscles,

   known as the _____

2. Mr. K also reports pain in the knee. You suspect an injury
    to the membrane that lines the joint cavity, a membrane
    called the   _____

3. You note that Mr. K has a significant amount of fat. Fat is
    contained in a type of connective tissue called   _____

4. Ms. J sustained a bloody nose in her wrestling match. Blood
    is a liquid form of the tissue classified as   _____

5. Ms. J also sustained a painful bump on her ankle in
    the same match. The swelling involved the superficial
    tissues and the fibrous covering of the bone, or the   _____

6. Mr. S was involved in a closely fought match when his
    opponent bent his ear back. Thankfully, the cartilage in
    his ear was able to spring back into shape. This kind of
    cartilage is called   _____

7. Later, Mr. S sustained a penetrating wound to his
    abdomen when his opponent accidentally threw him into
    the seating area. You fear that the wound may have penetrated
    the membrane that lines his abdomen, called the   _____

8. The wrestling coach comes over to talk to you during a
    break in the match. He has a question about his favorite
    shampoo. The advertisement stated that it contained
    collagen. He asks you which cells in the body synthesize
    collagen. These cells are called   _____

III. Short Essays

1. Compare and contrast connective and epithelial tissue membranes, and give an example of
   each. List at least one similarity and one difference in your answer.

   _____

   _____

   _____

2. Differentiate between epithelial tissue, connective tissue, and muscle in terms of the amount and composition of the extracellular matrix.

_____

_____

_____

Conceptual Thinking

1. Why is bone considered to be connective tissue? Define connective tissue in your answer.

_____

_____

_____

2. Which tissue, epithelial or connective, would be best suited to the following functions?
   a. cushioning the kidneys against a blow
   b. creating a virtually waterproof barrier between the body and the environment
   c. preventing toxins from entering the blood from the gastrointestinal tract

_____

_____

_____

Expanding Your Horizons

Text Box 4-1 talks about some of the possibilities and ethical dilemmas surrounding stem cell use. Although stem cells have enormous potential, the technical and political difficulties involved sometimes seem insurmountable. Indeed, it has proved difficult to find true stem cells that can differentiate into any cell type. Many alleged stem cell lines can only produce certain types of cells. Much research remains to be done regarding techniques to identify stem cells and the factors that cause differentiation into different cell types (say, a liver cell or a skin cell). You can learn more about the politics, difficulties, and potential of stem cell research in the following article.

Resource List

Lanza R, Rosenthal N. The Stem Cell Challenge. Sci Am 2004;290:92–100.

chapter 5

The Integumentary System

Overview

Because of its various properties, the skin can be classified as a membrane, an organ, or a system. The outermost layer of the skin is the **epidermis**. Beneath the epidermis is the **dermis** (the true skin), where glands and other accessory structures are mainly located. The **subcutaneous tissue** underlies the skin. It contains fat that serves as insulation. The accessory structures of the skin are the **sudoriferous** (sweat) **glands**, the oil-secreting **sebaceous glands**, **hair**, and **nails**.

The skin protects deeper tissues against drying and against invasion by harmful organisms. It regulates body temperature through evaporation of sweat and loss of heat at the surface. It collects information from the environment by means of sensory receptors.

The protein **keratin** in the epidermis thickens and protects the skin and makes up hair and nails. **Melanin** is the main pigment that gives the skin its color. It functions to filter out harmful ultraviolet radiation from the sun. Skin color is also influenced by the hemoglobin concentration and quantity of blood circulating in the surface blood vessels.

This chapter does not contain any particularly difficult material. However, you must be familiar with the different tissue types discussed in Chapter 4 to understand the structure and function of the integument.

Learning the Language: Word Anatomy

Complete the following table by writing the correct word part or meaning in the space provided. for each word part write a term that contains the word part.

Word Part	Meaning	Example
1. sub-	_____	_____
2. _____	dark, black	_____
3. _____	white	_____
4. hair	_____	_____
5. derm/o	_____	_____
6. _____	horny	_____
7. ap/o-	_____	_____

Addressing the Learning Outcomes

I. Writing Exercise

The learning outcomes for Chapter 5 are listed here. These learning outcomes provide an overview of the major topics covered in this chapter. On a separate piece of paper, try to write out an answer to each learning outcome. All of the answers can be found in the pages of the textbook. Outcomes 1, 2, and 3 are also addressed in the Coloring Atlas.

1. Name and describe the layers of the skin.
2. Describe the subcutaneous tissue.
3. Give the location and function of the accessory structures of the skin.
4. List the main functions of the skin.
5. Discuss the factors that contribute to skin color.
6. Show how word parts are used to build words related to the skin.

II. Labeling and Coloring Atlas

EXERCISE 5-1: The Skin (text Fig. 5-1)

INSTRUCTIONS

1. Write the names of the three skin layers in the numbered boxes 1–3.
2. Write the name of each labeled part on the numbered lines in different colors. Use a light color for structures 4 and 12. Use the same color for structures 15 and 16, for structures 13 and 14, and for structures 8 and 9.

3. Color the different structures on the diagram with the corresponding color. Try to color every structure in the figure with the appropriate color. For instance, structure number 8 is found in three locations.

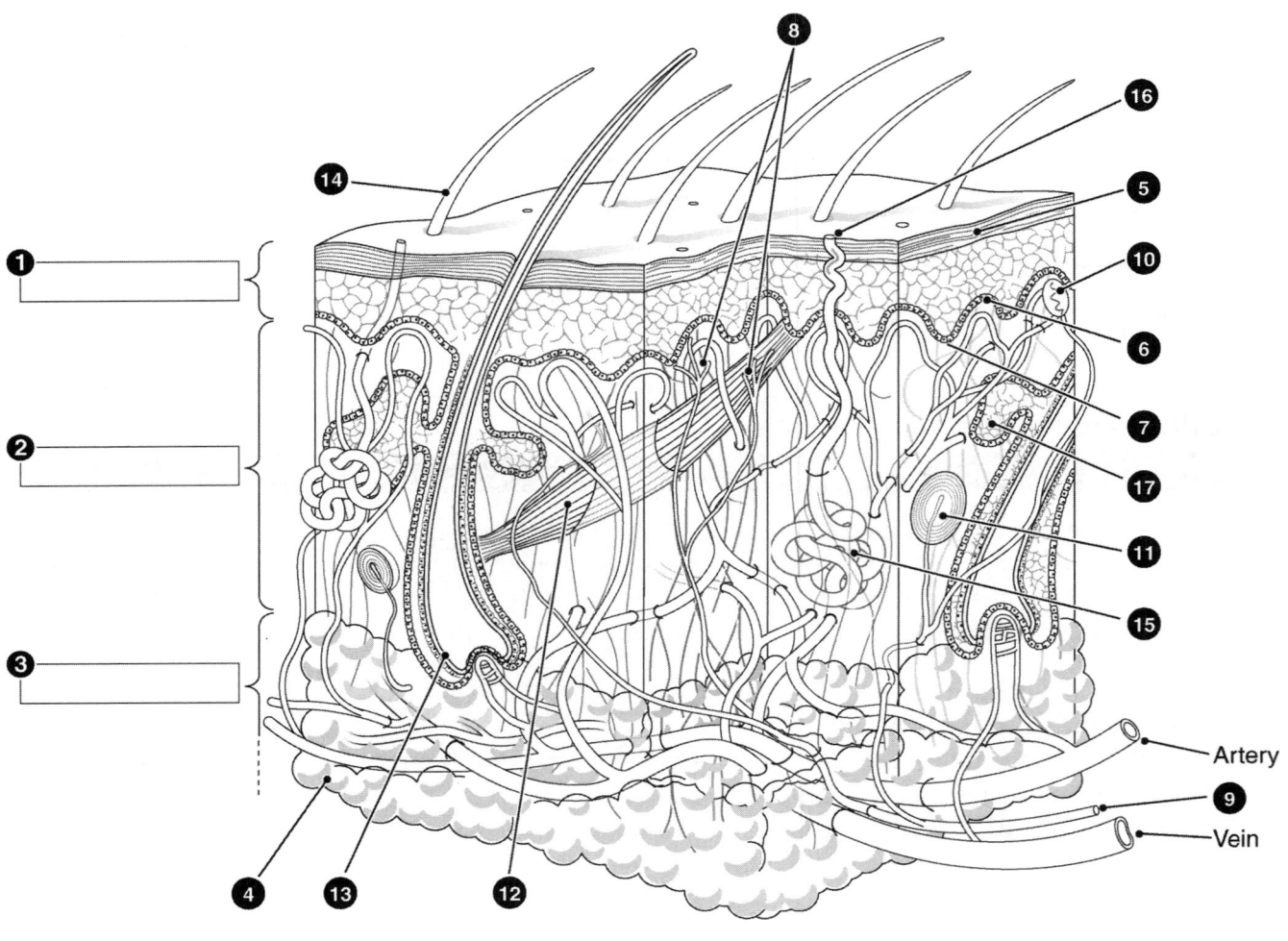

4. _____

5. _____

6. _____

7. _____

8. _____

9. _____

10. _____

11. _____

12. _____

13. _____

14. _____

15. _____

16. _____

17. _____

Making the Connections

The following concept map deals with the structural features of the skin. Complete the concept map by filling in the appropriate word or phrase that describes the indicated skin structure.

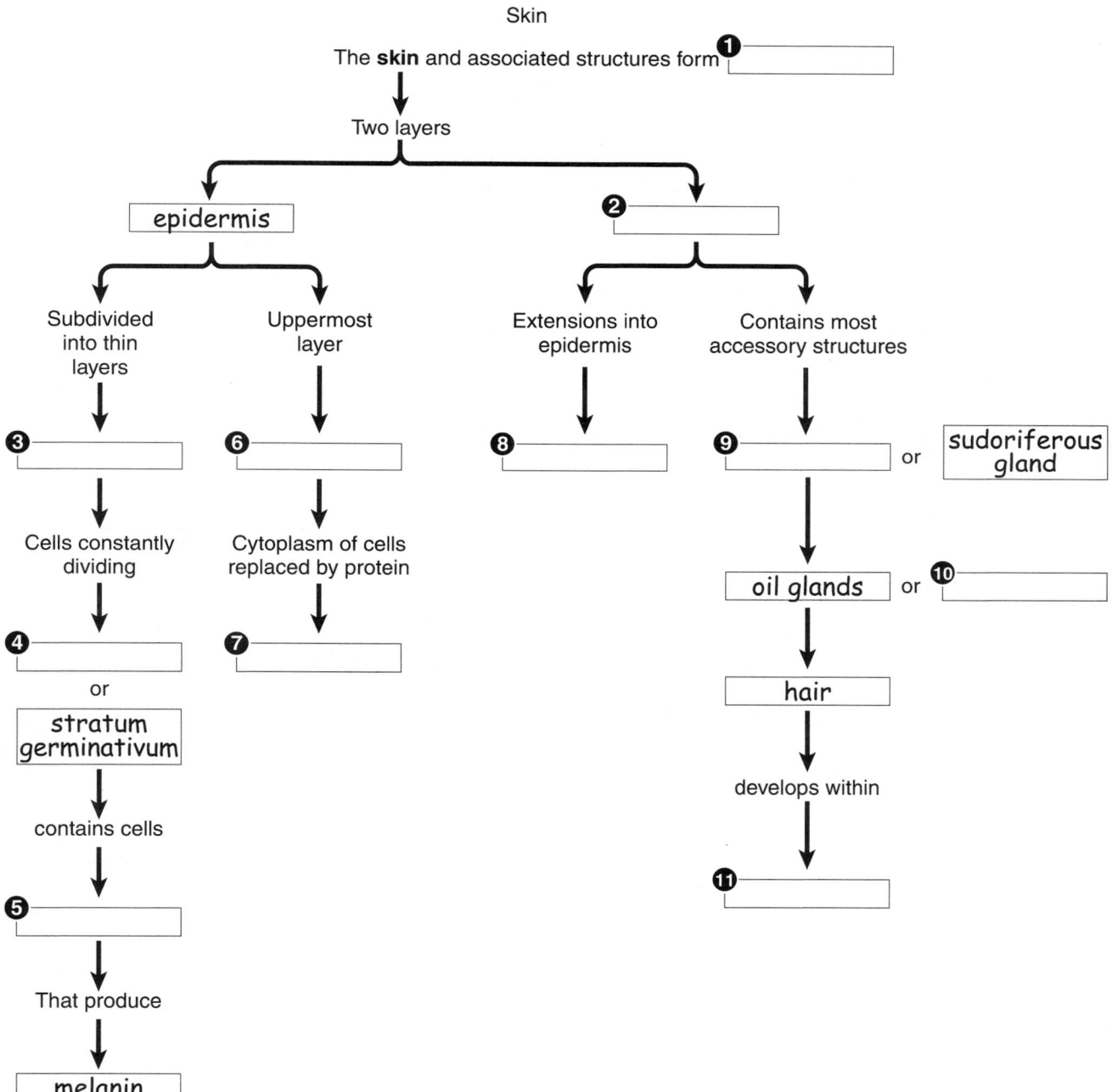

Testing Your Knowledge
Building Understanding

I. Matching Exercises

Matching only within each group, write the answers in the spaces provided.

➤ Group A

apocrine   eccrine   ceruminous   ciliary   sudoriferous

sebaceous   sebum   wax   vernix caseosa

1. A general term for any gland that produces sweat   _____

2. Sweat glands found throughout the skin that help cool

   the body   _____

3. Glands that are only found in the ear canal   _____

4. Excess activity of these glands contributes to acne vulgaris   _____

5. The product of ceruminous glands   _____

6. Sweat glands in the armpits and groin that become active at

   puberty   _____

7. Glands that are only found on the eyelids   _____

➤ Group B

melanocyte   integument   keratin   dermis   epidermis

stratum corneum   dermal papillae   stratum basale   subcutaneous tissue

1. A pigment-producing cell that becomes more active in

   the presence of ultraviolet light   _____

2. The protein in the epidermis that thickens and protects

   the skin   _____

3. The true skin, or corium   _____

4. The uppermost layer of skin, consisting of flat,

   keratin-filled cells   _____

5. Another name for the skin as a whole   _____

6. Portions of the dermis that extend into the epidermis   _____

7. The deepest layer of the epidermis, which contains

   living, dividing cells   _____

II. Multiple Choice

Select the best answer and write the letter of your choice in the blank.

1. New epidermal cells are produced by the: 1. _____
    a. dermis
    b. stratum corneum
    c. stratum basale
    d. subcutaneous layer
2. Which of the following glands is NOT a modified sweat gland?   2. _____
    a. mammary gland
    b. sebaceous gland
    c. ceruminous gland
    d. ciliary gland
3. Blood vessels become smaller to decrease blood flow. This
   decrease in size is called: 3. _____
    a. dilation
    b. constriction
    c. closure
    d. merger
4. Which of the following is NOT an accessory structure of the skin?   4. _____
    a. hair
    b. nails
    c. blood vessels
    d. sweat glands
5. A gland that produces ear wax is a(n):   5. _____
    a. ciliary gland
    b. ceruminous gland
    c. sudoriferous gland
    d. eccrine gland
6. Many babies are born with a cheesy covering known as: 6 _____
    a. keratin
    b. melanin
    c. cerumen
    d. vernix casseosa

III. Completion Exercise

Write the word or phrase that correctly completes each sentence.

1. The outer layer of the epidermis, which contains flat,

   keratin-filled cells, is called the   _____

2. Fingerprints are created by extensions of the dermis

   into the epidermis. These extensions are called   _____

3. The main pigment of the skin is   _____

4. The light-colored, proximal end of a nail that overlies the

   thicker, growing region is the   _____

5. The muscle attached to a hair follicle that produces a

   "goose bump" when it contracts is the   _____

6. The subcutaneous layer is also called the hypodermis or the   _____

7. The ceruminous glands and the ciliary glands are modified

   forms of   _____

8. Hair and nails are composed mainly of a protein named   _____

Understanding Concepts

I. True or False

For each question, write "T" for true or "F" for false in the blank to the left of each number. If a statement is false, correct it by replacing the underlined term and write the correct statement in the blanks below the question.

_____ 1. The nail cuticle, which seals the space between the nail plate and the skin above the nail root, is an extension of the stratum basale.

   _____

_____ 2. In cold weather, the blood vessels in the skin constrict to conserve heat.

   _____

_____ 3. Changes in temperature are detected by Meissner corpuscles.

   _____

_____ 4. Sebum is produced by sudoriferous glands.

   _____

_____ 5. The stratum corneum is the deepest layer of the epidermis.

   _____

II. Practical Applications

➤ Group A

Mr. B has experienced a fall in a downhill mountain biking competition. You are a first-aid volunteer at the competition and are the first person to the scene of the accident. Study each discussion. Then write the appropriate word or phrase in the space provided.

1. Mr. B has light scratches on his cheek. The scratches are not

   bleeding, indicating that they have only penetrated the

   uppermost layer of the epidermis, known as the   _____

2. A branch tore a long jagged wound in his right arm. The
   wound has penetrated into the tissue underneath the dermis,
   known as the superficial fascia or _____

3. The skin of Mr B's nose is very brown. The brown color reflects
   the presence of a pigment called _____

4. Mr. B has difficulties hearing your questions. You examine his
   ears, and discover that they are full of ear wax. Ear wax is
   synthesized by modified sweat glands called _____

5. You note that Mr B has a rather strong body odor. Body odor
   reflects the secretions of glands called _____

6. Mr B, like many young men, suffers from acne vulgaris. This skin
   disease, which is characterized by pimples and blackheads, involves
   infection of the oil-producing glands of the skin called the _____

III. Short Essays

1. Compare and contrast eccrine and apocrine sweat (sudoriferous) glands.

   _____

   _____

   _____

2. Describe the role that the skin plays in the regulation of body temperature.

   _____

   _____

   _____

Conceptual Thinking

1. Describe the location and structure of the different tissue types (epithelial, muscle, nervous,
   connective) present in the integumentary system.

   _____

   _____

   _____

   _____

   _____

Expanding Your Horizons

Why did different skin tones evolve? It is often thought that darker pigmentation (more melanin) has evolved to protect humans from skin cancer. However, because skin cancer occurs later in life (usually after reproduction), it cannot exert much evolutionary pressure. The advantages and disadvantages of darker skin tone are discussed in the following Scientific American article.

Resource List

Jablonski NG, Chaplin G. Skin deep. Sci Am 2002;287:74–81.

chapter 6

The Skeleton: Bones and Joints

Overview

The skeletal system protects and supports the body parts and serves as attachment points for the muscles, which furnish the power for movement. The bones also store calcium salts and are the site of blood cell production. The skeletal system includes approximately 206 bones; the number varies slightly according to age and the individual.

Although bone tissue contains a matrix of nonliving material, bones also contain living cells and have their own systems of blood vessels, lymphatic vessels, and nerves. Bone tissue may be either **spongy** or **compact**. Compact bone is found in the **diaphysis** (shaft) of long bones and in the outer layer of other bones. Spongy bone makes up the **epiphyses** (ends) of long bones and the center of other bones. **Red marrow**, present at the ends of long bones and the center of other bones, manufactures blood cells; **yellow marrow**, which is largely fat, is found in the central (medullary) cavities of the long bones.

Bone tissue is produced by cells called **osteoblasts**, which gradually convert cartilage to bone during development. The mature cells that maintain bone are called **osteocytes**, and the cells that break down (resorb) bone for remodeling and repair are the **osteoclasts**.

The skeleton is divided into two main groups of bones, the **axial skeleton** and the **appendicular skeleton**. The axial skeleton includes the skull, spinal column, ribs, and sternum. The appendicular skeleton consists of the bones of the upper and lower extremities, the shoulder girdle, and the pelvic girdle.

A **joint** is the region of union of two or more bones. Joints are classified into three main types on the basis of the material between the connecting bones. In **fibrous joints**, the bones are held together by fibrous connective tissue, and in **cartilaginous joints** the bones are joined by cartilage. In **synovial joints**, the material between the bones is synovial fluid, which is secreted by the synovial membrane lining the joint cavity. The bones in synovial joints are connected by ligaments. Synovial joints show the greatest degree of movement, and the six types of synovial joints allow for a variety of movements in different directions.

Learning the Language: Word Anatomy

Complete the following table by writing the correct word part or meaning in the space provided. For each word part, write a term that contains the word part.

Word Part	Meaning	Example
1. _____	near, beyond	_____
2. –clast	_____	_____
3. _____	rib	_____
4. amphi-	_____	_____
5. arthr/o-	_____	_____
6. _____	away from	_____
7. _____	around	_____
8. _____	toward, added to	_____
9. dia-	_____	_____
10. pariet/o-	_____	_____

Addressing the Learning Outcomes

I. Writing Exercise

The learning outcomes for Chapter 6 are listed below. These learning outcomes provide an overview of the major topics covered in this chapter. On a separate piece of paper, try to write out an answer to each learning outcome. All of the answers can be found in the pages of the textbook. Learning Outcomes 2, 8, 10, 11, 14, and 15 are also addressed in the Coloring Atlas.

1. List the functions of bones.
2. Describe the structure of a long bone.
3. Differentiate between compact bone and spongy bone with respect to structure and location.
4. Differentiate between red and yellow marrow with respect to function and location.
5. Name the three different types of cells in bone and describe the functions of each.
6. Explain how a long bone grows.
7. Name and describe various markings found on bones.
8. List the bones in the axial skeleton.
9. Explain the purpose of the infant fontanels.
10. Describe the normal curves of the spine and explain their purpose.
11. List the bones in the appendicular skeleton.
12. Compare the structure of the female pelvis and the male pelvis.
13. Describe how the skeleton changes with age.
14. Describe the three types of joints.
15. Describe the structure of a synovial joint and give six examples of synovial joints.
16. Demonstrate six types of movement that occur at synovial joints.
17. Show how word parts are used to build words related to the skeleton.

Exercise 6-1: The Skeleton (text Fig. 6-1)

Instructions

1. Write the name of each labeled part on the numbered lines in different colors. Use the same color for structures 24 and 25 and for structures 19 and 20.
2. Color the different structures on the diagram with the corresponding color. Try to color every structure in the figure with the appropriate color. For instance, structure number 3 is found in two locations.

1. _____

2. _____

3. _____

4. _____

5. _____

6. _____

7. _____

8. _____

9. _____

10. _____

11. _____

12. _____

13. _____

14. _____

15. _____

16. _____

17. _____

18. _____

19. _____

20. _____

21. _____

22. _____

23. _____

24. _____

25. _____

26. _____

EXERCISE 6-2: Structure of a Long Bone (text Fig. 6-2)

INSTRUCTIONS

1. Write the names of the three parts of a long bone in the numbered boxes 1–3.
2. Write the name of each labeled part on the numbered lines in different colors. Use a dark color for structure 5.
3. Color the different structures on the diagram with the corresponding color.

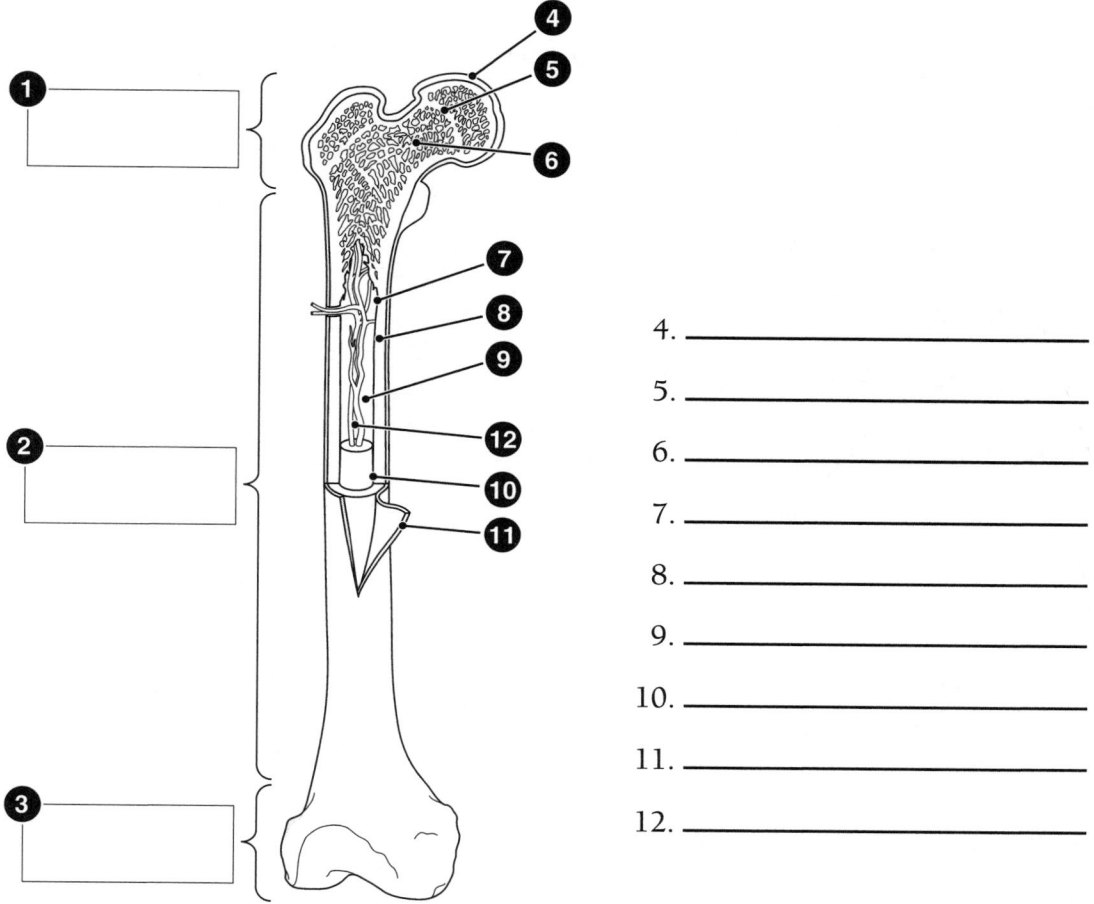

4. _____

5. _____

6. _____

7. _____

8. _____

9. _____

10. _____

11. _____

12. _____

EXERCISE 6-3: The Skull: Frontal View (text Fig. 6-5A)

INSTRUCTIONS

1. Color the boxes next to the names of the skull bones in different, light colors.
2. Color the skull bones in parts A, B, and C of the diagram with the corresponding color.
3. Label each of the following numbered bones and bone features. If you wish, you can use different dark colors to write the names and color or outline the corresponding part for all structures except structures 4, 9, and 12.

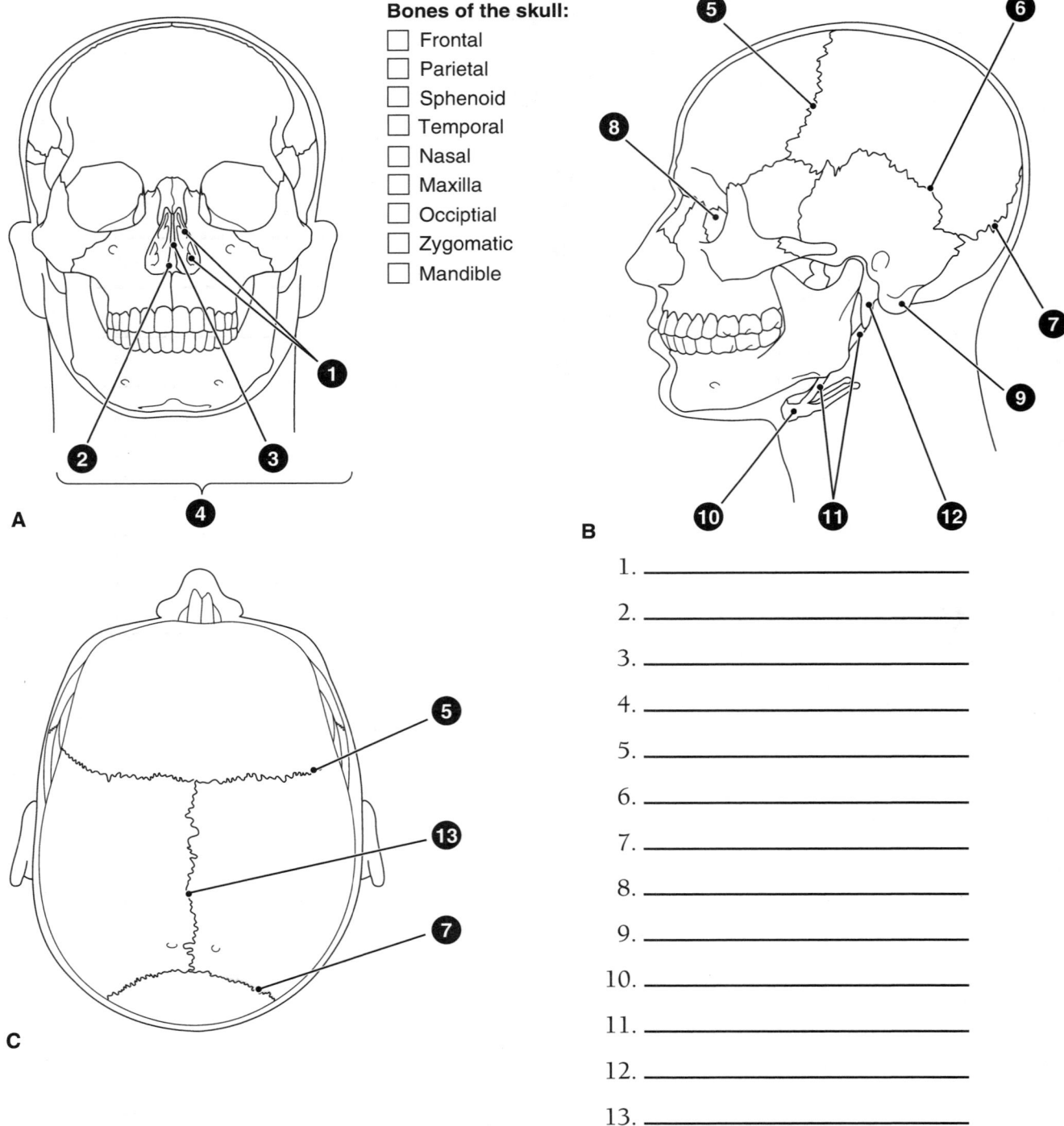

Bones of the skull:
☐ Frontal
☐ Parietal
☐ Sphenoid
☐ Temporal
☐ Nasal
☐ Maxilla
☐ Occiptial
☐ Zygomatic
☐ Mandible

A

B

C

1. _____
2. _____
3. _____
4. _____
5. _____
6. _____
7. _____
8. _____
9. _____
10. _____
11. _____
12. _____
13. _____

EXERCISE 6-4: The Skull: Inferior, Superior, and Sagittal Views (text Figs. 6-6, 6-7, and 6-8)

INSTRUCTIONS

1. Use the same colors you used in Exercise 6-3 to color the boxes next to the skull bone names.
2. Color the skull bones in parts A, B, and C of the diagram with the corresponding color.
3. Label each of the following numbered bones and bone features. If you wish, you can use different colors to write the name and color the corresponding part for all structures except structures 3, 5, and 8.

Bones of the skull:

☐ Frontal   ☐ Occipital
☐ Parietal   ☐ Zygomatic
☐ Temporal   ☐ Mandible
☐ Sphenoid   ☐ Maxilla

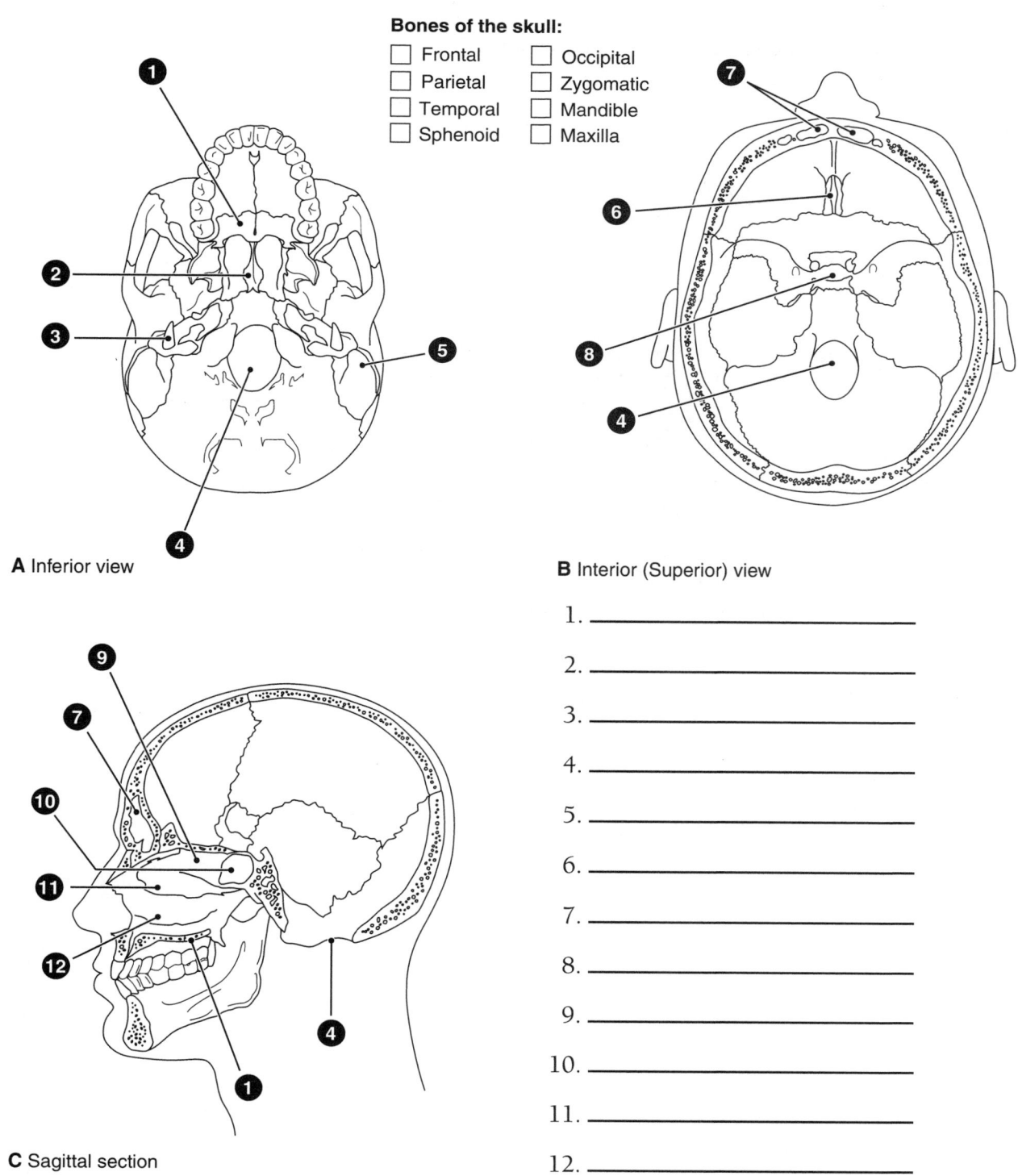

A Inferior view

B Interior (Superior) view

C Sagittal section

1. _____

2. _____

3. _____

4. _____

5. _____

6. _____

7. _____

8. _____

9. _____

10. _____

11. _____

12. _____

EXERCISE 6-5: Vertebral Column: Lateral View (text Fig. 6-10)

INSTRUCTIONS

1. Color each of the following bones the indicated color.
    a. cervical vertebrae—blue
    b. thoracic vertebrae—red
    c. lumbar vertebrae—green
    d. sacrum—yellow
    e. coccyx—violet
2. Label each of the indicated bones and bone parts.

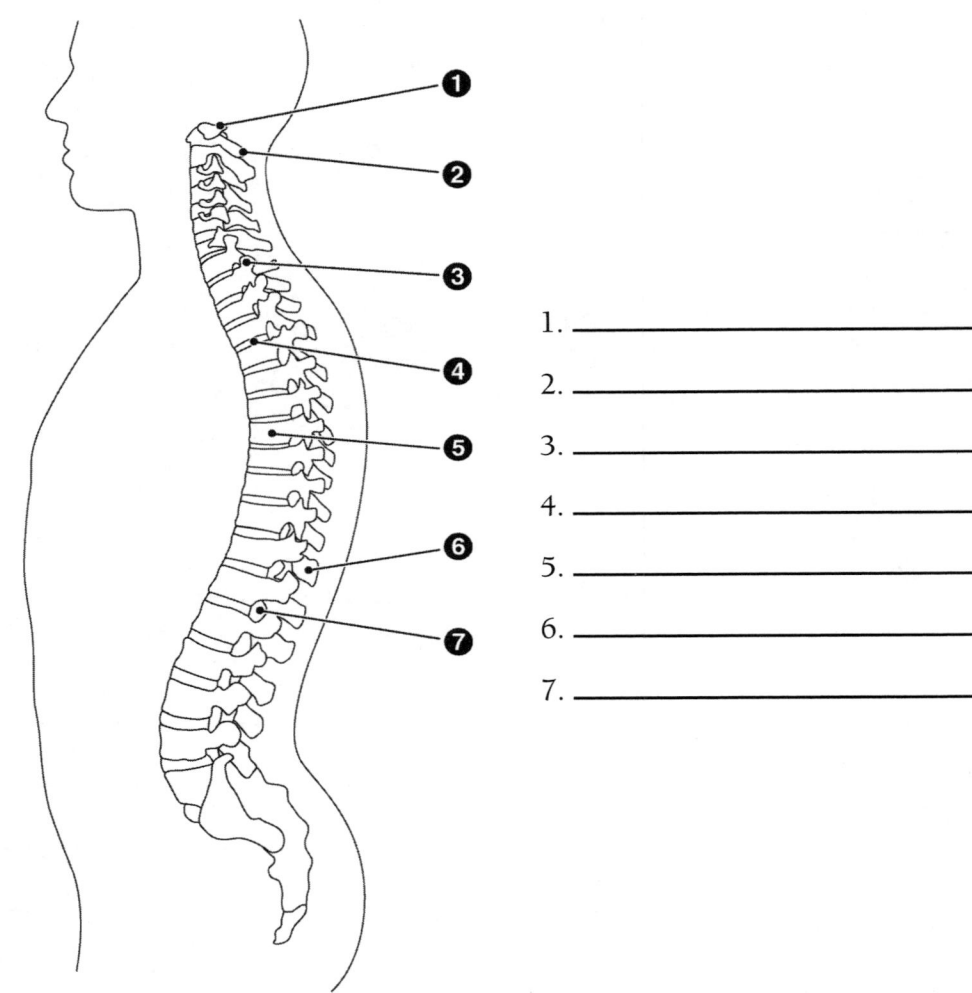

1. _____

2. _____

3. _____

4. _____

5. _____

6. _____

7. _____

EXERCISE 6-6: Vertebral Column: Anterior View (text Fig. 6-11)

INSTRUCTIONS

1. Write the name of each type of vertebra in the numbered boxes 1–3.
2. Write the name of each labeled part on the numbered lines in different colors.
3. Color the different structures on the diagram with the corresponding color.

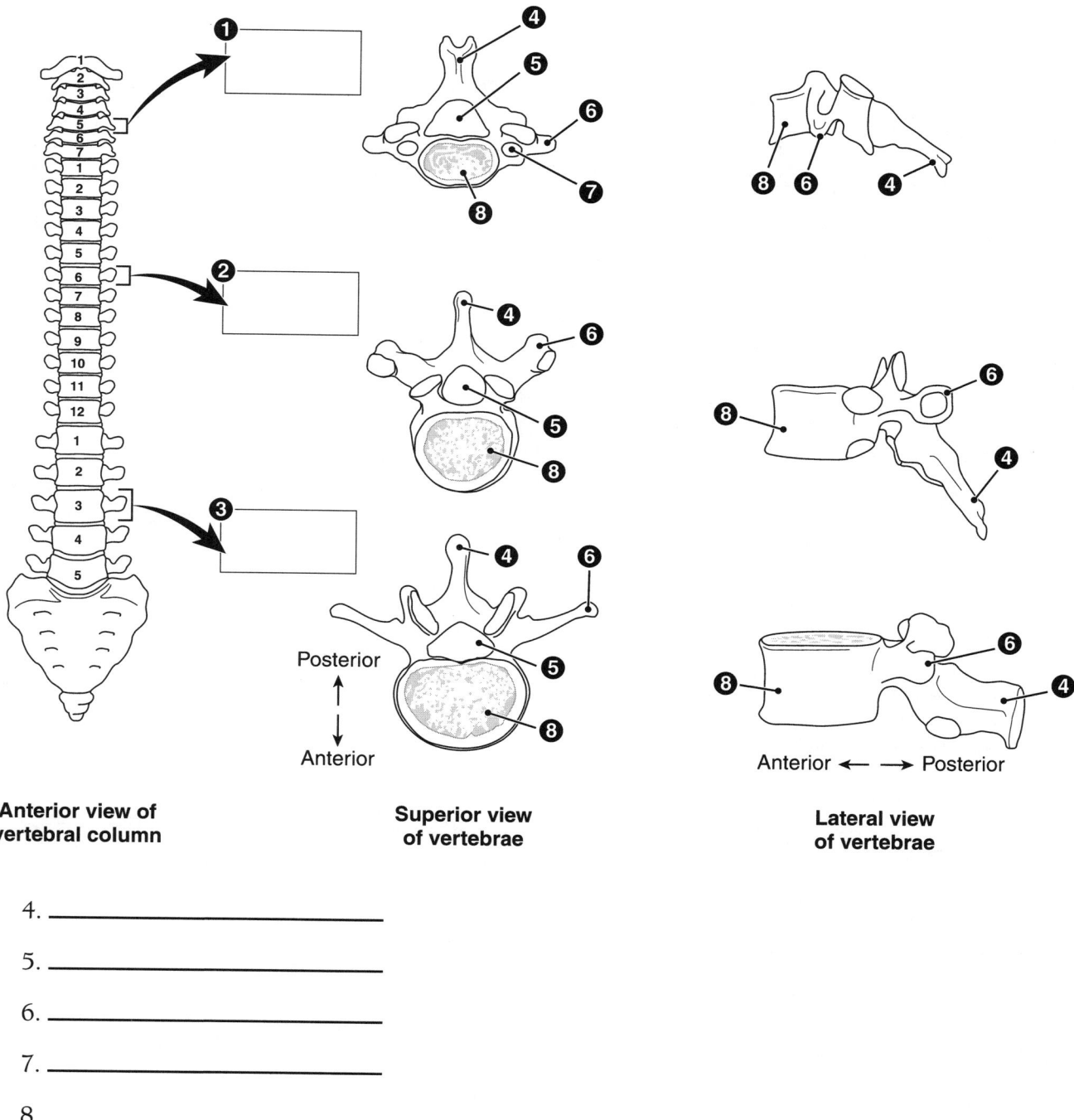

Anterior view of
vertebral column

Superior view
of vertebrae

Lateral view
of vertebrae

4. _____

5. _____

6. _____

7. _____

8. _____

EXERCISE 6-7: Bones of the Thorax: Anterior View (text Fig. 6-14)

INSTRUCTIONS

1. Write the name of each labeled part on the numbered lines in different colors. Structures 1, 3, 6, and 7 will not be colored, so write their names in black.
2. Color the different structures on the diagram with the corresponding color.

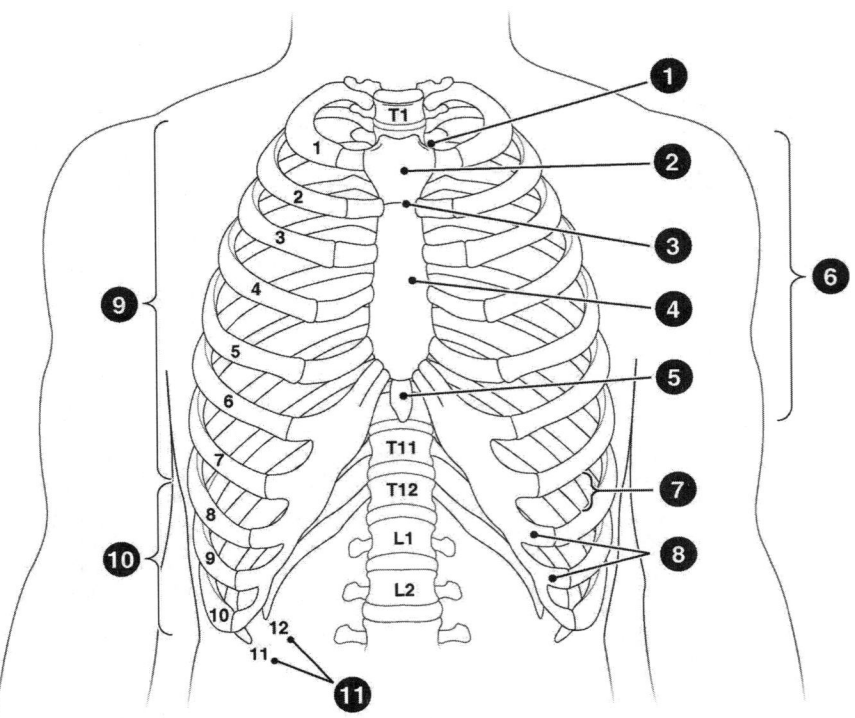

1. _____

2. _____

3. _____

4. _____

5. _____

6. _____

7. _____

8. _____

9. _____

10. _____

11. _____

EXERCISE 6-8: Bones of the Shoulder Girdle (text Fig. 6-15)

INSTRUCTIONS

1. Write the name of each labeled part on the numbered lines in different colors. Use the same color for all of the parts of the scapula.
2. Color the different structures on the diagram with the corresponding color.

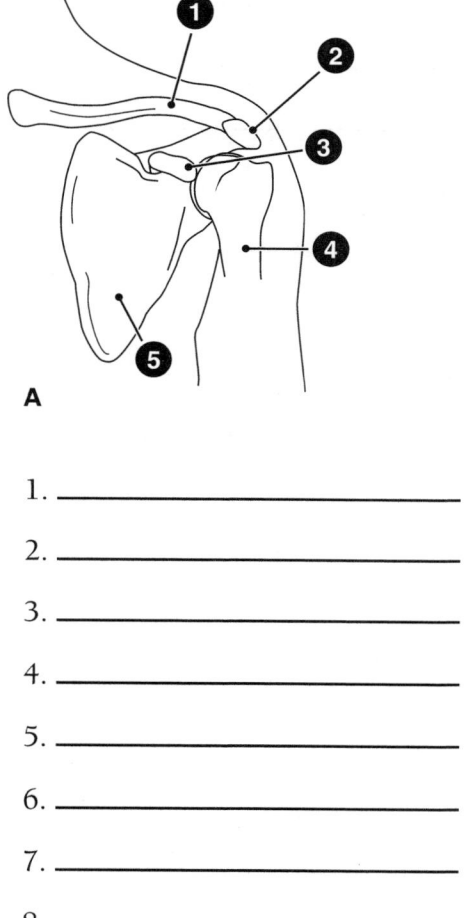
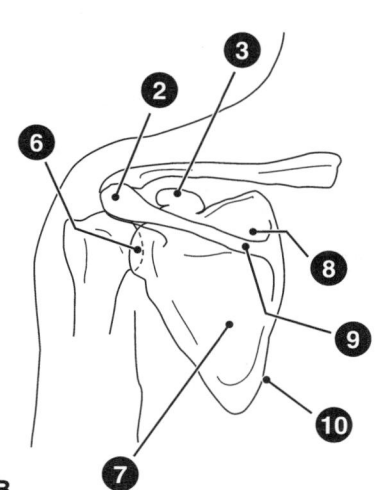

A   B

1. _____

2. _____

3. _____

4. _____

5. _____

6. _____

7. _____

8. _____

9. _____

10. _____

EXERCISE 6-9: Left Elbow: Lateral View (text Fig. 6-19)

INSTRUCTIONS

Label each of the indicated parts. The identity of parts 7 and 8 can be found in Figure 6-17.

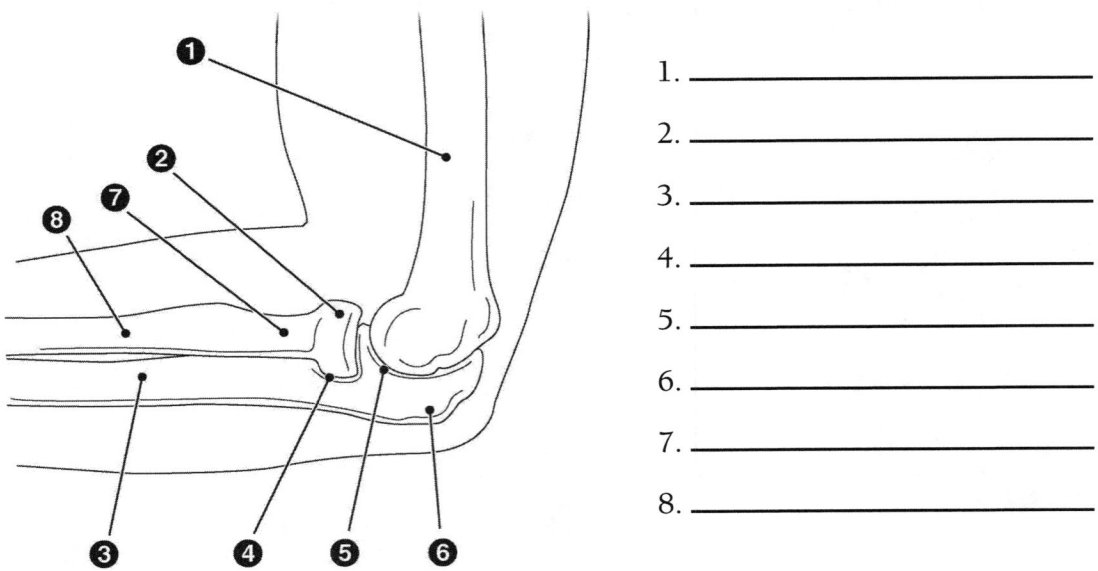

1. _____

2. _____

3. _____

4. _____

5. _____

6. _____

7. _____

8. _____

EXERCISE 6-10: Pelvic Bones (text Fig. 6-21)

INSTRUCTIONS

1. Color the boxes next to the names of the pelvic bones in different, light colors.
2. Color the pelvic bones in parts A and B of the diagram with the corresponding color.
3. Label each of the following numbered bones and bone features. If you wish, you can use different dark colors to write the names and color or outline the corresponding part for structures 1, 3, 8, and 10.

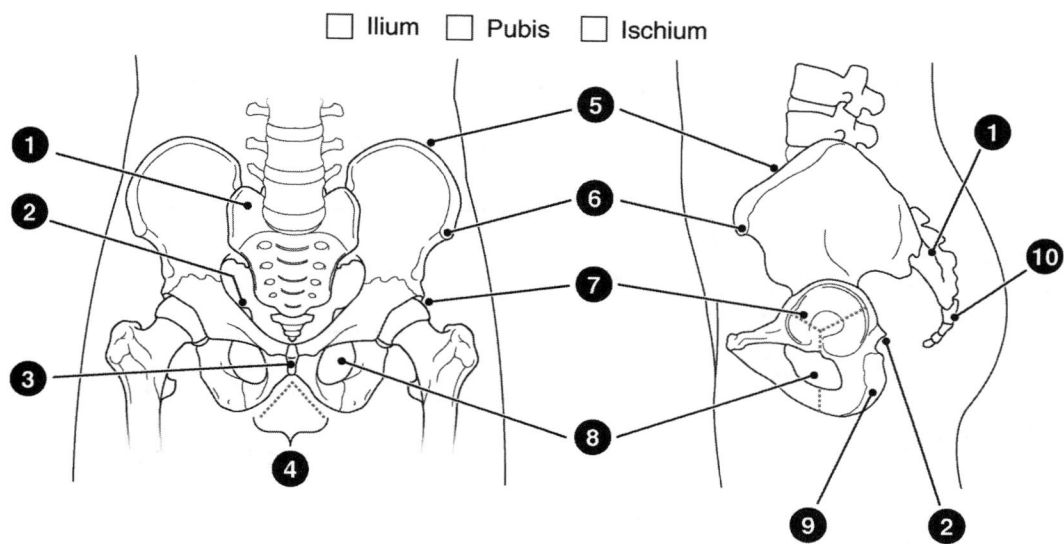

☐ Ilium   ☐ Pubis   ☐ Ischium

A Anterior view   **B** Lateral view

1. _____

2. _____

3. _____

4. _____

5. _____

6. _____

7. _____

8. _____

9. _____

10. _____

EXERCISE 6-11: The Knee Joint (text Fig. 6-27)

INSTRUCTIONS

1. Write the name of each labeled part on the numbered lines in different colors. Use a dark color for part 7, which can be outlined.
2. Color the different structures on the diagram with the corresponding color. Try to color every structure in the figure with the appropriate color. For instance, structure number 2 is found in two locations.

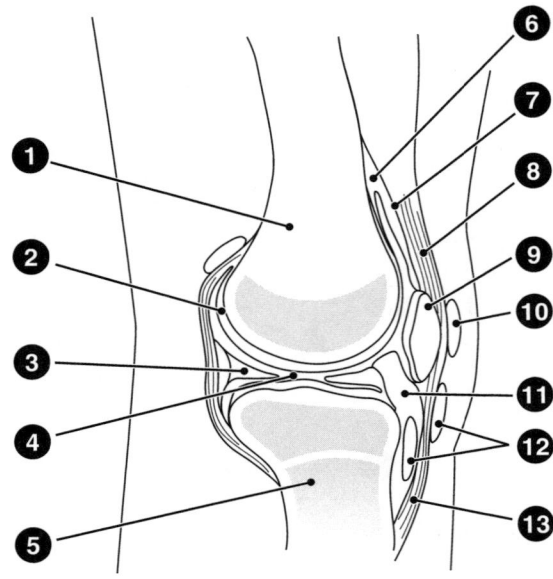

1. _____

2. _____

3. _____

4. _____

5. _____

6. _____

7. _____

8. _____

9. _____

10. _____

11. _____

12. _____

13. _____

EXERCISE 6-12: Movements at Synovial Joints (text Fig. 6-28)

INSTRUCTIONS

Label each of the illustrated motions with the correct term for that movement.

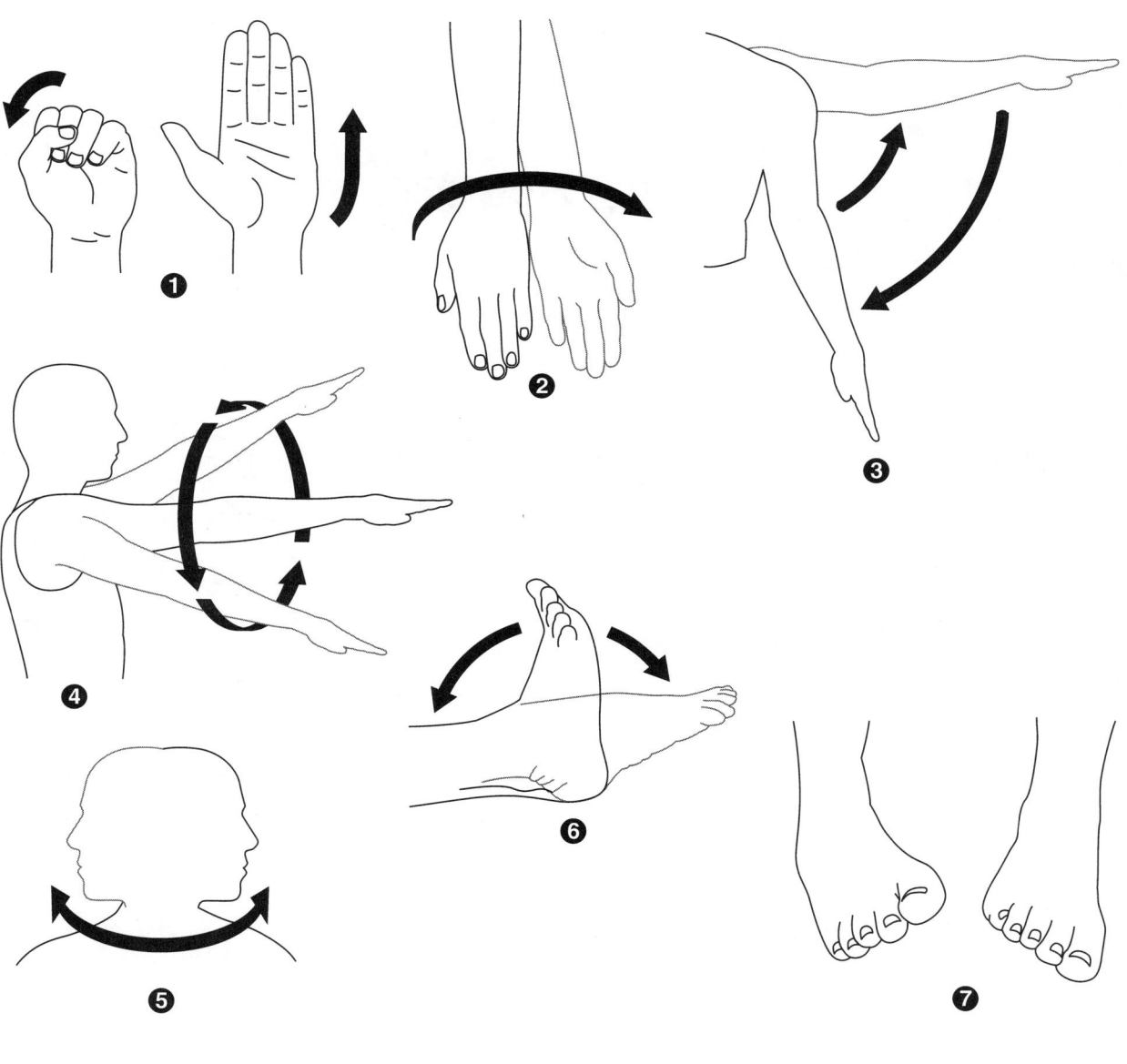

1. _____

2. _____

3. _____

4. _____

5. _____

6. _____

7. _____

EXERCISE 6-13: Types of Synovial Joints (text Table 6-3)

INSTRUCTIONS

Label each of the different types of synovial joints.

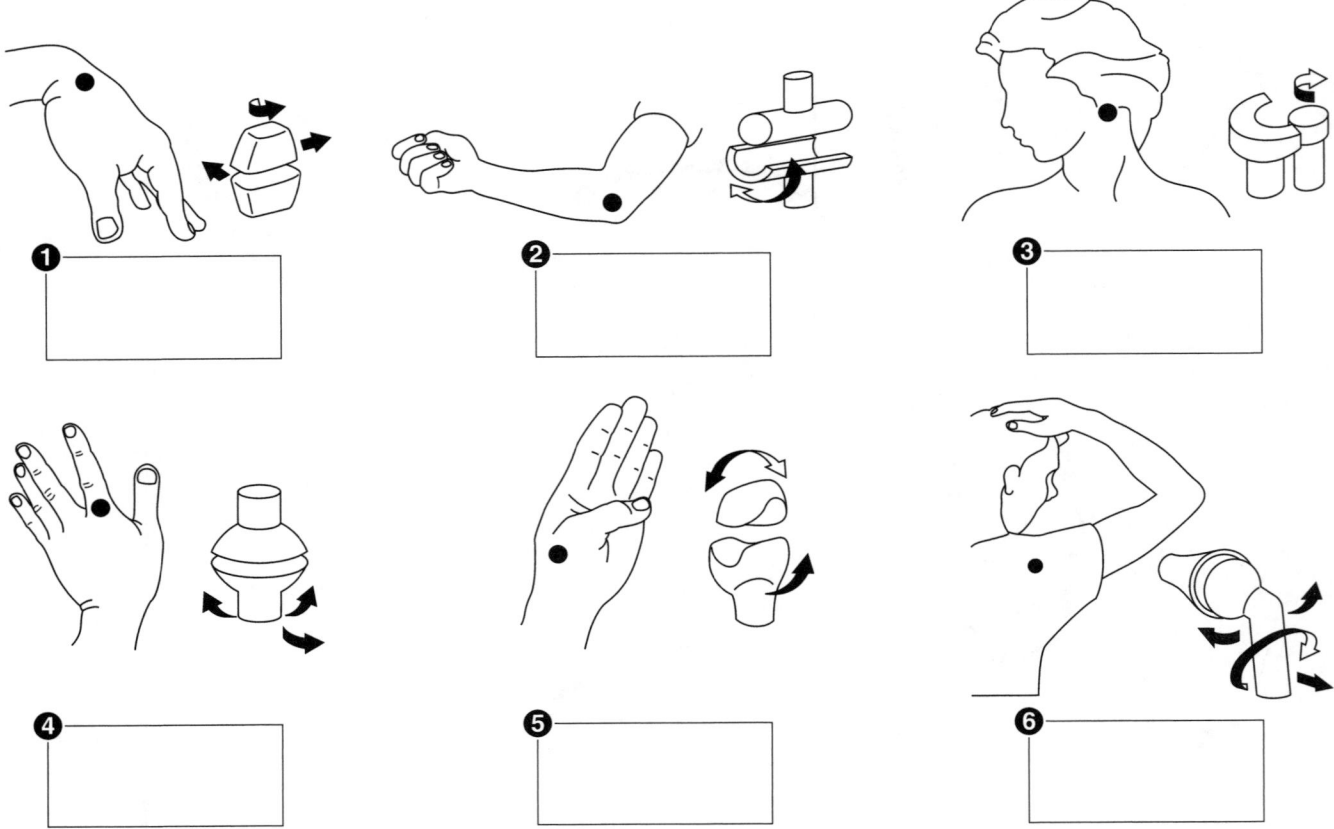

❶ _____

❷ _____

❸ _____

❹ _____

❺ _____

❻ _____

Making the Connections

The following concept map deals with bone structure. Complete the concept map by filling in the appropriate term or phrase that describes the indicated structure or process.

Optional Exercise: Make your own concept map, based on the different bone markings. Choose your own terms to incorporate into your map, or use the following list: bone markings, projections, depressions, head, process, condyle, crest, spine, foramen, sinus, fossa, meatus, sella turcica, mastoid sinus, foramen magnum, acromion, intervertebral foramina, supraspinous fossa, scapula spine. Try to find an example of each bone marking.

Bone Structure and Organization

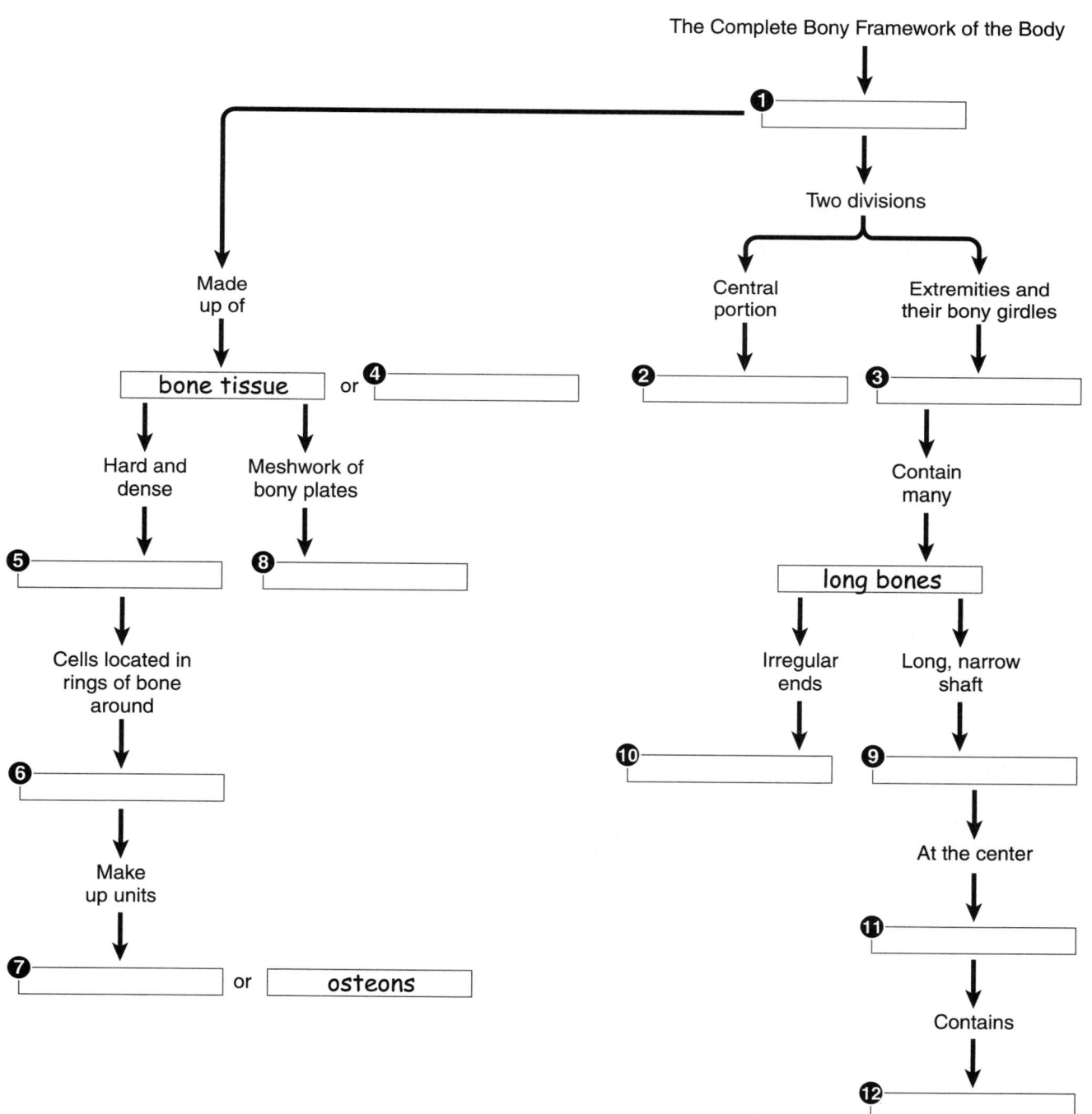

Testing Your Knowledge
Building Understanding

I. Matching Exercises

Matching only within each group, write the answers in the spaces provided.

➤ **Group A**

red marrow	diaphysis	epiphysis	medullary cavity	yellow marrow
periosteum	endosteum	spongy bone	osteon	

1. The fatty material found inside the central cavities of long bones _____

2. The shaft of a long bone _____

3. The tough connective tissue membrane that covers bones _____

4. The primary site of blood cell production _____

5. The end of a long bone _____

6. The type of bone tissue found at the end of long bones _____

7. The thin membrane that lines the central cavity of long bones _____

➤ **Group B**

osteoclast	osteoblast	osteocyte	crest	condyle
foramen	fossa	sinus	meatus	

1. A short channel or passageway _____

2. An air space found in some skull bones _____

3. A cell that resorbs bone matrix _____

4. A mature bone cell that is completely surrounded by hard bone tissue _____

5. A distinct border or ridge _____

6. A depression on a bone surface _____

7. A hole that permits the passage of a vessel or nerve _____

➤ **Group C**

parietal bone	temporal bone	frontal bone	hyoid bone	nasal bone
occipital bone	maxilla	mandible	sphenoid bone	zygomatic bone

1. The only movable bone of the skull _____

2. A bone of the upper jaw _____

3. The U-shaped bone lying just below the mandible _____

4. The bone that articulates with the parietal and temporal bones and forms the posterior inferior part of the cranium _____

5. The bone that forms the forehead

    _____

6. One of two slender bones that form the bridge of the nose

    _____

7. One of two large bones that articulate with the frontal bone
   and form the superior lateral portions of the cranium

    _____

8. The anatomical name for the cheekbone

    _____

➤ Group D

cervical region   thoracic region   lumbar region   coccyx

transverse process   intervertebral foramina

1. The site of attachment for spinal muscles on a vertebra

    _____

2. The second part of the vertebral column, made up of
   12 vertebrae

    _____

3. Spaces between the vertebrae that permit the passage of
   nerves

    _____

4. The most caudal part of the vertebral column

    _____

5. The region of the spine that contains the largest, strongest
   vertebrae

    _____

6. The region of the vertebral column made up of the first seven
   vertebrae

    _____

➤ Group E

floating ribs   true ribs   fontanel   costal   foramina

xiphoid process   manubrium   clavicular notch

1. The T-shaped, superior portion of the sternum

    _____

2. The portion of the sternum that is made of cartilage in
   children

    _____

3. An adjective that refers to the ribs

    _____

4. A soft spot in the infant skull that later closes

    _____

5. The last two pairs of ribs, which are very short and do not
   extend to the front of the body

    _____

6. The articulation between the sternum and the collarbone

    _____

7. Ribs that attach to the sternum by individual cartilagenous
   extensions

    _____

➤ **Group F**

olecranon	carpal bones	clavicle	ulna	radius
metacarpal bones	phalanges	scapula	humerus	

1. The anatomical name for the collarbone   _____

2. The five bones in the palm of the hand   _____

3. The medial forearm bone (in the anatomical position)   _____

4. The upper part of the ulna, which forms the point of the
   elbow   _____

5. The 14 small bones that form the framework of the fingers on
   each hand   _____

6. The bone located on the thumb side of the forearm   _____

7. The bone containing the supraspinous and infraspinous fossae   _____

➤ **Group G**

greater trochanter	patella	tibia	calcaneus	
fibula	ilium	ischium	acetabulum	pubis

1. The deep socket in the hip bone that holds the head of the
   femur   _____

2. The most inferior bone in the pelvis   _____

3. The lateral bone of the leg   _____

4. A bone that is wider and more flared in females   _____

5. The scientific name for the kneecap   _____

6. The largest of the tarsal bones; the heel bone   _____

7. The large, rounded projection at the upper and lateral portion
   of the femur   _____

➤ **Group H**

flexion	rotation	abduction	extension	adduction
supination	circumduction	dorsiflexion	plantar flexion	

1. A movement that increases the angle between two bones   _____

2. Movement away from the midline of the body   _____

3. Motion around a central axis   _____

4. A bending motion that decreases the angle between two parts   _____

5. Movement toward the midline of the body   _____

6. The act of turning the palm up or forward _____

7. The act of pointing the toes downward _____

➤ **Group I**

| articulation | diarthrosis | amphiarthrosis | synarthrosis | articular cartilage |

bursitis   bursa   joint capsule

1. Inflammation of a small sac near a joint _____

2. The region of union of two or more bones; a joint _____

3. A slightly movable joint _____

4. The connective tissue that encloses a joint and is continuous

   with the periosteum _____

5. Smooth connective tissue covering bone surfaces at synovial joints _____

6. A freely movable joint held together by ligaments _____

II. Multiple Choice

Select the best answer and write the letter of your choice in the blank.

1. The bone cells that synthesize new bone matrix are called: 1. _____
   a. osteoblasts
   b. osteocytes
   c. osteoclasts
   d. osteons

2. A suture is an example of an immovable joint also called a(n):   2. _____
   a. synovial joint
   b. diarthrosis
   c. synarthrosis
   d. amphiarthrosis

3. Which of the following is a projection?   3. _____
   a. process
   b. fossa
   c. foramen
   d. sinus

4. The back of the hard palate is formed by the: 4. _____
   a. vomer bone
   b. palatine bones
   c. hyoid bone
   d. mandible

5. The os coxae is a fused bone consisting of the ilium, ischium, and: 5. _____
   a. femur
   b. acetabulum
   c. sacrum
   d. pubis

6. The patella is the largest of a type of bone that develops within a tendon or a joint capsule. It is described as: 6. _____
   a. sesamoid
   b. axial
   c. tarsal
   d. symphysis

7. The shoulder girdle consists of the clavicle and the: 7. _____
   a. sternum
   b. tibia
   c. scapula
   d. os coxa

8. Ribs that individually attach to the sternum are called the: 8. _____
   a. false ribs
   b. floating ribs
   c. xiphoid ribs
   d. true ribs

9. The foramen magnum is: 9. _____
   a. a large hole in a hip bone near the symphysis pubis
   b. the curved rim along the top of the hip bone
   c. a hole between vertebrae that allows for passage of a spinal nerve
   d. a large opening at the base of the skull through which the spinal cord passes

10. Which of the following is an example of a cartilaginous joint?   10. _____
    a. condyloid
    b. pivot
    c. saddle
    d. pubic symphysis

III. Completion Exercise

Write the word or phrase that correctly completes each sentence.

1. The first cervical vertebra is called the   _____
2. The bat-shaped bone that extends behind the eyes and also forms part of the base of the skull is called the   _____
3. The bone located between the eyes that extends into the nasal cavity, eye sockets, and cranial floor is called the   _____
4. The hard bone matrix is composed mainly of salts of the element   _____
5. The part of the skull that encloses the brain is the   _____
6. A joint between bones of the skull is a(n)   _____
7. Pivot, hinge, and gliding joints are examples of freely movable joints, also called   _____
8. Swimming the overhead crawl requires a broad circular movement at the shoulder that is a combination of simpler movements. This combined motion is called   _____
9. When you bend your foot upward and walk on your heels, the motion is technically called   _____

10. In the embryo, most of the developing bones are made of _____
11. The type of bone tissue that makes up the shaft of a long bone is called _____
12. The skull, vertebrae, ribs, and sternum make up the division of the skeleton called the _____

Understanding Concepts

I. True or False

For each question, write "T" for true or "F" for false in the blank to the left of each number. If a statement is false, correct it by replacing the <u>underlined</u> term and write the correct statement in the blanks below the question.

_____ 1. The shaft of a long bone contains <u>yellow</u> marrow.

_____

_____ 2. The ethmoid bone is in the <u>axial</u> skeleton.

_____

_____ 3. Moving a bone toward the midline is <u>abduction</u>.

_____

_____ 4. The second cervical vertebra is called the <u>axis</u>.

_____

_____ 5. Increasing the angle at a joint is <u>extension</u>.

_____

_____ 6. There are <u>six</u> pairs of false ribs.

_____

_____ 7. A mature bone cell is an <u>osteocyte</u>.

_____

_____ 8. <u>Immovable</u> joints are called synovial joints.

_____

_____ 9. The ends of a long bone are composed mainly of <u>spongy</u> bone.

_____

_____ 10. In the anatomical position, the tibia is <u>medial</u> to the fibula.

_____

_____ 11. The medial malleolus is found at the distal end of the <u>fibula</u>.

_____

II. Practical Applications

➤ Group A

Ms. M, aged 67, experienced a serious fall at a recent bowling tournament. As a physician assistant trainee, you are responsible for her preliminary evaluation.

1. Her right forearm is bent at a peculiar angle. You suspect a fracture to the radius or to the _____

2. An x-ray reveals a broken radius as well as a number of fractures in the wrist bones, which are also called the _____

3. Ms. M also reports pain in the hip region. The hip joint consists of the femur and a deep socket called the _____

4. An x-ray reveals a crack in the "sitting bone" that supports the weight of the trunk when sitting. This bone is called the _____

5. The large number of fractures Ms. M sustained suggests that she has a bone disorder called osteoporosis. The physician prescribes a new medication designed to increase the activity of cells that synthesize new bone tissue. These cells are called _____

➤ Group B

Ms L, aged 23, suffers from rheumatoid arthritis, an inflammatory disease of the joints. She is at the clinic for her yearly checkup.

1. She experiences pain in the joints of her hands and fingers. The pain reflects overgrowth and inflammation of the membrane lining the joint cavities. This membrane is known as the _____

2. The pain is experienced primarily in freely moveable joints, which are known as synovial joints or _____

3. The bones in synovial joints are held together by bands of fibrous connective tissue called _____

4. The examining physician asks her to straighten her fingers. This movement, which increases the angle between the bones, is known as _____

5. Next, Ms L is asked to bend her foot upward at the ankle. This special movement at the ankle joint is known as _____

6. Ms L's range of motion has considerably diminished since her last appointment. The physician fears that the hyaline cartilage protecting the bone surface has been destroyed. This cartilage is known as the _____

III. Short Essays

1. What is the function of the fontanels?

_____

_____

_____

2. Describe the four curves of the adult spine and explain the purpose of these curves.

_____

_____

_____

3. What is the difference between true ribs, false ribs, and floating ribs?

_____

_____

_____

Conceptual Thinking

The following questions relate to the knee joint.

A. Classify the knee joint in terms of the **degree** of movement permitted.

_____

B. Classify the knee joint based on the **types** of movement permitted.

_____

C. Classify the knee joint in terms of the material between the adjoining bones.

_____

D. List the bones that articulate within the capsule of the knee joint.

_____

E. List the types of movement that can occur at the knee joint.

_____

Expanding Your Horizons

The human skeleton has evolved from that of four-legged animals. Unfortunately, the adaptation is far from perfect; thus, our upright posture causes problems like backache and knee injuries. If you could design the human skeleton from scratch, what would you change? The following Scientific American article suggests some improvements.

Resource List

Olshansky JS, Carnes BA, Butler RN. If humans were built to last. Sci Am 2001;284:50–55.

chapter 7

The Muscular System

Overview

There are three basic types of muscle tissue: skeletal, smooth, and cardiac. This chapter focuses on **skeletal muscle**, which is usually attached to bones. Skeletal muscle is also called **voluntary muscle**, because it is normally under conscious control. The muscular system is composed of more than 650 individual muscles.

Skeletal muscles are activated by electrical impulses from the nervous system. A nerve fiber makes contact with a muscle cell at the **neuromuscular junction**. The neurotransmitter **acetylcholine** transmits the signal from the neuron to the muscle cell by producing an electrical change called the **action potential** in the muscle cell membrane. The action potential causes the release of **calcium** from the endoplasmic reticulum into the muscle cell cytoplasm. Calcium enables two types of intracellular filaments inside the muscle cell, made of **actin** and **myosin**, to contact each other. The myosin filaments pull the actin filaments closer together, resulting in muscle contraction. **ATP** is the direct source of energy for the contraction. To manufacture ATP, the cell must have adequate supplies of **glucose** and **oxygen** delivered by the blood. A reserve supply of glucose is stored in muscle cells in the form of **glycogen**. Additional oxygen is stored by a muscle cell pigment called myoglobin.

When muscles do not receive enough oxygen, as during strenuous activity, they can produce a small amount of ATP and continue to function for a short period. As a result, however, the cells produce **lactic acid**, which may contribute to muscle fatigue. A person must then rest and continue to inhale oxygen, which is used to convert the lactic acid into other substances. The amount of oxygen needed for this purpose is referred to as the **oxygen debt**.

Muscles usually work in groups to execute a body movement. The muscle that produces a given movement is called the **prime mover**; the muscle that produces the opposite action is the **antagonist**.

Muscles act with the bones of the skeleton as lever systems, in which the joint is the pivot point or fulcrum. Exercise and proper body mechanics help maintain muscle health and effectiveness. Continued activity delays the undesirable effects of aging.

This chapter contains some challenging concepts, particularly with respect to muscle contractions, and many muscles to memorize. Try to learn the muscle names and actions by using your own body. You should be familiar with the different movements and the anatomy of joints from Chapter 6 before you tackle this chapter.

Learning the Language: Word Anatomy

Word Part	Meaning	Example
1._____	muscle	_____
2. brachi/o	_____	_____
3. _____	nutrition, nurture	_____
4. erg/o	_____	_____
5. metr/o	_____	_____
6. _____	four	_____
7. _____	tone, tension	_____
8. _____	flesh	_____
9. vas/o	_____	_____
10. iso-	_____	_____

Addressing the Learning Outcomes

I. Writing Exercise

The learning outcomes for Chapter 7 are listed below. These learning outcomes provide an overview of the major topics covered in this chapter. On a separate piece of paper, try to write out an answer to each learning outcome. All of the answers can be found in the pages of the textbook. Learning Outcomes 3, 9, and 12 are also addressed in the Coloring Atlas.

1. Compare the three types of muscle tissue.
2. Describe three functions of skeletal muscle.
3. Briefly describe how skeletal muscles contract.
4. List the substances needed in muscle contraction and describe the function of each.
5. Define the term "oxygen debt."
6. Describe three compounds stored in muscle that are used to generate energy in highly active muscle cells.
7. Cite the effects of exercise on muscles.
8. Compare isotonic and isometric contractions.
9. Explain how muscles work in pairs to produce movement.
10. Compare the workings of muscles and bones to lever systems.
11. Explain how muscles are named.
12. Name some of the major muscles in each muscle group and describe the main function of each.
13. Describe how muscles change with age.
14. Show how word parts are used to build words related to the muscular system.

II. Labeling and Coloring Atlas

EXERCISE 7-1: Structure of a Skeletal Muscle (text Fig. 7-1)

INSTRUCTIONS

Label each of the indicated parts.

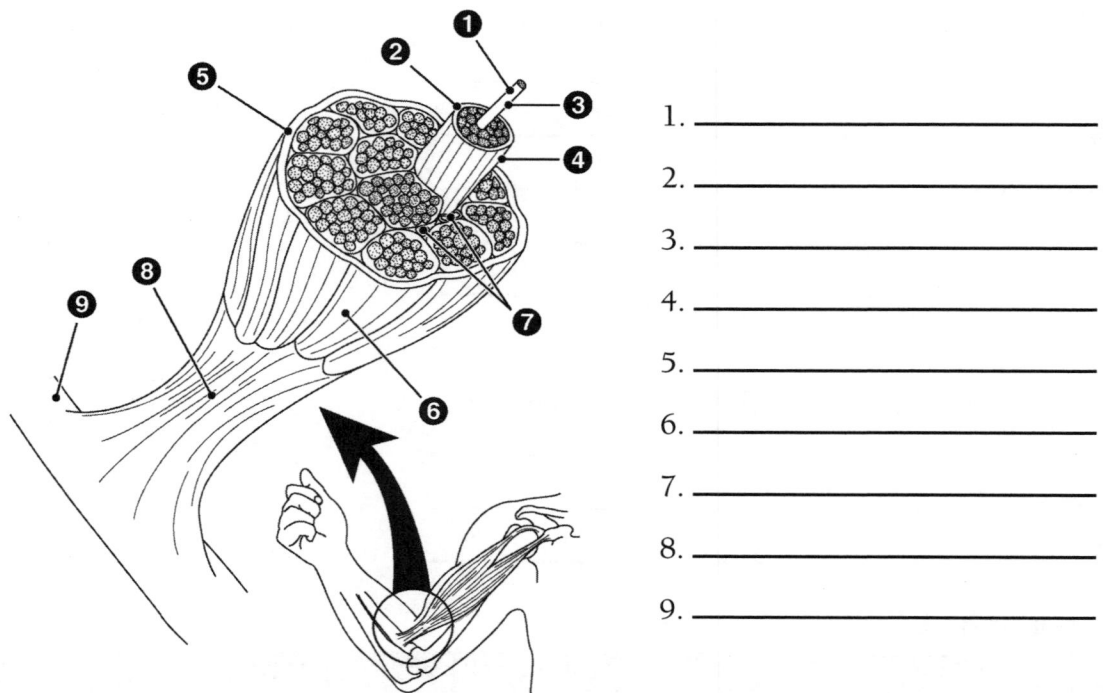

1. _____
2. _____
3. _____
4. _____
5. _____
6. _____
7. _____
8. _____
9. _____

EXERCISE 7-2: Neuromuscular Junction (text Fig. 7-3)

INSTRUCTIONS

Label each of the indicated parts.

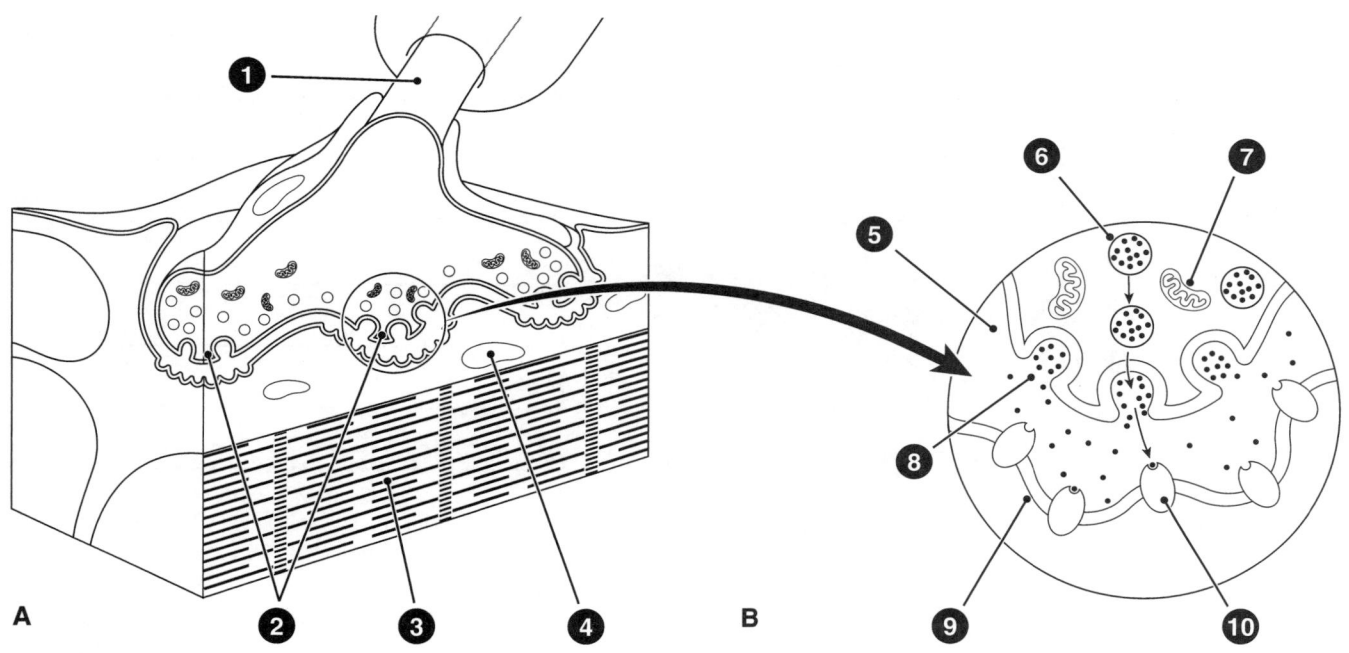

1. _____

2. _____

3. _____

4. _____

5. _____

6. _____

7. _____

8. _____

9. _____

10. _____

EXERCISE 7-3: Muscle Attachment to Bones (text Fig. 7-7)

INSTRUCTIONS

Label each of the indicated parts.

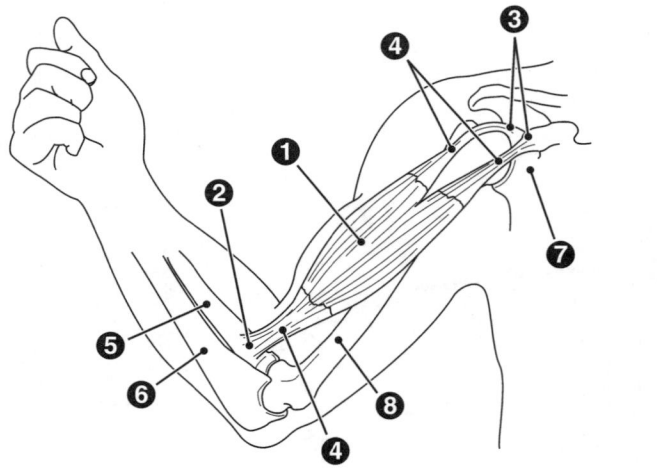

1. _____

2. _____

3. _____

4. _____

5. _____

6. _____

7. _____

8. _____

EXERCISE 7-4: Superficial Muscles: Anterior View (text Fig. 7-9)

INSTRUCTIONS

1. Write the name of each labeled muscle on the numbered lines in different colors.
2. Color the different muscles on the diagram with the corresponding color.

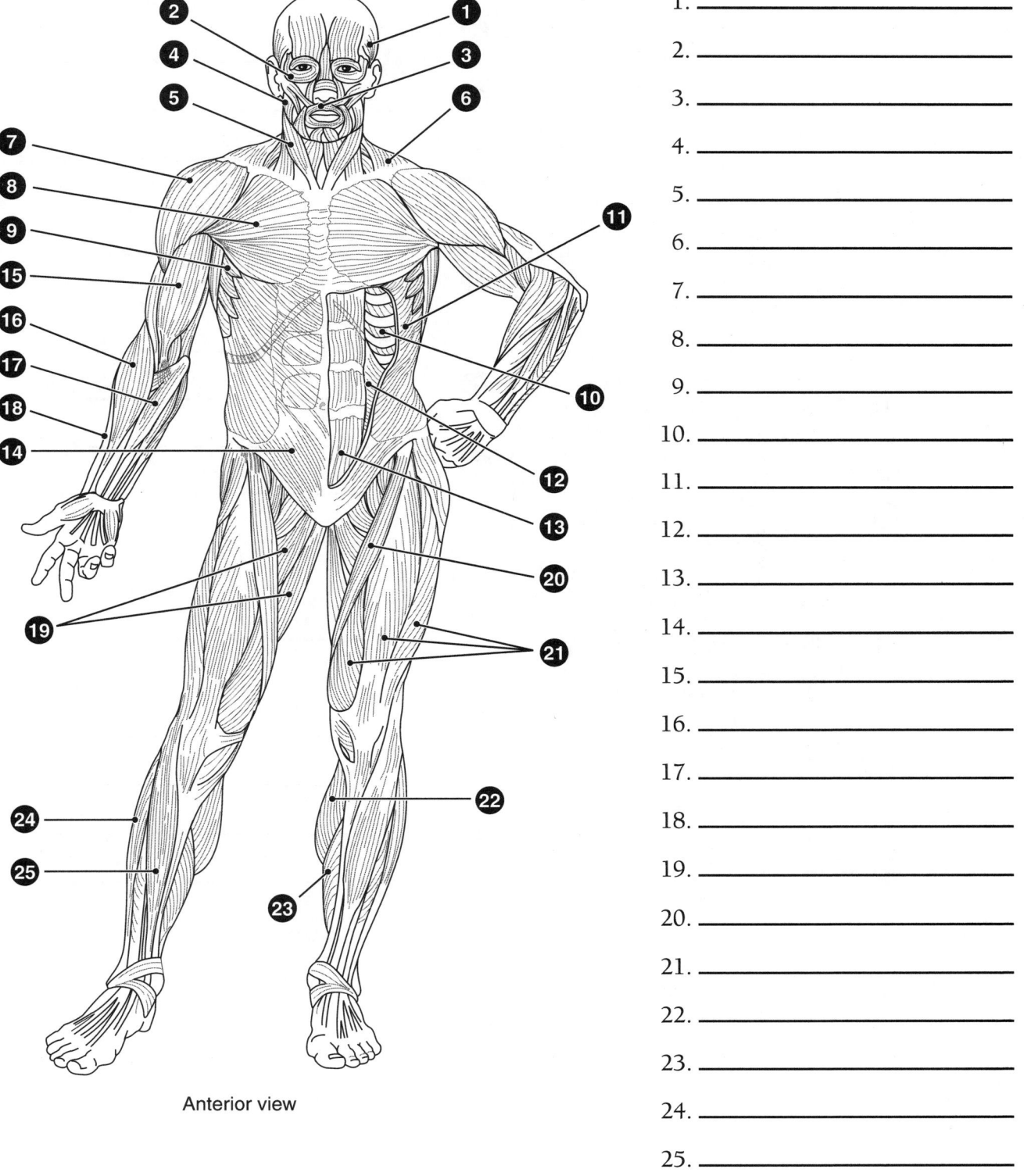

Anterior view

1. _____

2. _____

3. _____

4. _____

5. _____

6. _____

7. _____

8. _____

9. _____

10. _____

11. _____

12. _____

13. _____

14. _____

15. _____

16. _____

17. _____

18. _____

19. _____

20. _____

21. _____

22. _____

23. _____

24. _____

25. _____

EXERCISE 7-5: Superficial Muscles: Posterior View (text Fig. 7-10)

INSTRUCTIONS

1. Write the name of each labeled muscle or tendon on the numbered lines in different colors. If possible, use the same color you used for the muscle in Exercise 7-4.
2. Color the different muscles and tendons on the diagram with the corresponding color.

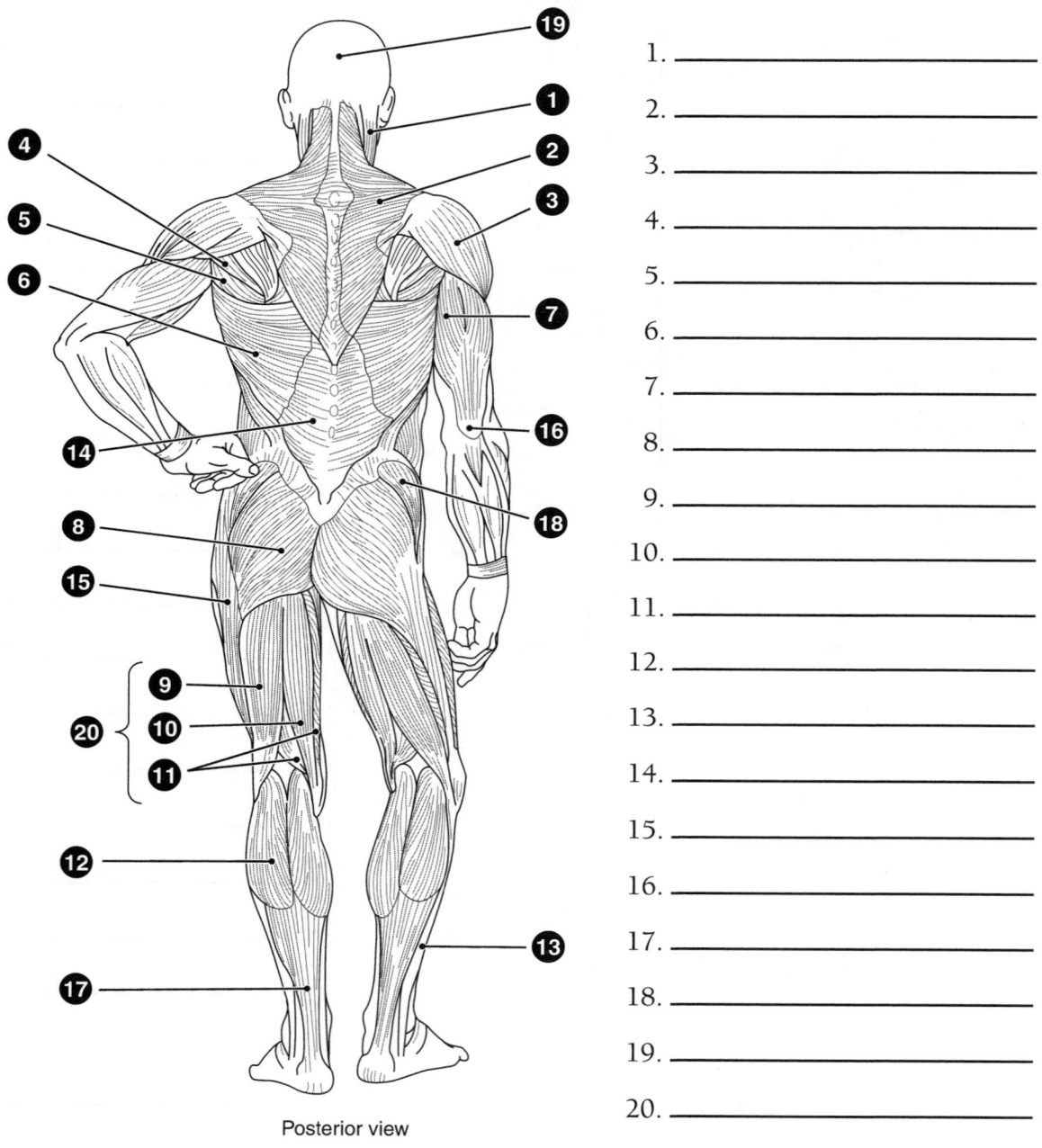

Posterior view

1. _____

2. _____

3. _____

4. _____

5. _____

6. _____

7. _____

8. _____

9. _____

10. _____

11. _____

12. _____

13. _____

14. _____

15. _____

16. _____

17. _____

18. _____

19. _____

20. _____

EXERCISE 7-6: Muscles of the Head (text Fig. 7-11)

INSTRUCTIONS

1. Write the name of each labeled muscle or tendon on the numbered lines in different colors. If possible, use the same color you used for the muscle in Exercise 7-4.
2. Color the different muscles and tendons on the diagram with the corresponding color.

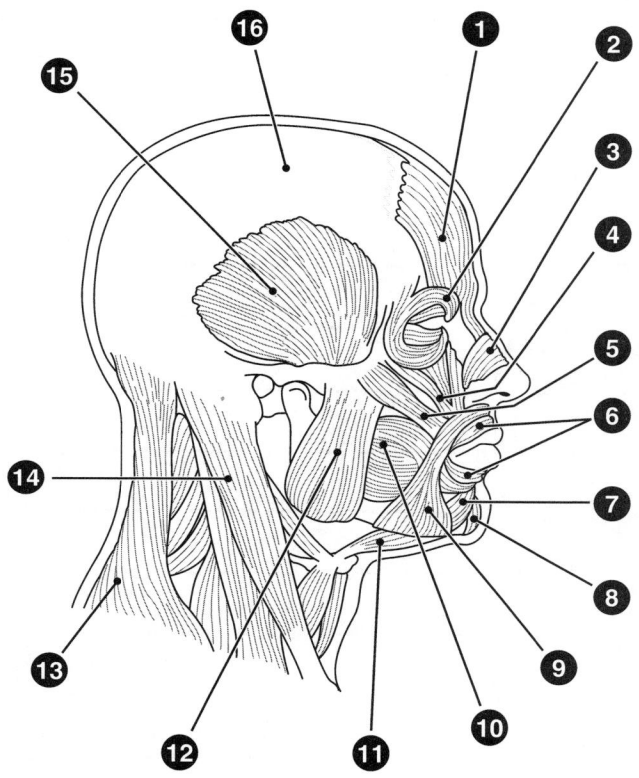

1. _____

2. _____

3. _____

4. _____

5. _____

6. _____

7. _____

8. _____

9. _____

10. _____

11. _____

12. _____

13. _____

14. _____

15. _____

16. _____

EXERCISE 7-7: Muscles of the Thigh: Anterior View (text Fig. 7-16A)

INSTRUCTIONS

1. Write the name of each labeled muscle, tendon, or bone on the numbered lines in different colors. If possible, use the same color you used for the muscle in Exercise 7-4.
2. Color the different structures on the diagram with the corresponding color.

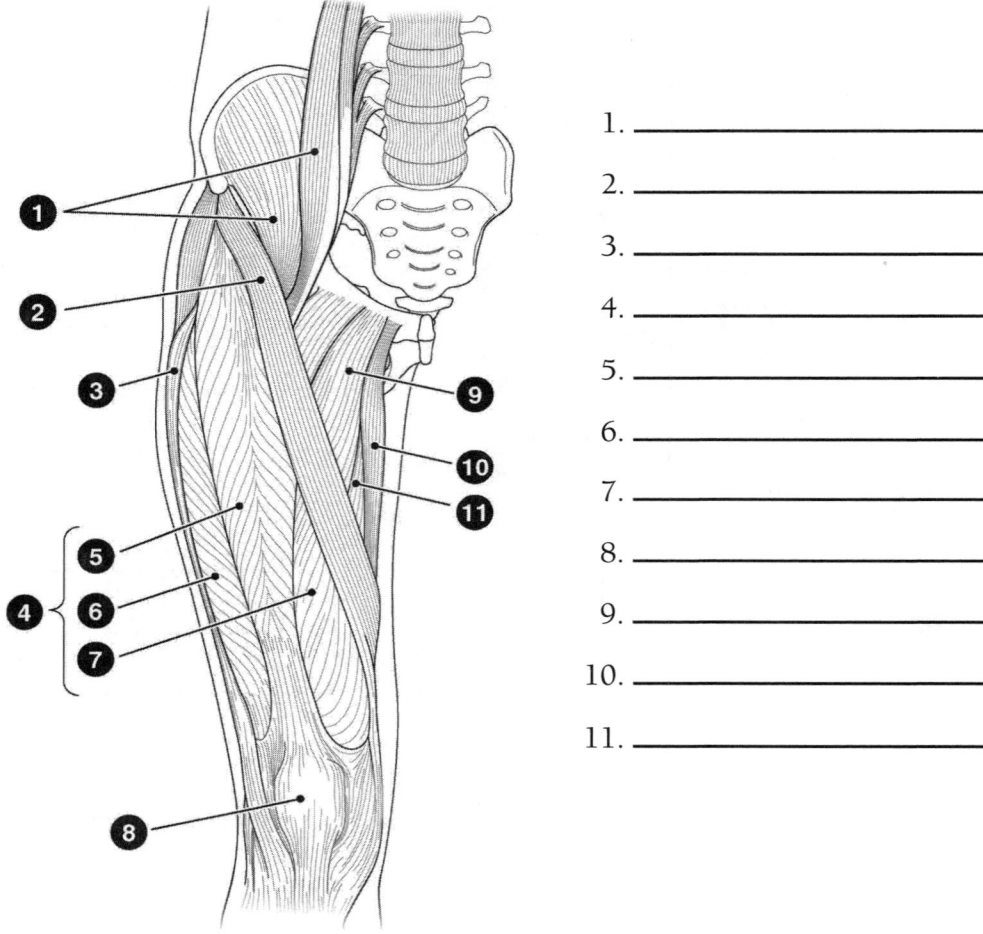

1. _____

2. _____

3. _____

4. _____

5. _____

6. _____

7. _____

8. _____

9. _____

10. _____

11. _____

Making the Connections

The following concept map deals with substances and structures required for muscle contraction. Each pair of terms is linked together by a connecting phrase into a sentence. The sentence should be read in the direction of the arrow. Complete the concept map by filling in the appropriate term or phrase. There is one right answer for each term. However, there are many correct answers for the connecting phrases. Write the connecting phrases beside the appropriate number (where space permits) or on a separate piece of paper.

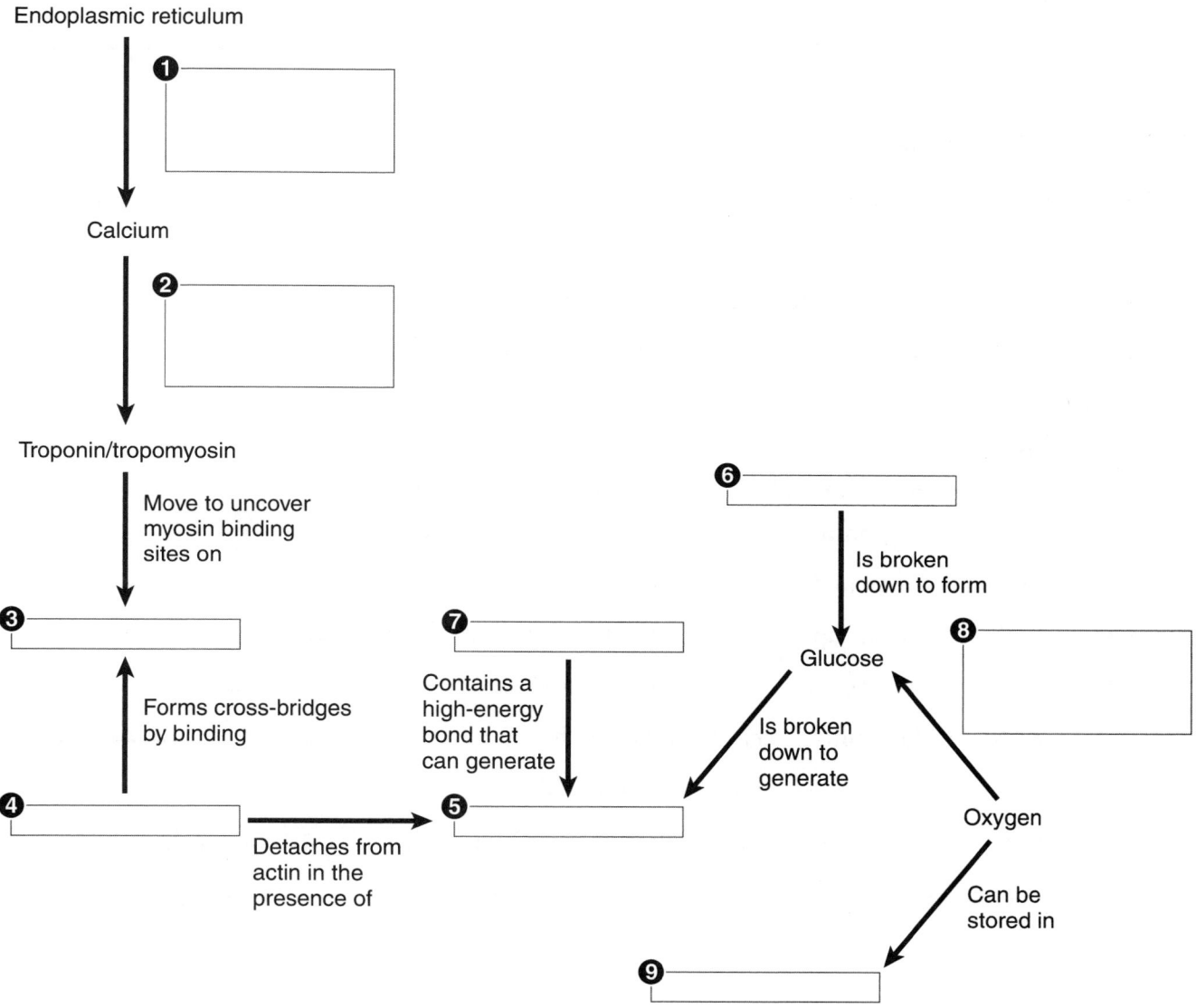

Optional Exercise: Make your own concept map, based on the events of muscle contraction. Choose your own terms to incorporate into your map, or use the following list: neuron, acetylcholine, neuromuscular junction, synaptic cleft, motor end plate, myosin, actin, endoplasmic reticulum, calcium, sarcomere, troponin/tropomyosin, ATP.

Testing Your Knowledge
Building Understanding

I. Matching Exercises

Matching only within each group, write the answers in the spaces provided.

➤ **Group A**

cardiac muscle	skeletal muscle	smooth muscle	fascicle	
endomysium	perimysium	epimysium	tendon	ligament

1. A cord-like structure that attaches a muscle to bone   _____

2. A bundle of muscle fibers   _____

3. A connective tissue layer surrounding muscle fiber bundles   _____

4. Muscle under voluntary control   _____

5. The only muscle type that does not have visible striations   _____

6. An involuntary muscle containing intercalated disks   _____

7. The innermost layer of the deep fascia that surrounds the

   entire muscle   _____

➤ **Group B**

synaptic cleft	motor end plate	motor unit	actin	ATP
myosin	troponin	sarcomere	calcium	

1. The immediate source of energy for muscle contraction   _____

2. The protein that makes up muscle's lighter, thin filaments   _____

3. The protein that interacts with actin to form a cross-bridge   _____

4. The membrane of the muscle cell that binds ACh   _____

5. The space between the neuron and the muscle cell   _____

6. A single neuron and all of the muscle fibers it stimulates   _____

7. A protein that binds calcium during muscle contraction   _____

➤ **Group C**

origin	insertion	prime mover	antagonist	synergist
lactic acid	aponeurosis	glycogen	creatine phosphate	myoglobin

1. A muscle acting as a helper to accomplish a particular

   movement   _____

2. The compound that stores oxygen in muscle cells   _____

3. The compound that accumulates during anaerobic

   metabolism   _____

4. The muscle attachment joined to a moving part of the body   _____

5. A compound similar to ATP that can be used to generate ATP   _____

6. The muscle attachment joined to a more fixed part of the body   _____

7. The muscle that produces a given movement   _____

8. A polysaccharide that can be used to generate glucose   _____

➤ **Group D**

sternocleidomastoid	buccinator	masseter	trapezius	orbicularis oris
deltoid		rotator cuff	latissimus dorsi	orbicularis oculi

1. The muscle capping the shoulder and upper arm   _____

2. A deep muscle group that supports the shoulder joint   _____

3. A muscle that closes the eye   _____

4. The muscle that makes up the fleshy part of the cheek   _____

5. A muscle that closes the jaw   _____

6. A muscle on the side of the neck that flexes the head   _____

7. A triangular muscle on the back of the neck and the upper back that extends the head   _____

➤ **Group E**

triceps brachii	serratus anterior	brachioradialis	biceps brachii	
intercostals	levator ani	erector spinae	latissimus dorsi	trapezius

1. A large muscle of the middle and lower back that inserts in the humerus and extends the arm at the shoulder behind the back   _____

2. The muscle in the pelvic floor that aids in defecation   _____

3. A muscle on the front of the arm that flexes the elbow and supinates the hand   _____

4. The large muscle on the back of the arm that extends the elbow   _____

5. A chest muscle inferior to the axilla that moves the scapula forward   _____

6. A deep muscle that extends the vertebral column   _____

7. Muscles between the ribs that can enlarge the thoracic cavity   _____

➤ Group F

rectus abdominis	transversus abdominis	gluteus maximus	gluteus medius
iliopsoas	adductor longus	gracilis	biceps femoris rectus femoris

1. Part of the quadriceps femoris muscle _____

2. The muscle that forms much of the fleshy part of the buttock _____

3. A deep muscle of the buttock that abducts the thigh _____

4. A vertical muscle covering the anterior surface of the

    abdomen _____

5. A muscle that aids in pressing the thighs together _____

6. A muscle extending from the pubic bone to the tibia that

    adducts the thigh at the hip _____

7. A powerful flexor of the thigh that arises from the ilium _____

➤ Group G

sartorius	gastrocnemius	soleus	peroneus longus
tibialis anterior	quadriceps femoris	semimembranosus	flexor digitorum group

1. The thin muscle that travels down and across the medial

    surface of the thigh _____

2. The chief muscle of the calf of the leg _____

3. The muscle that inverts and dorsiflexes the foot _____

4. Muscles that flex the toes _____

5. The muscle that everts the foot _____

6. A deep muscle that plantarflexes the foot at the ankle _____

II. Multiple Choice

Select the best answer and write the letter of your choice in the blank.

1. Which of the following statements is NOT true of skeletal muscle?   1. _____
    a. The cells are long and threadlike.
    b. It is involuntary.
    c. It is described as striated.
    d. The cells are multinucleated.

2. When muscles and bones act together in the body as a lever system, the
   pivot point or fulcrum of the system is the: 2. _____
    a. joint
    b. tendon
    c. ligament
    d. myoglobin

3. The quadriceps muscles act to: 3. _____
    a. flex the thigh
    b. extend the leg
    c. adduct the leg
    d. abduct the thigh

4. Which of the following is NOT a muscle of the hamstring group?   4. _____
    a. biceps femoris
    b. rectus femoris
    c. semimembranosus
    d. semitendinosus

5. The connective tissue layer around individual muscle fibers is called the: 5. _____
    a. epimysium
    b. perimysium
    c. superficial fascia
    d. endomysium

6. During muscle contraction, ATP binds to: 6. _____
    a. tropomyosin
    b. myosin
    c. actin
    d. troponin

III. Completion Exercise

Write the word or phrase that correctly completes each sentence.

1. Normally, muscles are in a partially contracted state, even when not in use. This state of mild constant tension is called   _____

2. The hemoglobin-like compound that stores oxygen in muscle is   _____

3. The muscle attachment that is usually relatively fixed is called its   _____

4. A contraction that generates tension but does not shorten the muscle is called   _____

5. The band of connective tissue that attaches the gastrocnemius muscle to the heel is the   _____

6. The muscles of the pelvic floor together form the   _____

7. A muscle that must relax during a given movement is called the   _____

8. The muscular partition between the thoracic and abdominal cavities is the   _____

9. A superficial muscle of the neck and upper back acts at the shoulder. This muscle is the   _____

10. The large muscle of the upper chest that flexes the arm across the body is the   _____

11. The muscle responsible for dorsiflexion and inversion of the foot is the   _____

Understanding Concepts

I. True or False

For each question, write "T" for true or "F" for false in the blank to the left of each number. If a statement is false, correct it by replacing the underlined term and write the correct statement in the blank below the question.

_____ 1. The triceps brachii flexes the arm at the elbow.

_____

_____ 2. Muscles enter into oxygen debt when they are functioning anaerobically.

_____

_____ 3. In an isometric contraction, muscle tension increases but the muscle does not shorten.

_____

_____ 4. The neurotransmitter used at the neuromuscular junction is norepinephrine.

_____

_____ 5. A contracting subunit of skeletal muscle is called a cross-bridge.

_____

_____ 6. The storage form of glucose is called creatine phosphate.

_____

_____ 7. The element that binds to the troponin and tropomyosin complex is calcium.

_____

II. Practical Applications

Study each discussion. Then write the appropriate word or phrase in the space provided.

➤ Group A

Ms. J is sitting at her desk studying for her anatomy final examination.

1. She has excellent posture, with her back straight. The deep back muscle responsible for her erect posture is the _____

2. Despite her excellent posture, Ms. J has a muscle spasm that has fixed her head in a flexed, rotated position. The muscle that flexes and rotates the head is the _____

3. Ms. J has a cheerful disposition, and she likes to whistle while she works. The cheek muscle involved in whistling is the _____

4. Ms. J is furiously writing notes, and her hand is flexed around the pen. The muscle groups that flex the hand are called the _____

5. After several hours of intense studying, Ms. J takes a break. Stretching, she straightens her leg at the knee joint. The muscle that accomplishes this action is the _____

➤ **Group B**

Mr. L, aged 72, is a retired concert pianist.

1. He reports numbness and weakness in his right hand. He can no longer flex and extend his fingers rapidly enough to play Rachmaninoff. The muscles that extend the fingers are the _____
2. Mr. L also experiences pain when he sits. He has lost muscle mass in the muscle forming the fleshy part of the buttock, known as the _____
3. The healthcare worker recommends that he undertakes a regular exercise program, incorporating stretching, aerobic exercise, and resistance training. This type of varied program is called interval training, or _____
4. Mr. L asks if the resistance training will give him bigger muscles. He is told that his muscle cells may increase in size, a change called _____

III. Short Essays

1. Mr. Q has embarked on an exercise program based solely on jogging. Name three distinct changes that will occur in his muscles.

   _____

   _____

   _____

2. Ms. L sustained an embarrassing (but relatively painless) fall. Mr. L is staring with his mouth open. Ms. L asks him to activate two muscles to close his jaw. Name these two muscles.

   _____

Conceptual Thinking

1. Ms. S is competing in an endurance event at the Olympics. She is consuming a special herbal product that reputedly degrades lactic acid in the absence of oxygen. Explain the potential benefit of this product, discussing the production and effects of lactic acid.

   _____

   _____

   _____

2. While attending the ballet, you notice a dancer raising her heels to stand on her tip-toes.
   A. What is the name of this action (*i.e.*, adduction)? _____
   B. What is the prime mover for this action? _____

    C. Name a synergistic muscle involved in this action. ———————————
    D. Name an antagonist muscle involved. ———————————
    E. Which class of lever is represented by this action? ———————————
    F. Name the fulcrum and resistance, and describe the relative
       positions of the fulcrum, resistance, and effort. ———————————

———————————————————————————

———————————————————————————

Expanding Your Horizons

Are world-class athletes born or made? It is no coincidence that athletic performance tends to run in families. Genetic influences on muscular function are discussed in an article in Scientific American (Resource 1). This information could be used to screen for elite athletes—perhaps children of the future will know which sports they can excel in based on their genetic profile. This possibility is discussed in a special Scientific American issue entitled "Building the Elite Athlete" (Resource 2).

Resource List

Andersen JL, Schjerling P, Saltin B. Muscle, genes and athletic performance. Sci Am 2000;283:48–55.
Taubes G. Toward Molecular Talent Scouting. Scientific American Presents: Building the Elite Athlete 2000;11:26–31.

chapter 8

The Nervous System: The Spinal Cord and Spinal Nerves

Overview

The nervous system is the body's coordinating system, receiving, sorting, and controlling responses to both internal and external changes (stimuli). The nervous system as a whole is divided structurally into the **central nervous system (CNS)**, made up of the brain and the spinal cord, and the **peripheral nervous system (PNS)**, made up of the cranial and spinal nerves. The PNS connects all parts of the body with the CNS. The brain and cranial nerves are the subject of Chapter 10. Functionally, the nervous system is divided into the somatic (voluntary) system and the autonomic (involuntary) system.

The nervous system functions by means of the **nerve impulse**, an electrical current or **action potential** that spreads along the membrane of the **neuron** (nerve cell). Each neuron is composed of a cell body and nerve fibers, which are threadlike extensions from the cell body. A **dendrite** is a fiber that carries impulses toward the cell body, and an **axon** is a fiber that carries impulses away from the cell body. Some axons are covered with a sheath of fatty material called **myelin**, which insulates the fiber and speeds conduction along the fiber. In the PNS, nerve cell fibers are collected in bundles to form **nerves**. Bundles of fibers in the CNS are called **tracts**.

Nerve cells make contact at a junction called a **synapse**. Here, a nerve impulse travels across a very narrow cleft between the cells by means of a chemical referred to as a **neurotransmitter**. Neurotransmitters are released from axons of presynaptic cells to be picked up by receptors in the membranes of responding cells, the postsynaptic cells.

A neuron may be classified as either a sensory (afferent) type, which carries impulses toward the central nervous system, or a motor (efferent) type, which carries impulses away from the central nervous system. **Interneurons** are connecting neurons within the central nervous system.

The basic functional pathway of the nervous system is the **reflex arc**, in which an impulse travels from a receptor, along a sensory neuron to a synapse or synapses in the central nervous system, and then along a motor neuron to an effector organ that carries out a response. The spinal cord carries impulses to and from the brain. It is also a center for simple reflex activities in which responses are coordinated within the cord.

The **autonomic nervous system** controls unconscious activities. This system regulates the actions of glands, smooth muscle, and the heart muscle. The autonomic nervous system has two divisions, the **sympathetic nervous system** and the **parasympathetic nervous system**, which generally have opposite effects on a given organ.

Learning the Language: Word Anatomy

Word Part	Meaning	Example
1._____	sheath	_____
2. re-	_____	_____
3._____	four	_____
4. soma-	_____	_____
5._____	nerve, nervous tissue	_____
6._____	remove	_____
7. aut/o	_____	_____
8. post-	_____	_____

Addressing the Learning Outcomes

I. Writing Exercise

The learning outcomes for Chapter 8 are listed below. These learning outcomes provide an overview of the major topics covered in this chapter. On a separate piece of paper, try to write out an answer to each learning outcome. All of the answers can be found in the pages of the textbook. Learning Outcomes 2, 7, 8, 10, 11, and 13 are also addressed in the Coloring Atlas.

1. Describe the organization of the nervous system according to structure and function.
2. Describe the structure of a neuron.
3. Describe how neuron fibers are built into a nerve.
4. Explain the purpose of neuroglia.
5. Diagram and describe the steps in an action potential.
6. Briefly describe the transmission of a nerve impulse.
7. Explain the role of myelin in nerve conduction.
8. Briefly describe transmission at a synapse.
9. Define *neurotransmitter* and give several examples of neurotransmitters.

10. Describe the distribution of gray and white matter in the spinal cord.
11. List the components of a reflex arc.
12. Define a simple reflex and give several examples of reflexes.
13. Describe and name the spinal nerves and three of their main plexuses.
14. Compare the location and functions of the sympathetic and parasympathetic nervous systems.
15. Show how word parts are used to build words related to the nervous system.

II. Labeling and Coloring Atlas

EXERCISE 8-1: Anatomic Divisions of the Nervous System (text Fig. 8-1)
Label the parts and divisions of the nervous system shown below.

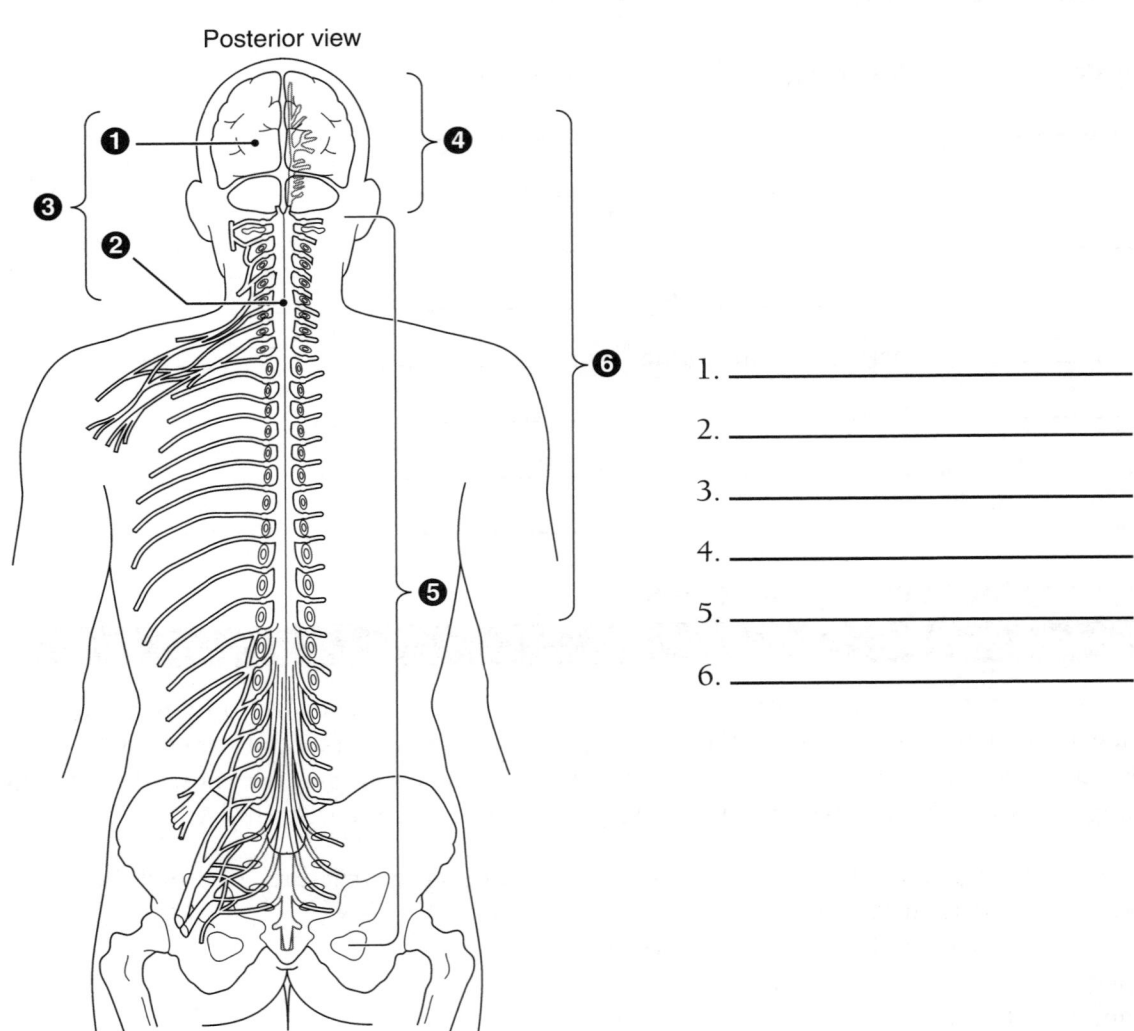

Posterior view

1. _____

2. _____

3. _____

4. _____

5. _____

6. _____

EXERCISE 8-2: The Motor Neuron (text Fig. 8-2)

INSTRUCTIONS

1. Write the name of each labeled part on the numbered lines in different colors. Structures 4–6 will not be colored, so write their names in black.
2. Color the different structures on the diagram with the corresponding color.
3. Add large arrows showing the direction the nerve impulse will travel, from the dendrites to the muscle.

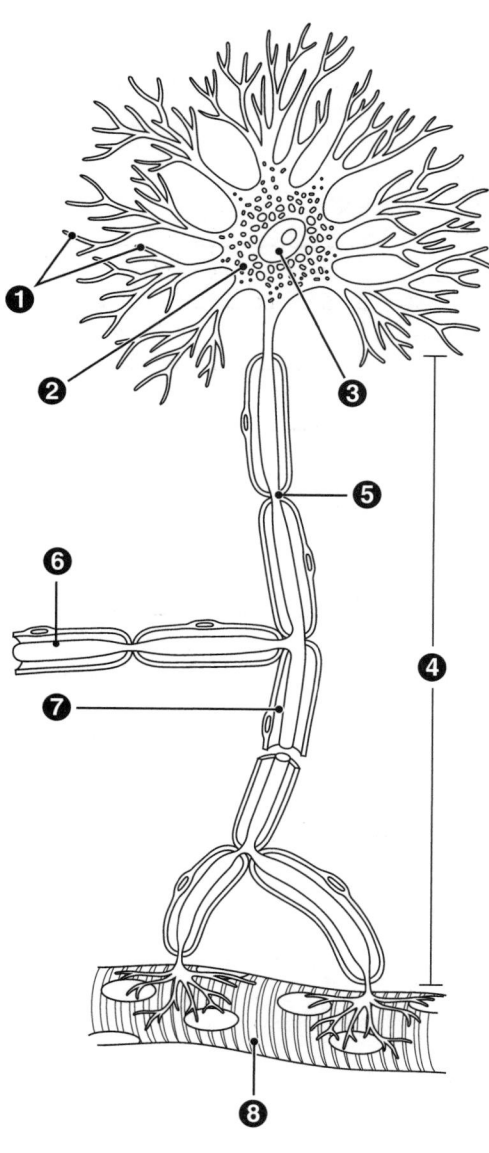

1. _____

2. _____

3. _____

4. _____

5. _____

6. _____

7. _____

8. _____

EXERCISE 8-3: Formation of a Myelin Sheath (text Fig. 8-4)

INSTRUCTIONS

1. Write the name of each labeled part on the numbered lines in different colors. Structures 4 and 7 to 9 will not be colored, so write their names in black.
2. Color the different structures on the diagram with the corresponding color. Make sure you color the structure in all parts of the diagram. For instance, structure 3 is visible in three locations.

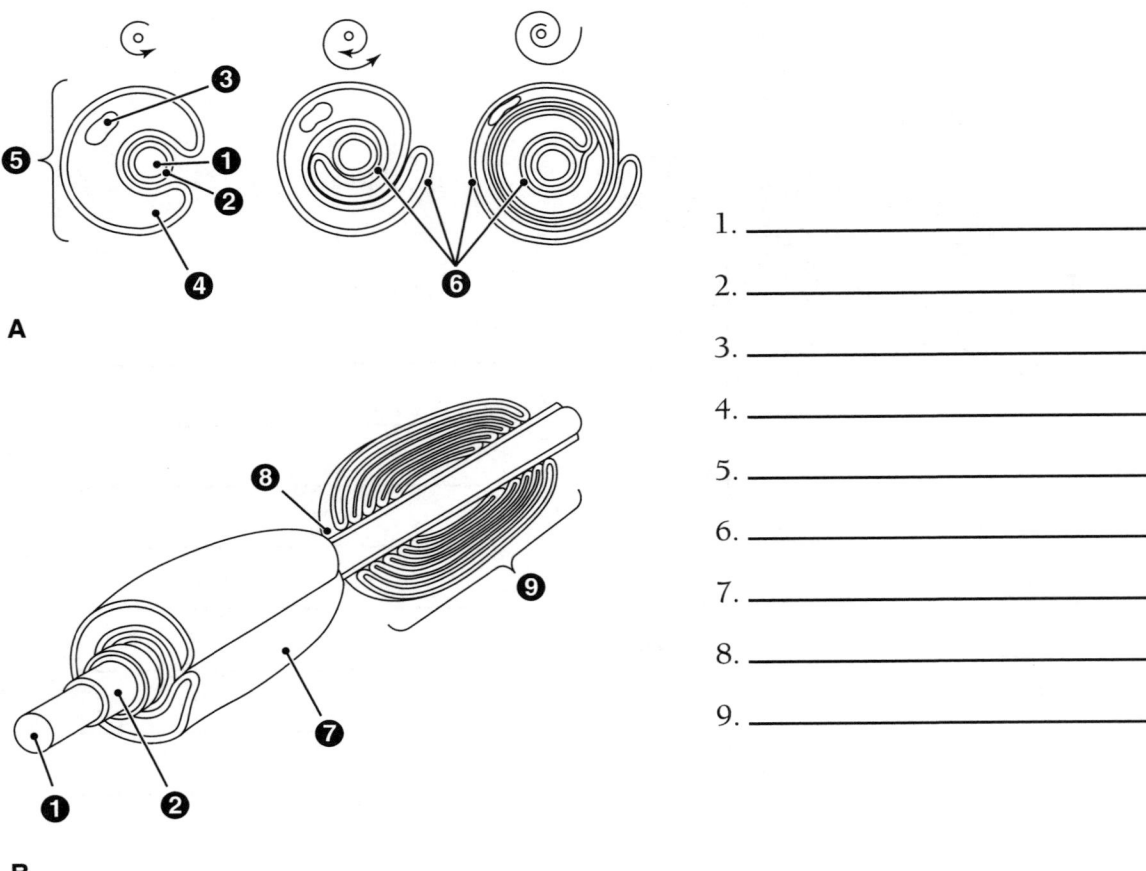

1. _____

2. _____

3. _____

4. _____

5. _____

6. _____

7. _____

8. _____

9. _____

EXERCISE 8-4: A Synapse (text Fig. 8-9)
Label the parts of the synapse shown below.

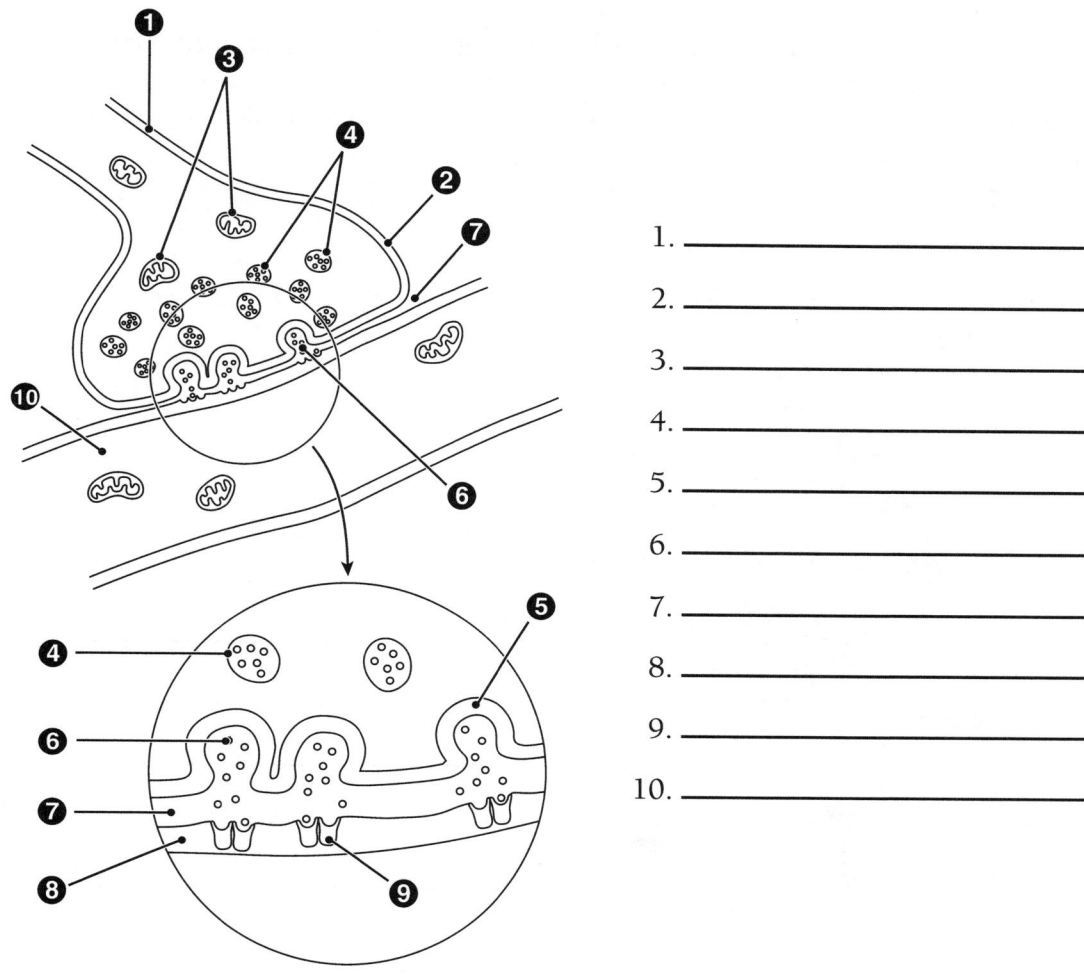

1. _____

2. _____

3. _____

4. _____

5. _____

6. _____

7. _____

8. _____

9. _____

10. _____

EXERCISE 8-5: Spinal Cord and Spinal Nerves (text Fig. 8-11)

INSTRUCTIONS

1. Label the parts of the CNS (structures 1–5).
2. Spinal nerves are named based on the site they emerge from the spinal cord. Write the names of the nerve groups on the appropriate line (lines 6–10).
3. Some of the anterior branches of the spinal nerves interlace to form plexuses. Identify the plexuses (structures 11–13).
4. Label the specific nerves (structures 14–20).

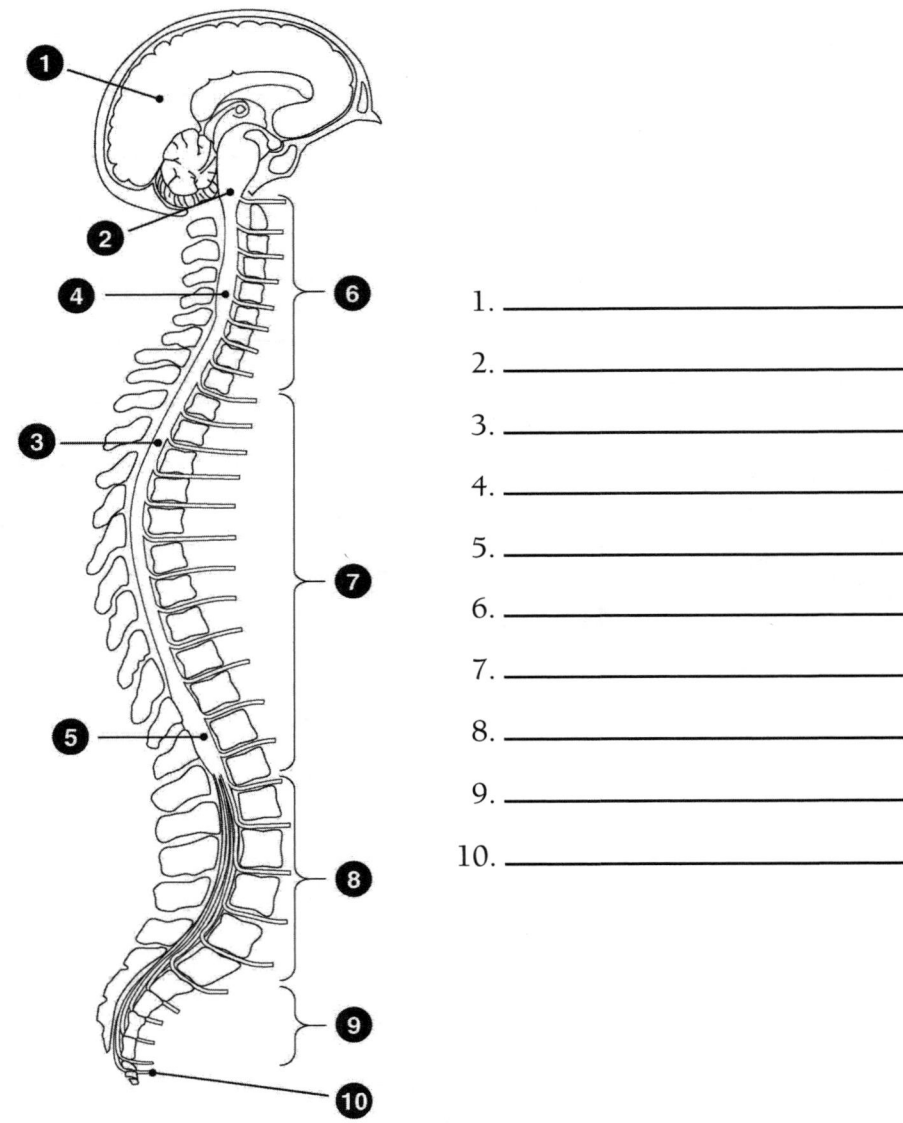

1. _____

2. _____

3. _____

4. _____

5. _____

6. _____

7. _____

8. _____

9. _____

10. _____

A

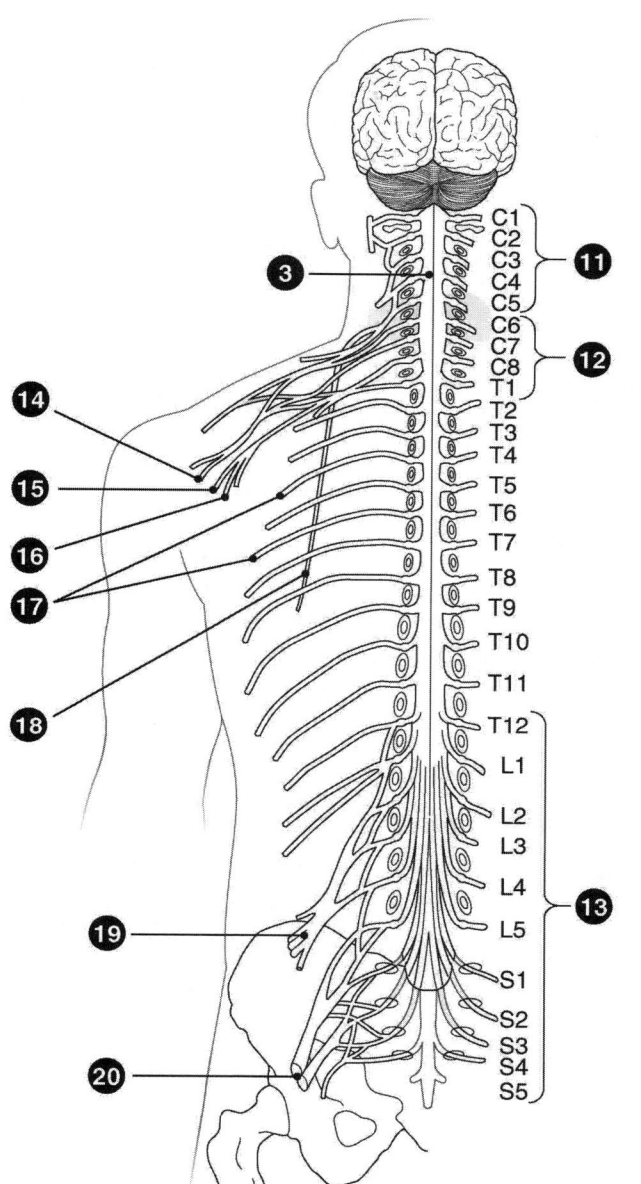

C1
C2
C3
C4
C5
C6
C7
C8
T1
T2
T3
T4
T5
T6
T7
T8
T9
T10
T11
T12
L1
L2
L3
L4
L5
S1
S2
S3
S4
S5

B

11. _____

12. _____

13. _____

14. _____

15. _____

16. _____

17. _____

18. _____

19. _____

20. _____

EXERCISE 8-6: Spinal Cord (text Fig. 8-11A)

INSTRUCTIONS

1. Write the name of each labeled part on the numbered lines. Use the following color scheme:
   - 1 and 2: red
   - 3, 4, 9: different dark colors
   - 5: pink
   - 6: any light color
   - 7: light blue
   - 10: medium blue
   - 11: purple
2. Color or outline the different structures on the diagram with the corresponding color.

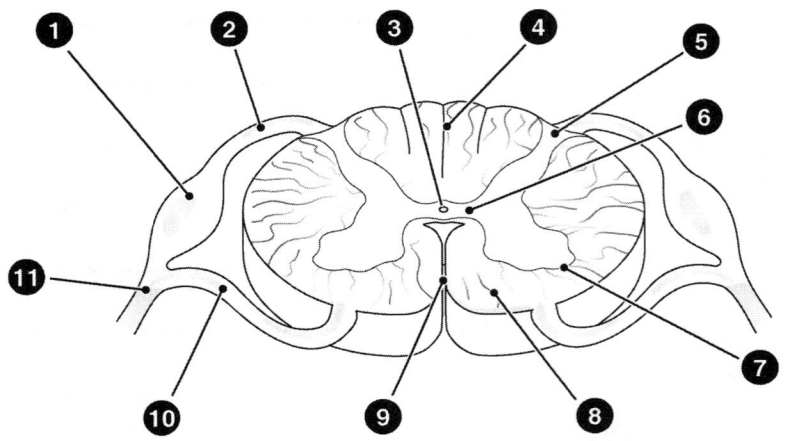

1. _____
2. _____
3. _____
4. _____
5. _____
6. _____
7. _____
8. _____
9. _____
10. _____
11. _____

EXERCISE 8-7: Reflex Arc (text Fig. 8-13)

INSTRUCTIONS

1. Write the names of the five components of a reflex arc on the numbered lines 1 to 5 in different colors, and color the components with the appropriate color. Follow the color scheme provided below.

2. Write the names of the parts of the spinal cord on numbered lines 6 to 12 in different colors, and color the structures with the appropriate color. Follow the color scheme provided below.
   Color Scheme
   - 1, 2, 6, 7, 8: red
   - 3: green
   - 4, 10: medium blue
   - 5: purple
   - 9: do not color (write name in black)
   - 11: pink
   - 12: light blue

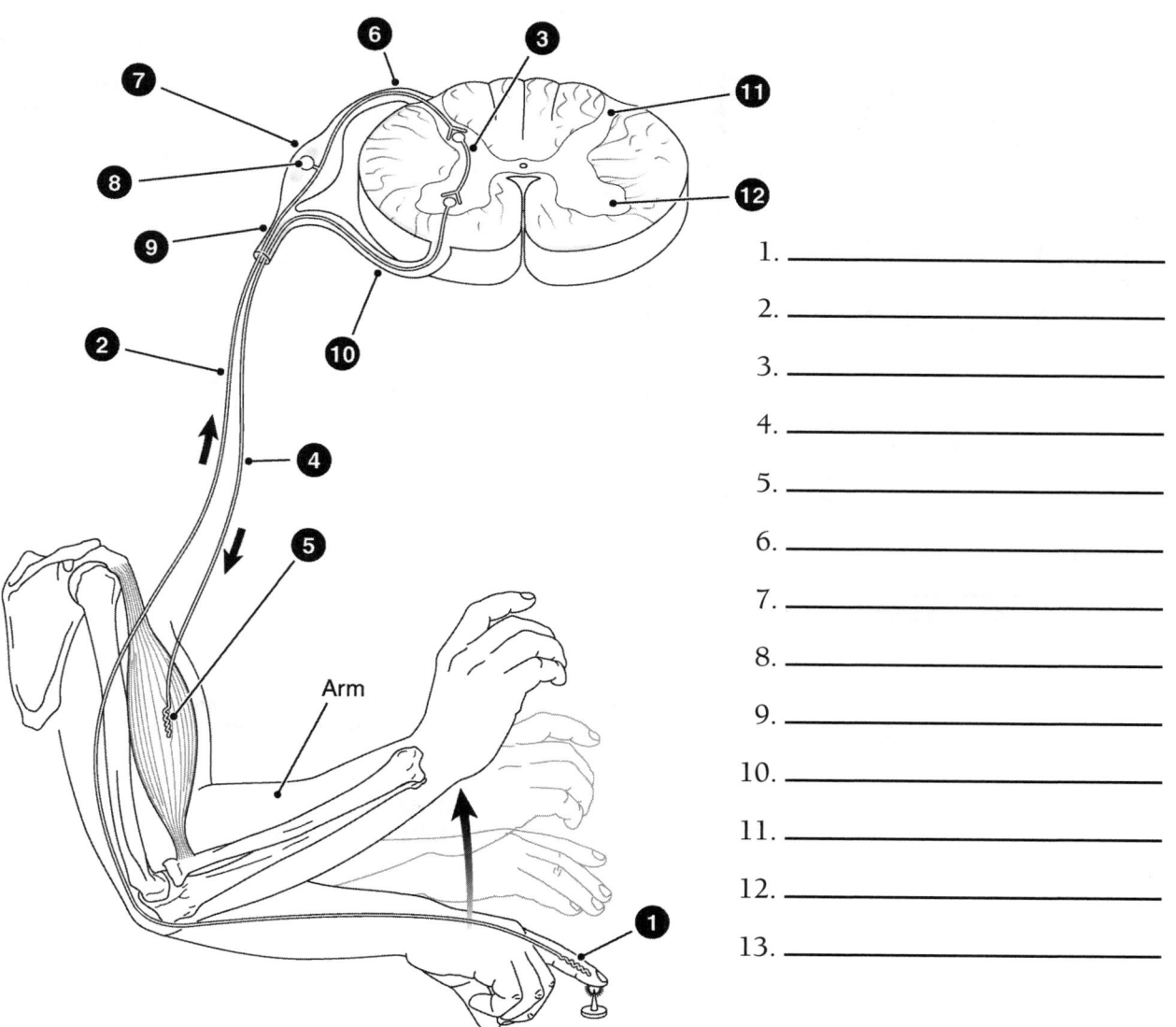

Arm

1. _____
2. _____
3. _____
4. _____
5. _____
6. _____
7. _____
8. _____
9. _____
10. _____
11. _____
12. _____
13. _____

Making the Connections

The following concept map deals with the organization of the nervous system. Each pair of terms is linked together by a connecting phrase into a sentence. The sentence should be read in the direction of the arrow. Complete the concept map by filling in the appropriate term or phrase. There is one right answer for each term. However, there are many correct answers for the connecting phrases (2, 8, 9, and 12). Write the connecting phrases beside the appropriate number (where space permits) or on a separate piece of paper.

Optional Exercise: Make your own concept map, based on the structures of the spinal cord and the components of a reflex arc. Choose your own terms to incorporate into your map, or use the following list: dorsal root ganglion, gray matter, white matter, ventral root ganglion, afferent fibers, efferent fibers, sensory fibers, motor fibers, receptor, muscle, gland, effector.

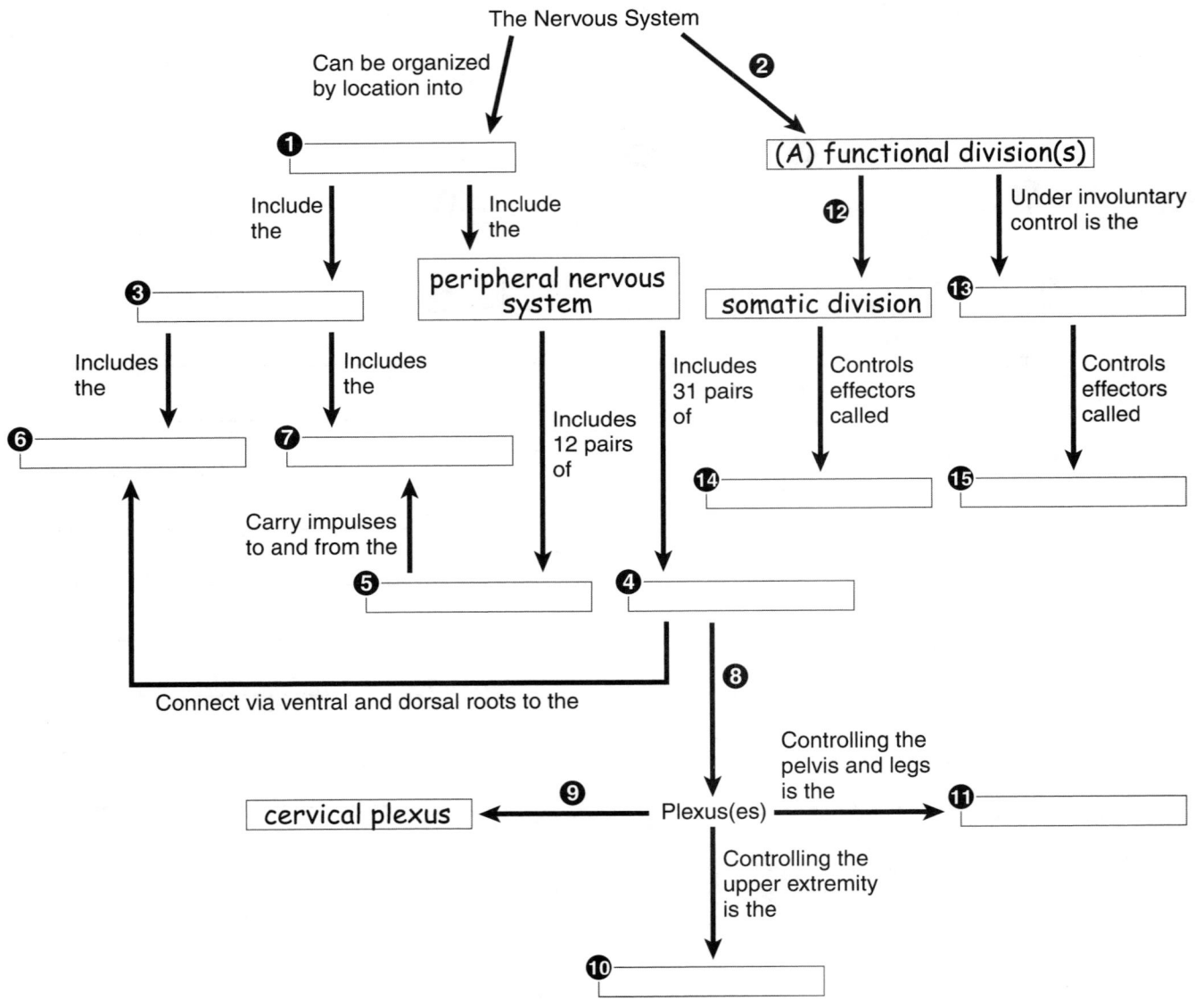

Testing Your Knowledge
Building Understanding

I. Matching Exercises

Matching only within each group, write the answers in the spaces provided.

➤ **Group A**

nerve	central nervous system	peripheral nervous system
somatic nervous system	sympathetic nervous system	parasympathetic nervous system
neuron	effector	

1. The system that promotes the fight-or-flight response   _____

2. The system that stimulates the activity of the digestive tract   _____

3. The structural division of the nervous system that includes the brain   _____

4. The structural division of the nervous system that includes the cranial nerves   _____

5. The scientific name for a nerve cell   _____

6. A bundle of nerve cell fibers located outside the central nervous system   _____

➤ **Group B**

dendrite	neurilemma	axon	white matter	gray matter
node	ganglion	efferent	afferent	tract

1. The term for neurons that carry impulses toward the CNS   _____

2. A nerve cell fiber that carries impulses away from the cell body   _____

3. A collection of neuron cell bodies located outside the CNS   _____

4. The part of a neuron that receives a stimulus   _____

5. The sheath around some neuron fibers that aids in regeneration   _____

6. A gap in the neuron sheath   _____

7. The portion of the spinal cord made up of myelinated axons   _____

➤ **Group C**

depolarization	action potential	repolarization	Na^+	K^+
neurotransmitter	neuroglia	reflex	motor nerve	mixed nerve

1. A chemical that carries an impulse across a synapse   _____

2. The support cells of the nervous system   _____

3. A nerve containing afferent and efferent fibers _____

4. The result of positive ions entering the neuron _____

5. A sudden change in membrane potential that is transmitted

   along axons _____

6. A simple, automatic response that involves few neurons _____

7. The ion that leaves the neuron to cause repolarization _____

➤ **Group D**

brachial plexus   sciatic nerve   cervical plexus   thoracolumbar

craniosacral   terminal ganglia   adrenergic   cholinergic   collateral ganglia

1. The network of nerves that supplies the neck muscles _____

2. Term that describes the sympathetic portion of the autonomic

   nervous system, based on where it originates _____

3. The largest branch of the lumbosacral plexus _____

4. The network of nerves that supplies the upper extremities _____

5. Term that describes the parasympathetic portion of the

   autonomic nervous system, based on where it originates _____

6. Adjective for a response activated by the neurotransmitter

   epinephrine _____

7. The celiac, superior mesenteric, and inferior mesenteric

   ganglia make up the _____

II. Multiple Choice

Select the best answer and write the letter of your choice in the blank.

1. The skin region supplied by a single spinal nerve is called a(n):   1. _____
   a. dermatome
   b. ganglion
   c. plexus
   d. synapse
2. The voluntary nervous system controls: 2. _____
   a. visceral muscle
   b. skeletal muscle
   c. glands
   d. cardiac muscle
3. Which of the following are effectors of the nervous system?   3. _____
   a. sensory neurons and ganglia
   b. muscles and glands

  c. synapses and dendrites

  d. receptors and neurotransmitters

4. Cell bodies of sensory neurons are collected in ganglia in the: 4. _____

  a. dorsal root of the spinal cord

  b. sympathetic chain

  c. ventral root of the spinal cord

  d. effector organ

5. Which of the following substances is a neurotransmitter?   5. _____

  a. myelin

  b. actin

  c. epinephrine

  d. sebum

6. White matter contains   6. _____

  a. neuronal cell bodies

  b. myelinated axons

  c. unmyelinated axons

  d. cerebrospinal fluid

7. Neurons that relay impulses within the spinal cord are called: 7. _____

  a. afferent neurons

  b. motor neurons

  c. interneurons

  d. mixed nerves

III. Completion Exercise

Write the word or phrase that correctly completes each sentence.

1. Fibers that carry impulses toward the neuron cell body are called   _____

2. The portion of the spinal cord made up of cell bodies and unmyelinated axons is called the   _____

3. The fatty material that covers some axons is called   _____

4. Dilation of the bronchial tubes is increased by the part of the autonomic nervous system called the   _____

5. The junction between two neurons is called a(n)   _____

6. The network of spinal nerves that supplies the pelvis and legs is the   _____

7. The brain and spinal cord together are referred to as the   _____

8. The neurotransmitter used at cholinergic synapses is   _____

9. The small channel in the center of the spinal cord that contains cerebrospinal fluid is the   _____

10. A nerve cell is also called a(n)   _____

11. The bridge of gray matter connecting the right and left horns of the spinal cord is the   _____

Understanding Concepts

I. True or False

For each question, write "T" for true or "F" for false in the blank to the left of each number. If a statement is false, correct it by replacing the underlined term and write the correct statement in the blanks below the question.

_____ 1. Motor impulses leave the <u>dorsal</u> horn of the spinal cord.

_____

_____ 2. <u>An axon</u> carries impulses toward the neuron cell body.

_____

_____ 3. A <u>tract</u> is a bundle of neuron fibers within the central nervous system.

_____

_____ 4. The <u>parasympathetic</u> system has terminal ganglia.

_____

_____ 5. The <u>brachial plexus</u> controls the shoulder and arm.

_____

_____ 6. The parasympathetic system is <u>adrenergic</u>.

_____

_____ 7. The spinal nerves are part of the <u>central</u> nervous system.

_____

_____ 8. Neurotransmitters bind to specific proteins on the postsynaptic cells called <u>transporters.</u>

_____

_____ 9. At a synapse, a neurotransmitter is released from the <u>postsynaptic</u> cell.

_____

_____ 10. A reflex arc that passes through the spinal cord but not the brain is called a <u>spinal</u> reflex.

_____

II. Practical Applications

Study each discussion. Then write the appropriate word or phrase in the space provided.

1. Mr. W, a patient with diabetes mellitus for 10 years, reported pain and numbness of his feet. In observing Mr. W walk, the physician noted there was weakness in the muscles responsible for dorsiflexion of the foot. These symptoms are caused by a degenerative disorder of nerves to the extremities. The nerves that supply the foot are found in a plexus called the _____

2. The physician pricked Mr. W's foot with a needle. Mr. W did not feel the needle prick, suggesting that there was a problem with the nerves that carry impulses to the brain. These nerves are called _____

3. The physician tapped below Mr. W's knee to elicit a knee-jerk response. The tendon she struck was the _____

4. The effector in this reflex arc is the _____

III. Short Essays

1. List the events that occur in an action potential.

_____

_____

_____

2. What are neuroglia, and what are some of their functions?

_____

_____

_____

Conceptual Thinking

1. Ms. J is teaching English in Japan. She dines on a local delicacy called pufferfish, and soon thereafter her lips go numb. She later discovers that pufferfish contain a toxin that blocks sodium channels. Explain why her lips are numb.

_____

_____

_____

2. Dopamine is a neurotransmitter involved in feelings of pleasure. Cocaine blocks the reuptake of dopamine. Use this information to discuss how cocaine affects mood.

_____

_____

_____

Expanding Your Horizons

Paralysis resulting from spinal cord injuries is generally thought to be irreversible, because neurons in the central nervous system do not easily regenerate. However, there is new hope for patients with spinal cord injuries. New therapies are discussed in a recent Scientific American article.

Resource List

McDonald JW. Repairing the damaged spinal cord. Sci Am 1999;281:64–73.

chapter 9

The Nervous System: The Brain and Cranial Nerves

Overview

The brain consists of the two cerebral hemispheres, the diencephalon, the brain stem, and the cerebellum. Each cerebral hemisphere is covered by a layer of gray matter, the **cerebral cortex**, which is further divided into four lobes (the frontal, parietal, temporal, and occipital lobes). Specific functions have been localized to the different lobes. For instance, the interpretation of visual images is performed by an area of the occipital lobe. The diencephalon consists of the **thalamus**, an important relay station for sensory impulses, and the **hypothalamus**, which plays an important role in homeostasis. The brain stem links the spinal cord to the brain and regulates many involuntary functions necessary for life, whereas the cerebellum is involved in coordination and balance. The **limbic system** is not found in a specific brain division. It consists of several structures located between the cerebrum and diencephalon that are involved in emotion, learning, and memory.

The brain and spinal cord are covered by three layers of fibrous membranes called the **meninges**. The **cerebrospinal fluid** (CSF) also protects the brain and spinal cord by providing support and cushioning. The CSF is produced by the choroid plexuses (capillary networks) in four ventricles (spaces) within the brain.

Connected with the brain are 12 pairs of **cranial nerves**, most of which supply structures in the head. Most of these, like all the spinal nerves, are mixed nerves containing both sensory and motor fibers. A few of the cranial nerves contain only sensory fibers, whereas others are motor in function.

Learning the Language: Word Anatomy

Word Part	Meaning	Example
1. _____	cut	_____
2. chori/o-	_____	_____
3. _____	tongue	_____
4. encephal/o-	_____	_____
5. cerebr/o-	_____	_____
6. _____	opposed, against	_____
7. _____	lateral, side	_____
8. gyr/o	_____	_____

Addressing the Learning Outcomes

I. Writing Exercise

The learning outcomes for Chapter 9 are listed below. These learning outcomes provide an overview of the major topics covered in this chapter. On a separate piece of paper, try to write out an answer to each learning outcome. All of the answers can be found in the pages of the textbook. Learning Outcomes 1–7 and 10 are also addressed in the Coloring Atlas.

1. Give the location and functions of the four main divisions of the brain.
2. Name and describe the three meninges.
3. Cite the function of cerebrospinal fluid and describe where and how this fluid is formed.
4. Name and locate the lobes of the cerebral hemispheres.
5. Cite one function of the cerebral cortex in each lobe of the cerebrum.
6. Name two divisions of the diencephalon and cite the functions of each.
7. Locate the three subdivisions of the brain stem and give the functions of each.
8. Describe the cerebellum and cite its functions.
9. Name some techniques used to study the brain.
10. Cite the names and functions of the 12 cranial nerves.
11. Show how word parts are used to build words related to the nervous system.

II. Labeling and Coloring Atlas

EXERCISE 9-1: Brain: Sagittal Section (text Fig. 9-1)

INSTRUCTIONS

1. Write the names of the four labeled brain divisions in lines 1 to 4, using four different colors. Use red for 2 and blue for 3. DO NOT COLOR THE DIAGRAM YET.
2. Write the name of each labeled structure on the appropriate numbered line in different colors. Use different shades of red for structures 5 and 6 and different shades of blue for structures 8–10.
3. Color each structure on the diagram with the appropriate color.

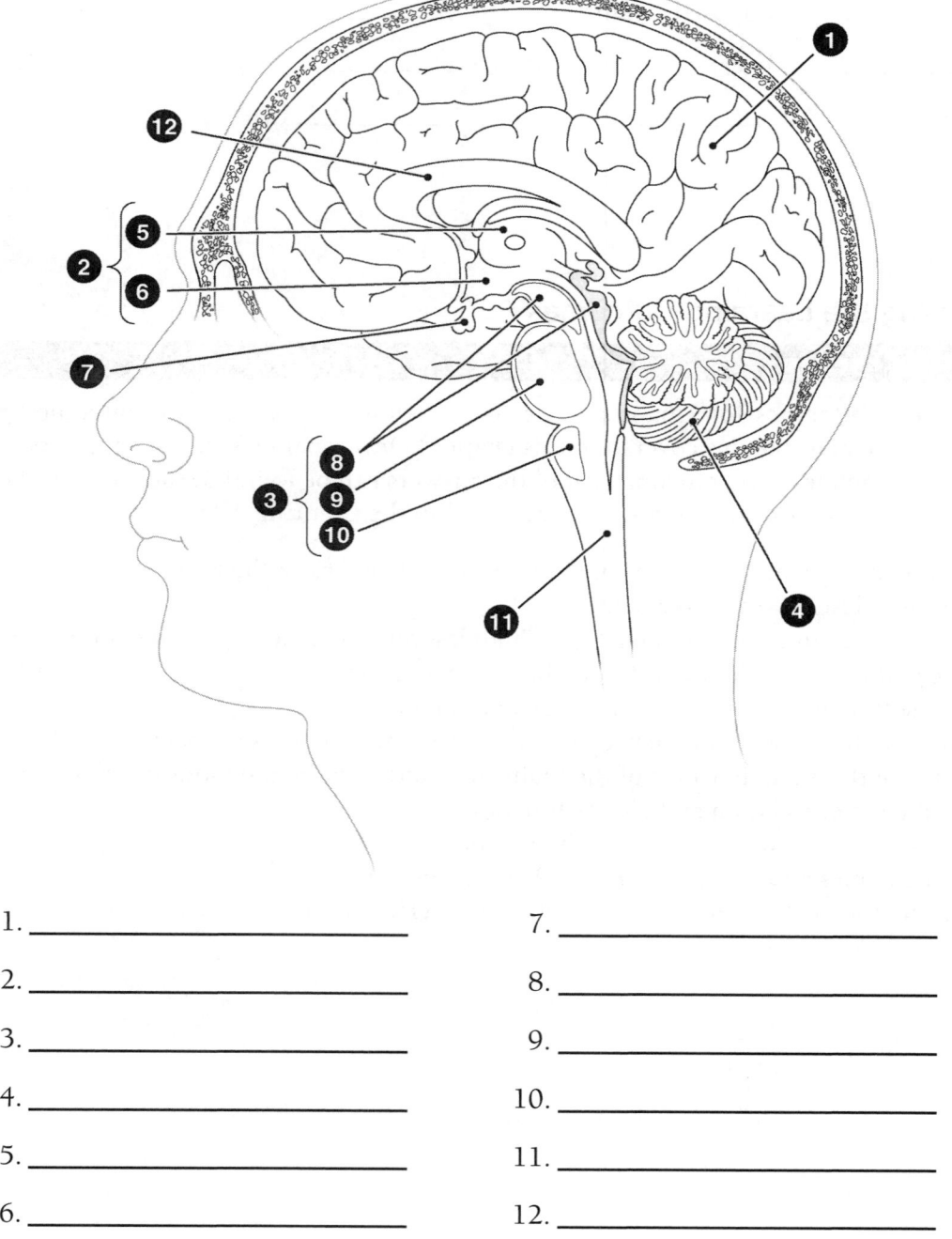

1. _____

2. _____

3. _____

4. _____

5. _____

6. _____

7. _____

8. _____

9. _____

10. _____

11. _____

12. _____

EXERCISE 9-2: Meninges and Related Parts (text Fig. 9-3)

INSTRUCTIONS

1. Write the name of each labeled part on the numbered lines in different colors. Use the same color for structures 7 and 8. Write the names of structures 4, 10, and 12 in black.
2. Color the structures on the diagram with the corresponding color. Do not color structures 4, 10, and 12.

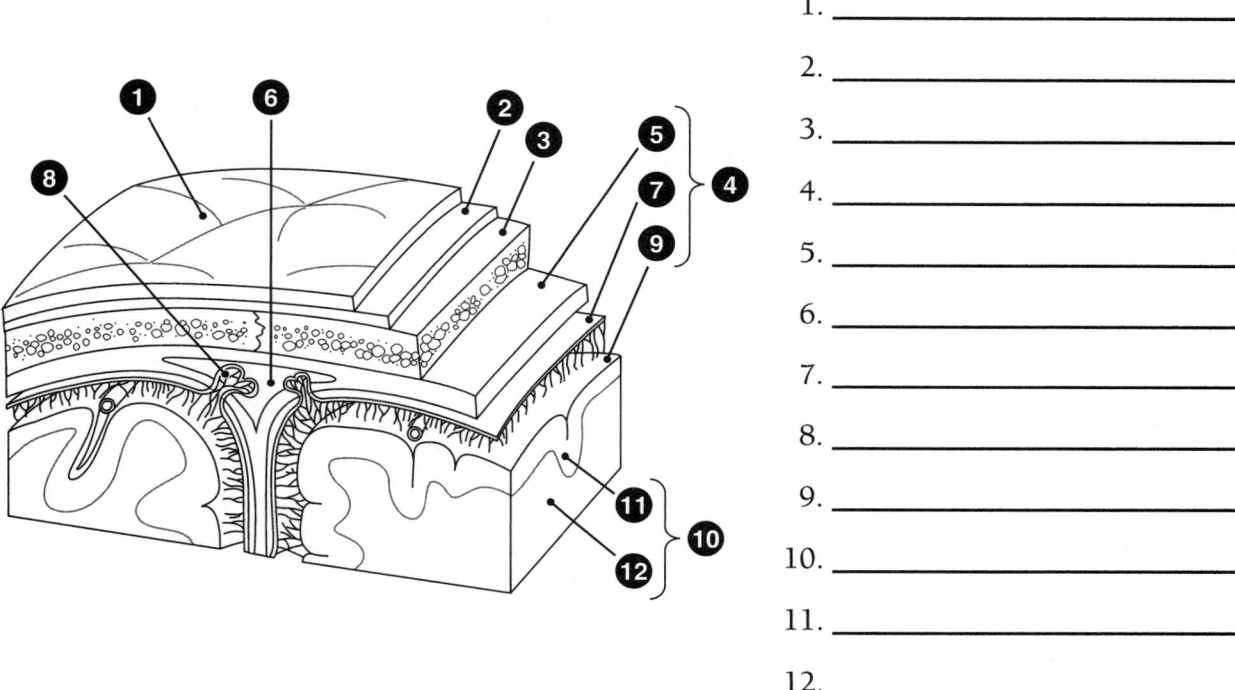

1. _____

2. _____

3. _____

4. _____

5. _____

6. _____

7. _____

8. _____

9. _____

10. _____

11. _____

12. _____

EXERCISE 9-3: Flow of Cerebrospinal Fluid (text Fig. 9-4)

INSTRUCTIONS

1. Write the name of each labeled part on the numbered lines in different colors. Use light colors for structures 5–12.
2. Color the structures on the diagram with the corresponding color. The boundaries between structures 5–12 (inclusive) are not always well defined. For instance, structure 6 is continuous with structure 7. You can overlap your colors to signify this fact.
3. Draw arrows to indicate the direction of CSF flow.

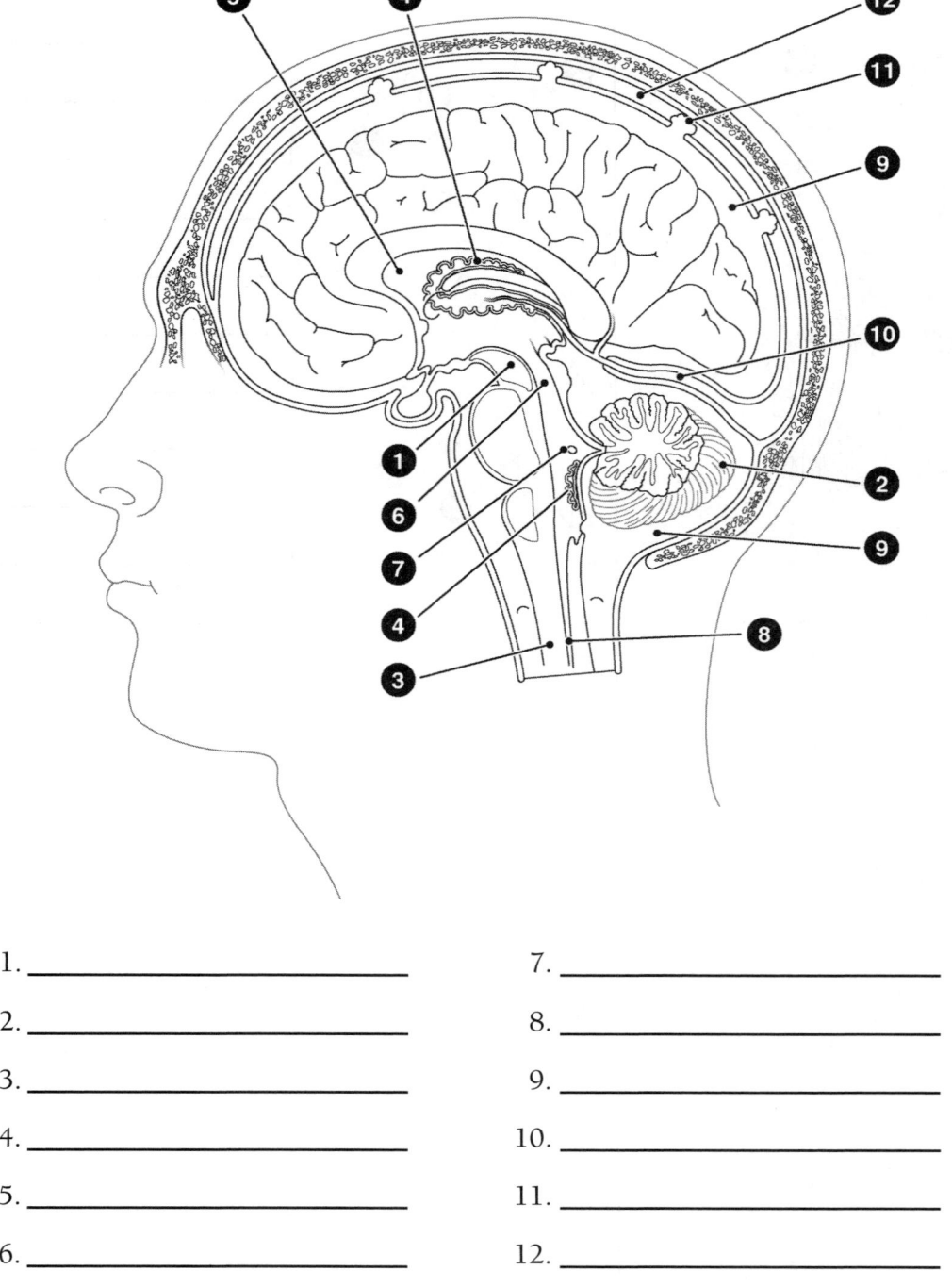

1. _____

2. _____

3. _____

4. _____

5. _____

6. _____

7. _____

8. _____

9. _____

10. _____

11. _____

12. _____

EXERCISE 9-4: Ventricles of the Brain (text Fig. 9-5)

INSTRUCTIONS

1. Write the name of each labeled part on the numbered lines in different colors. Write the names of structures 5, 6, and 9 in black, because they will not be colored.
2. Color the structures on the diagram with the corresponding color (except for structures 5, 6, and 9). The boundaries between structures are not always well defined. For instance, structure 2 is continuous with structure 4. You can overlap your colors to signify this fact.

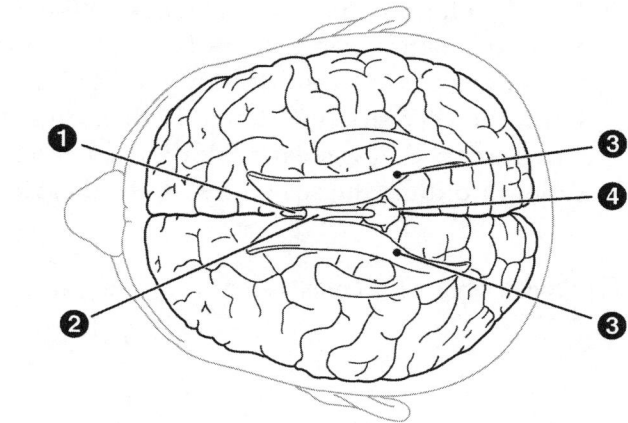

1. _____

2. _____

3. _____

4. _____

5. _____

6. _____

7. _____

8. _____

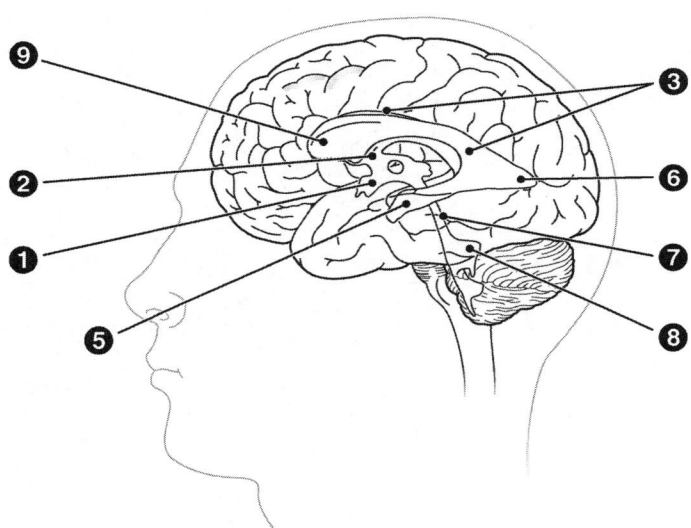

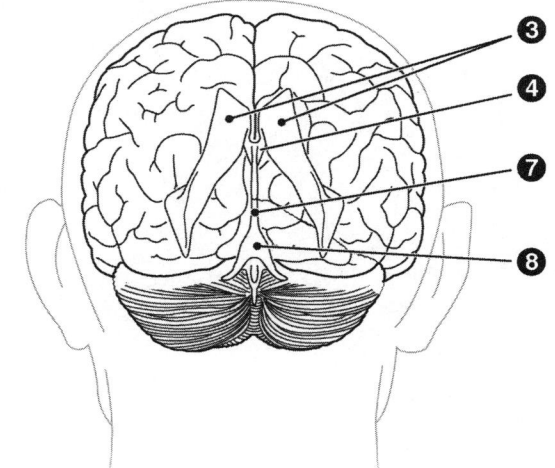

EXERCISE 9-5: Functional Areas of the Cerebral Cortex (text Fig. 9-8)

INSTRUCTIONS

1. Color the boxes next to the cerebral lobe names as follows: frontal lobe, pink; parietal lobe, light purple; temporal lobe, light blue; occipital lobe, light green.
2. Lightly color the four cerebral lobes on the diagram with the appropriate colors.
3. Write the names of structures 1–9 on the appropriate lines in different colors. For all structures except for 3, use a darker color than the one used for the corresponding cerebral lobe. For instance, a structure found in the frontal lobe could be colored red. Use the same color for structures 6–8. Use a dark color for structure 3.
4. Color or outline the structures on the diagram with the corresponding color.

☐ Frontal lobe   ☐ Parietal lobe   ☐ Temporal lobe   ☐ Occipital lobe

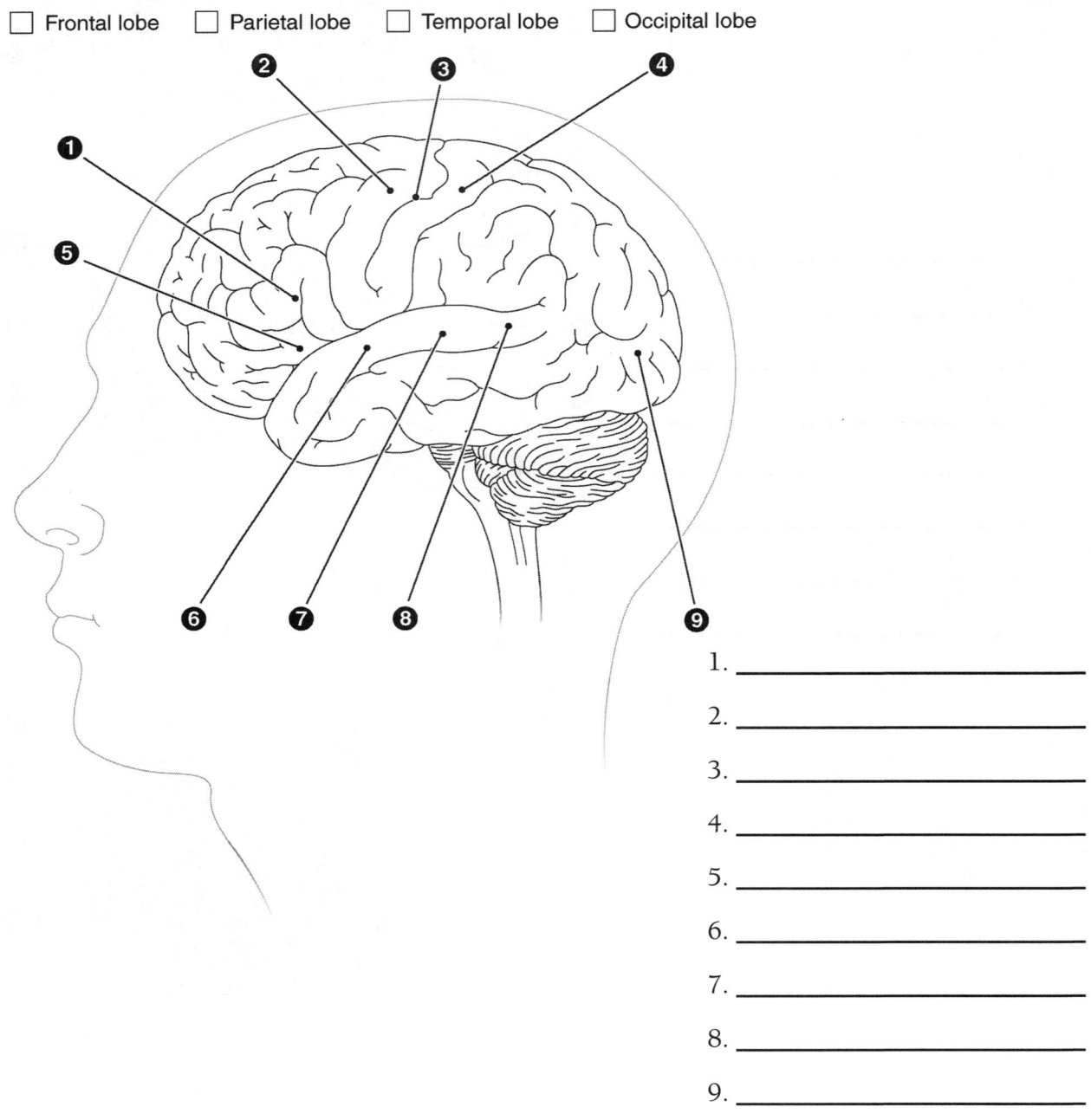

1. _____

2. _____

3. _____

4. _____

5. _____

6. _____

7. _____

8. _____

9. _____

EXERCISE 9-6: Cranial Nerves (text Fig. 9-14)

INSTRUCTIONS

1. Write the number and name of each labeled cranial nerve on the numbered lines in different colors. Use the same color for structures 1 and 2.
2. Color the nerves on the diagram with the corresponding color.

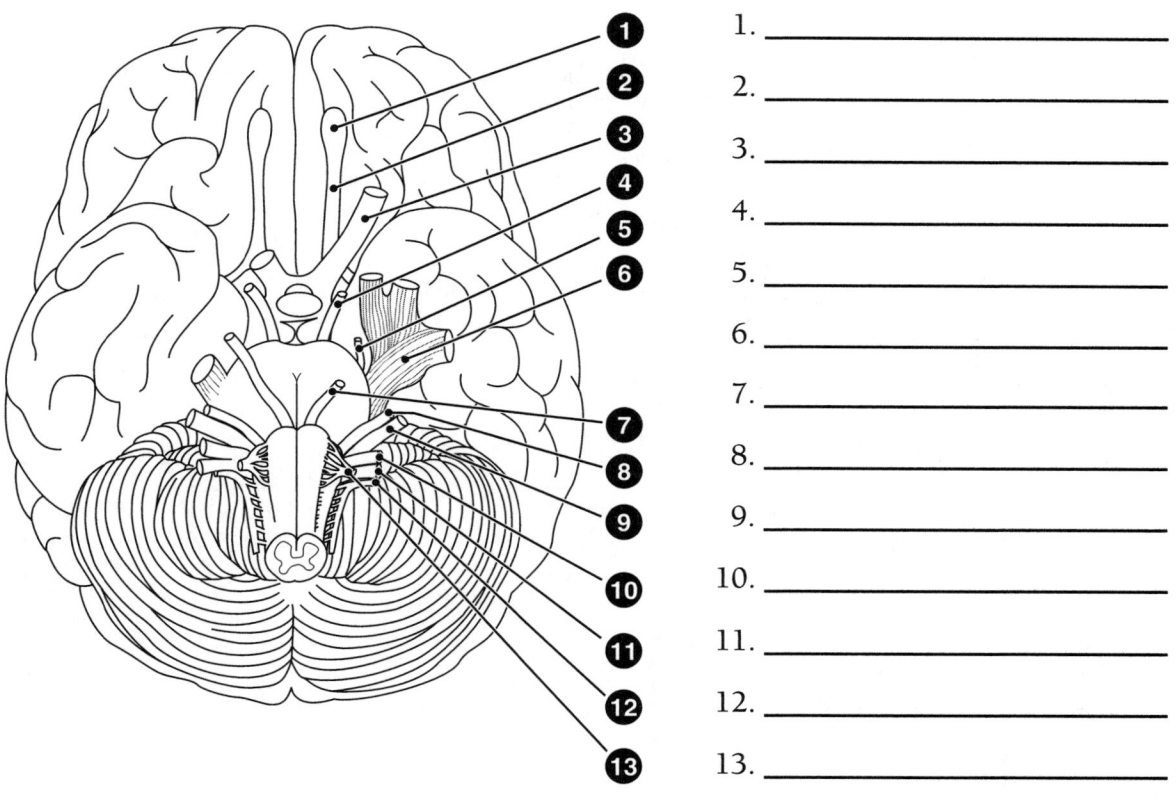

1. _____
2. _____
3. _____
4. _____
5. _____
6. _____
7. _____
8. _____
9. _____
10. _____
11. _____
12. _____
13. _____

Making the Connections

The following concept map deals with the structure of the brain. Each pair of terms is linked together by a connecting phrase into a sentence. The sentence should be read in the direction of the arrow. Complete the concept map by filling in the appropriate term or phrase. There is one right answer for each term. However, there are many correct answers for the connecting phrases (4, 8, 11, 14, 17). Write the connecting phrases beside the appropriate number (where space permits) or on a separate piece of paper. There are many other connections that could be made on this map. For instance, how could you connect the structures 2 and 16? Can you add more terms to the map?

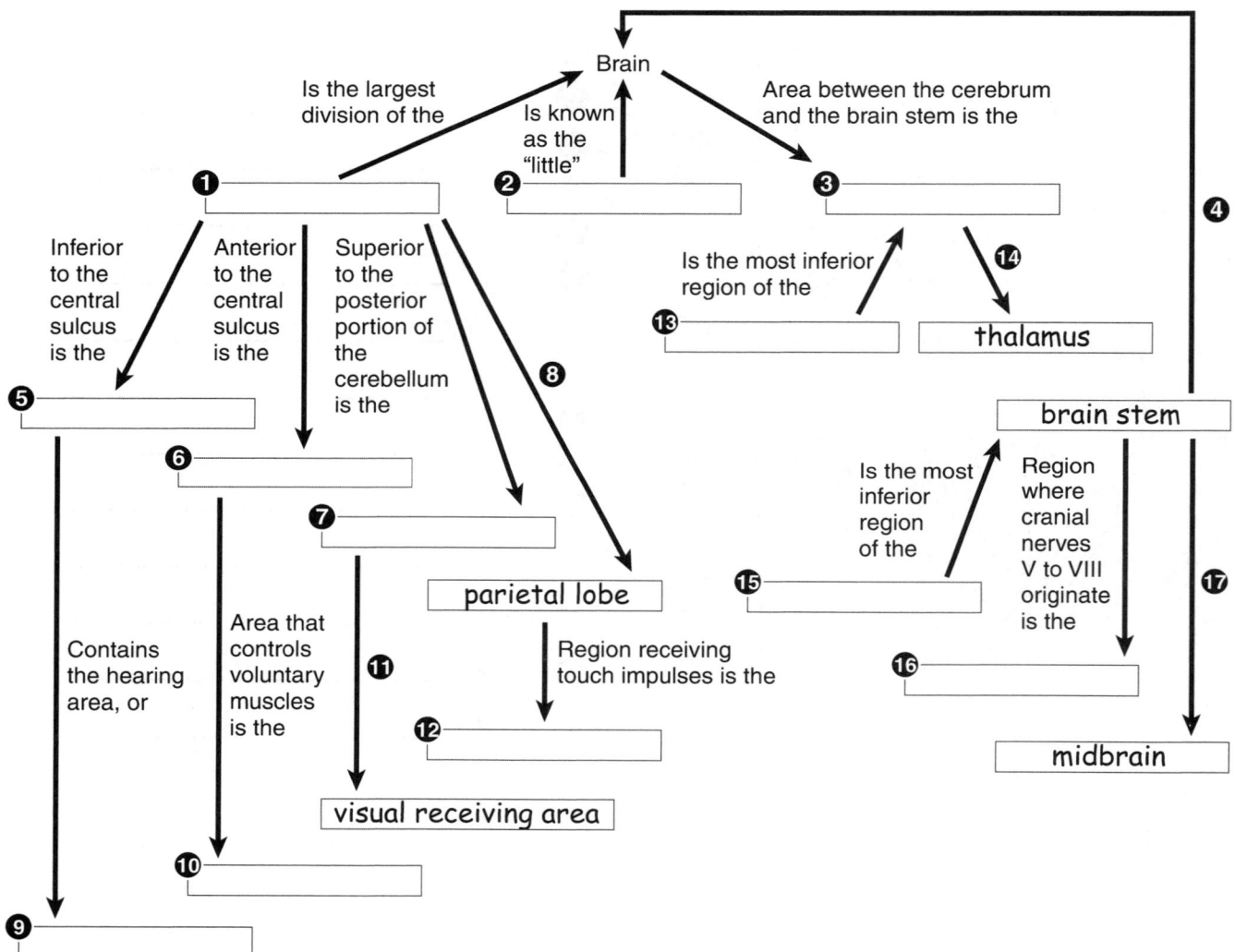

Optional Exercise: Make your own concept map, based on structures involved in the synthesis and movement of cerebrospinal fluid. Choose your own terms to incorporate into your map, or use the following list: ventricle, choroid plexus, lateral ventricles, third ventricle, fourth ventricle, foramina, horns, cerebral aqueduct, spinal cord, cerebrospinal fluid, dural sinuses, subarachnoid space, arachnoid villi.

Testing Your Knowledge
Building Understanding

I. Matching Exercises

Matching only within each group, write the answers in the spaces provided.

➤ **Group A**

dura mater	pia mater	arachnoid	choroid plexus	cerebral aqueduct
subarachnoid space		arachnoid villi	ventricle	dural sinus

1. The web-like middle meningeal layer _____

2. Venous channel between the two outermost meninges _____

3. The innermost layer of the meninges, the delicate membrane in which there are many blood vessels _____

4. The area in which cerebrospinal fluid collects before its return to the blood _____

5. The vascular network in a ventricle that forms cerebrospinal fluid _____

6. The projections in the dural sinuses through which cerebrospinal fluid is returned to the blood _____

7. The outermost layer of the meninges, which is the thickest and toughest _____

➤ **Group B**

gyrus	central sulcus	lateral sulcus	basal ganglia
dopamine	corpus callosum	internal capsule	cortex

1. A shallow groove that separates the temporal lobe from the frontal and parietal lobes _____

2. Masses of gray matter deep within the cerebrum that help regulate body movement and the muscles of facial expression _____

3. A band of white matter that carries impulses between the cerebrum and the brain stem _____

4. An elevated portion of the cerebral cortex _____

5. The thin layer of gray matter on the surface of the cerebrum _____

6. A band of myelinated fibers that bridges the two cerebral hemispheres _____

7. The neurotransmitter used by the basal nuclei neurons _____

➤ Group C

lobe	hemisphere	medulla oblongata	pons
cerebrum	diencephalon	cerebellum	midbrain

1. Each half of the cerebrum   _____

2. The portion of the brain stem composed of myelinated nerve fibers that connects to the cerebellum   _____

3. An individual subdivision of the cerebrum that regulates specific functions   _____

4. The part of the brain between the pons and the spinal cord   _____

5. The portion of the brain that contains the thalamus and hypothalamus   _____

6. The superior portion of the brain stem   _____

7. The largest part of the brain   _____

➤ Group D

thalamus	hypothalamus	limbic system	parietal lobe	
temporal lobe	occipital lobe	frontal lobe	vasomotor center	cardiac center

1. Nuclei that regulate the contraction of smooth muscle in blood vessel walls   _____

2. The region of the diencephalon that acts as a relay center for sensory stimuli   _____

3. The region consisting of portions of the cerebrum and diencephalon that is involved in emotional states and behavior   _____

4. The portion of the cerebral cortex where visual impulses from the retina are interpreted   _____

5. The portion of the cerebral cortex where auditory impulses are interpreted   _____

6. Location of a sensory area for interpretation of pain, touch, and temperature   _____

7. The lobe controlling voluntary muscles   _____

➤ **Group E**

optic nerve	vagus nerve	glossopharyngeal nerve
trochlear nerve	abducens nerve	vestibulocochlear nerve
facial nerve	trigeminal nerve	accessory nerve

1. A motor nerve controlling the trapezius, sternocleidomastoid,

   and larynx muscles   _____

2. The nerve that controls contraction of a single eye muscle _____

3. The nerve that carries visual impulses from the eye to the brain _____

4. The most important sensory nerve of the face and head   _____

5. The nerve that supplies most of the organs in the thoracic and

   abdominal cavities   _____

6. The nerve that supplies the muscles of facial expression   _____

7. The nerve that carries sensory impulses for hearing and

   equilibrium   _____

II. Multiple Choice

Select the best answer and write the letter of your choice in the blank.

1. The shallow goove lying between the frontal and parietal lobe is the: 1. _____
   a. lateral sulcus
   b. central sulcus
   c. longitudinal fissure
   d. basal nuclei
2. The dura mater is: 2. _____
   a. the innermost layer of the meninges
   b. the outermost layer of the meninges
   c. the network of vessels that produces cerebrospinal fluid
   d. the part of the brain that connects with the spinal cord
3. Impulses for the sense of taste travel to the: 3. _____
   a. parietal lobe
   b. temporal lobe
   c. hippocampus
   d. occipital lobe
4. The cerebrospinal fluid is formed in the: 4. _____
   a. cerebral aqueduct
   b. central sulcus
   c. choroid plexus
   d. internal capsule
5. The abducens nerve supplies the: 5. _____
   a. eye
   b. ear and pharynx

      c. face and salivary gland

      d. tongue and pharynx

6. The reticular formation is: 6. _____

      a. a region of the limbic system that controls wakefulness and sleep

      b. a deep groove that divides the cerebral hemispheres

      c. the part of the temporal lobe concerned with the sense of smell

      d. the fifth lobe of the cerebrum

III. Completion Exercise

Write the word or phrase that correctly completes each sentence.

1. The four chambers within the brain where cerebrospinal fluid is produced are the   _____

2. Sounds are interpreted in the area of the temporal lobe called the   _____

3. The region of the diencephalon that helps maintain homeostasis (*e.g.*, water balance, appetite, and body temperature) and controls the autonomic nervous system is the   _____

4. The storage of information to be recalled at a later time is called   _____

5. Records of the electrical activity of the brain can be made with an instrument called a(n)   _____

6. Extensions of the lateral ventricles into the cerebral lobes are called   _____

7. Except for the first two pairs, all the cranial nerves arise from the   _____

8. The three layers of membranes that surround the brain and spinal cord are called the   _____

9. The clear liquid that helps to support and protect the brain and spinal cord is   _____

10. The number of pairs of cranial nerves is   _____

11. The area of the brain stem concerned with eye-tracking reflexes involved in reading is the   _____

12. The middle portion of the cerebellum is called the   _____

Understanding Concepts

I. True or False

Each of the following statements is false. Correct each statement by replacing the underlined word or phrase and write the correct statement in the blank provided.

———— 1. The <u>pia mater</u> is the middle layer of the meninges.

———————————————————————————————————

———— 2. The interventricular foramina form channels between the lateral ventricles and the <u>fourth ventricle</u>.

———————————————————————————————————

———— 3. The primary motor cortex is found in the <u>parietal lobe</u>.

———————————————————————————————————

———— 4. The <u>internal capsule</u> consists of myelinated fibers linking the cerebral hemispheres with the brain stem.

———————————————————————————————————

———— 5. The <u>parietal lobe</u> lies posterior to the central sulcus and superior to the occipital lobe.

———————————————————————————————————

———— 6. The raised areas on the surface of the cerebrum are called <u>gyri</u>.

———————————————————————————————————

———— 7. Smell impulses are carried by the <u>third</u> cranial nerve.

———————————————————————————————————

———— 8. The <u>hypoglossal</u> nerve transmits sensory information from the tongue.

———————————————————————————————————

II. Practical Applications

Study each discussion. Then write the appropriate word or phrase in the space provided.

1. Mr. B, age 87, drove his car into a ditch. When the paramedics arrived, he was unable to speak, a disorder called ————————————————

2. Mr. B also experienced paralysis on his right side, indicating a problem within the largest division of the brain, the ————————————————

3. The right side of Mr. B's face droops, and he cannot control his facial expressions. The facial muscles are controlled by the cranial nerve numbered _____

4. A computed tomography (CT) scan at the hospital revealed the rupture of a cerebral blood vessel, The rupture occurred in the left side of the brain. The anatomical name for the left side of the brain is the left _____

5. Mr. B's speech disorder indicates that the bleed affected his motor speech area, also called _____

III. Short Essays

1. Describe the structures that protect the brain and spinal cord.

_____

_____

_____

2. List some functions of the structures in the diencephalon.

_____

_____

_____

3. List the name, number, and sensory information conveyed for each of the purely sensory cranial nerves.

_____

_____

_____

Conceptual Thinking

1. Describe the journey of cerebrospinal fluid (CSF), beginning with its synthesis and ending with its entry into the circulatory system.

_____

_____

_____

_____

Expanding Your Horizons

Do you use herbal supplements like ginkgo biloba to boost your learning power? As discussed in a Scientific American article (Resource 1), ginkgo biloba does boost memory—to the same extent as a candy bar! Mental exercise may be the best way to improve your academic performance (Resource 2).

Resource List

Gold PE, Cahill L, Wenk GL. The lowdown on Ginkgo biloba. Sci Am 2003;288:86–91.
Holloway M. The mutable brain. Sci Am 2003;289:78–85.

chapter 10

The Sensory System

Overview

The sensory system enables us to detect changes taking place both internally and externally. These changes are detected by specialized structures called **receptors**. Any change that acts on a receptor to produce a response in the nervous system is termed a stimulus. The **special senses**, so called because the receptors are limited to a few specialized sense organs in the head, include the senses of vision, hearing, equilibrium, taste, and smell. The receptors of the eye are the **rods** and **cones** located in the retina. The receptors for both hearing (the **organ of Corti**) and equilibrium (the **vestibule** and **semicircular canals**) are located within the inner ear. Receptors for the chemical senses of taste and smell are located on the tongue and in the upper part of the nose, respectively. The **general senses** are scattered throughout the body; they respond to touch, pressure, temperature, pain, and position. Receptors for the sense of position, known as **proprioceptors**, are found in muscles, tendons, and joints. The nerve impulses generated in a receptor cell by a stimulus must be carried to the central nervous system by way of a **sensory** (afferent) neuron. Here, the information is processed and a suitable response is made.

This chapter is quite challenging, because it contains difficult concepts and large amounts of detail. You can use concept maps to assemble all of the details into easy-to-remember frameworks.

Learning the Language: Word Anatomy

Complete the following table by writing the correct word part or meaning in the space provided.
For each word part, write a term that contains the word part.

Word Part	Meaning	Example
1. presby-	_____	_____
2. _____	stone	_____
3. kine	_____	_____
4. narc/o	_____	_____
5. _____	drum	_____
6. _____	yellow	_____
7. propri/o-	_____	_____
8. _____	pain	_____
9. -esthesia	_____	_____
10. _____	hearing	_____

Addressing the Learning Outcomes

I. Writing Exercise

The learning outcomes for Chapter 10 are listed below. These learning outcomes provide an overview of the major topics covered in this chapter. On a separate piece of paper, try to write out an answer to each learning outcome. All of the answers can be found in the pages of the textbook. Learning Outcomes 3, 4, 7, 8, 9, 10, and 11 are also addressed in the Coloring Atlas.

1. Describe the function of the sensory system.
2. Differentiate between the special and general senses and give examples of each.
3. Describe the structure of the eye.
4. List and describe the structures that protect the eye.
5. Define *refraction* and list the refractive parts of the eye.
6. Differentiate between the rods and the cones of the eye.
7. Compare the functions of the extrinsic and intrinsic muscles of the eye.
8. Describe the nerve supply to the eye.
9. Describe the three divisions of the ear.
10. Describe the receptor for hearing and explain how it functions.
11. Compare static and dynamic equilibrium and describe the location and function of these receptors.
12. Explain the function of proprioceptors.
13. List several methods for treatment of pain.
14. Describe sensory adaptation and explain its value.
15. Show how word parts are used to build words related to the sensory system (see Word Anatomy at the end of the chapter).

II. Labeling and Coloring Atlas

EXERCISE 10-1: The Lacrimal Apparatus (text Fig. 10-2)
Label the indicated parts.

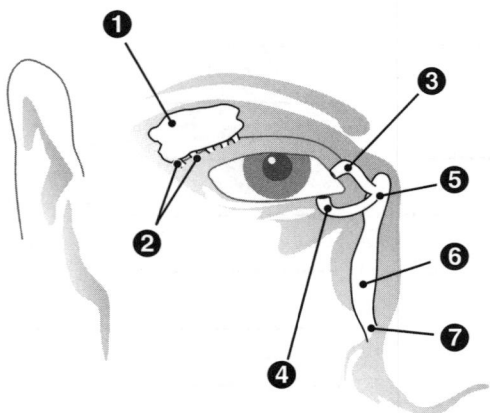

1. _____

2. _____

3. _____

4. _____

5. _____

6. _____

7. _____

EXERCISE 10-2: The Eye (text Fig. 10-3)

INSTRUCTIONS

1. Write the name of each labeled part on the numbered lines in different colors. Use the same color for structures 3 and 4 and structures 6–9 (inclusive). Write the name of structure 1 in black, because it will not be colored.
2. Color the different structures on the diagram with the corresponding color. Some structures are present in more than one location on the diagram. Try to color all of a particular structure in the appropriate color. For instance, only one of the suspensory ligaments is labeled, but color both suspensory ligaments.

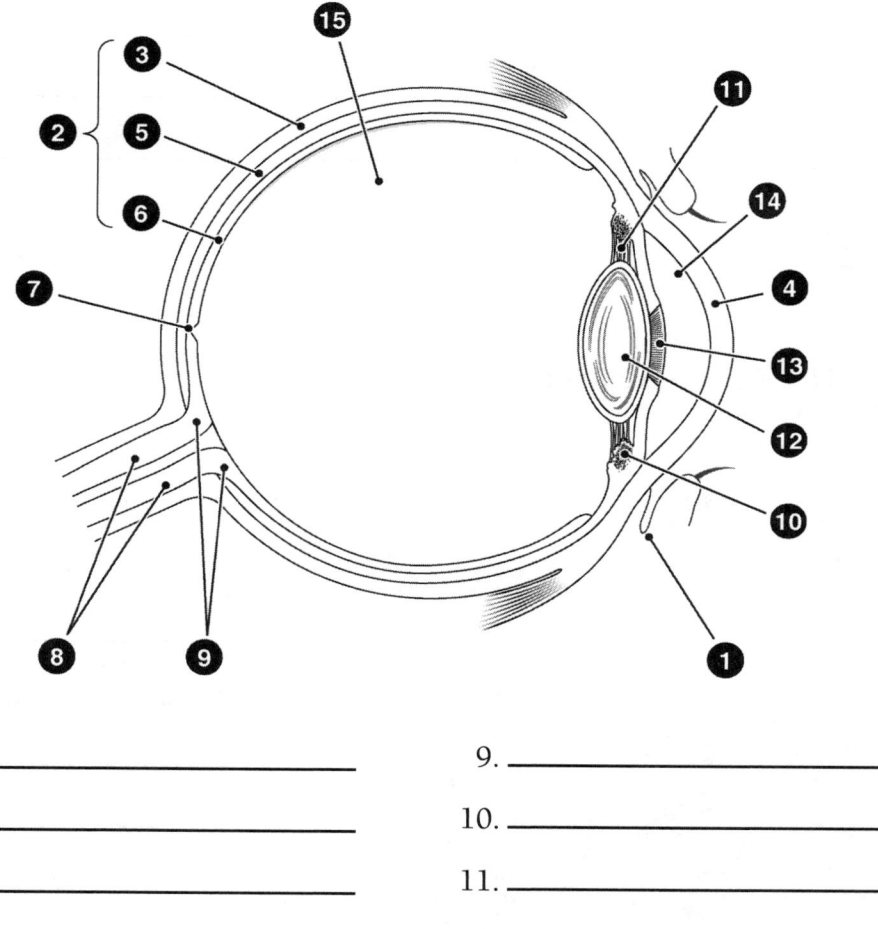

1. _____
2. _____
3. _____
4. _____
5. _____
6. _____
7. _____
8. _____

9. _____
10. _____
11. _____
12. _____
13. _____
14. _____
15. _____

EXERCISE 10-3: Extrinsic Muscles of the Eye (text Fig. 10-6)

INSTRUCTIONS

1. Write the name of each labeled muscle on the numbered lines in different colors.
2. Color the different muscles on the diagram with the corresponding color.

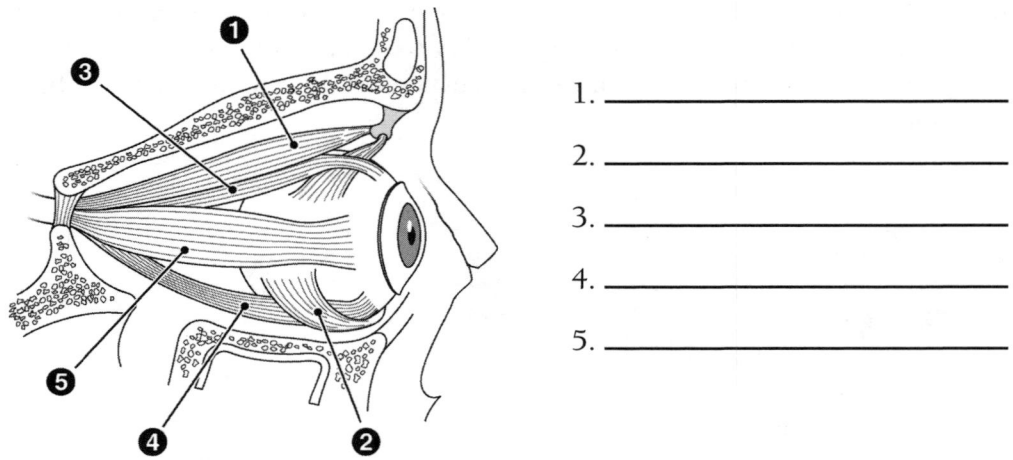

1. _____

2. _____

3. _____

4. _____

5. _____

EXERCISE 10-4: Nerves of the Eye (text Fig. 10-10)

Label the indicated nerves.

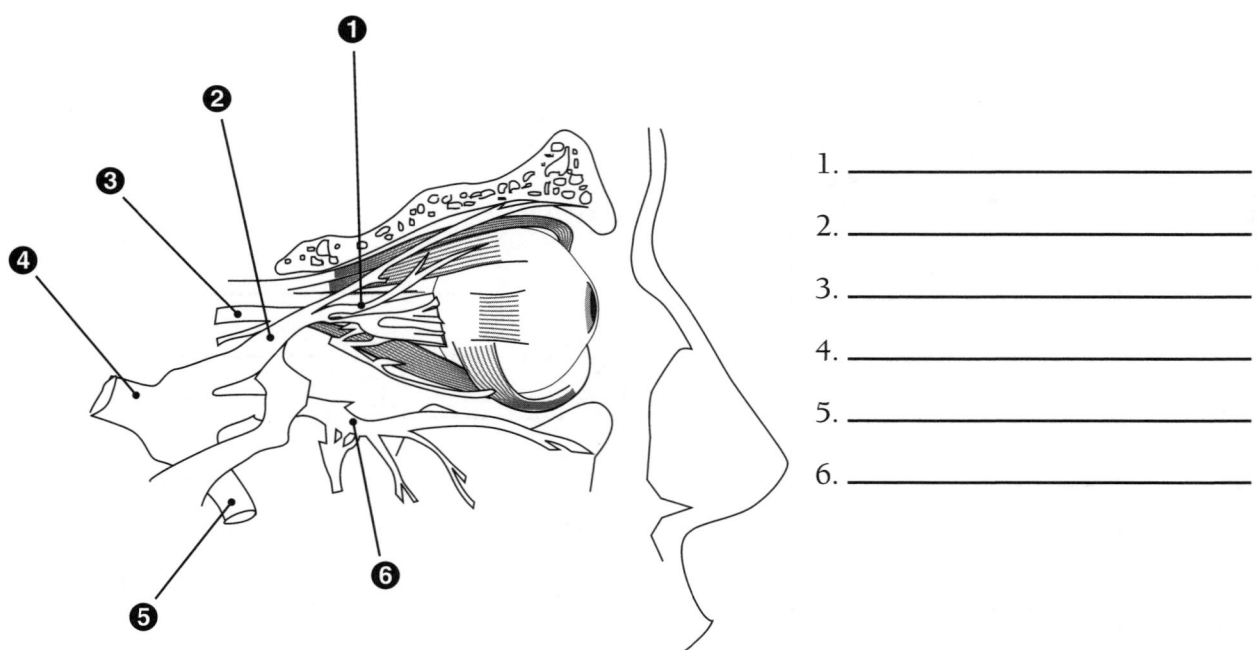

1. _____

2. _____

3. _____

4. _____

5. _____

6. _____

EXERCISE 10-5: The Ear (text Fig. 10-11)

INSTRUCTIONS

1. Write the names of the three ear divisions on the appropriate lines (1–3).
2. Write the names of the labeled parts on the numbered lines in different colors. Use black for structures 12–14, because they will not be colored.
3. Color each part with the corresponding color (except for parts 12–14).

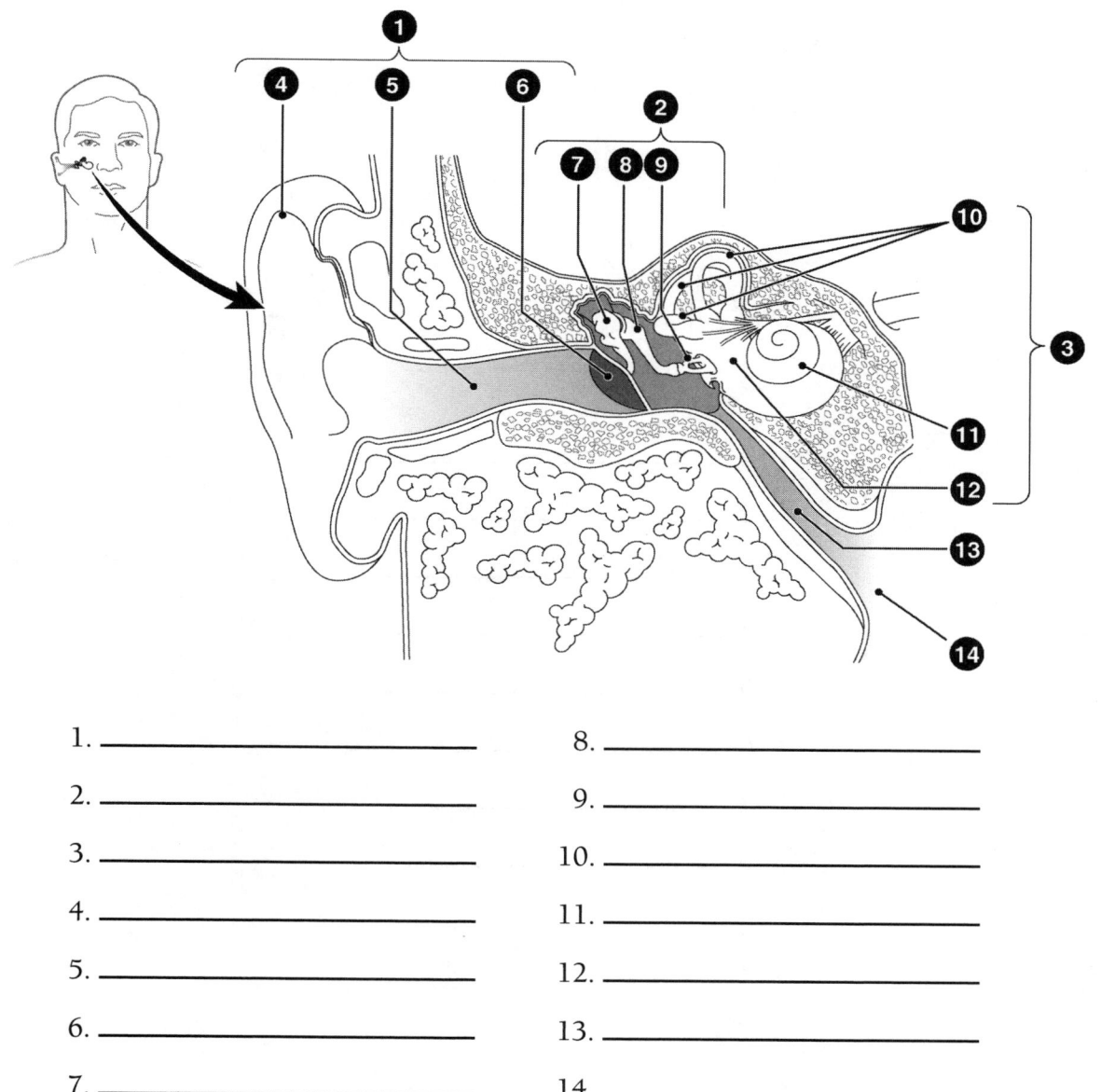

1. _____

2. _____

3. _____

4. _____

5. _____

6. _____

7. _____

8. _____

9. _____

10. _____

11. _____

12. _____

13. _____

14. _____

EXERCISE 10-6: The Inner Ear (text Fig. 10-13)
Label the indicated parts.

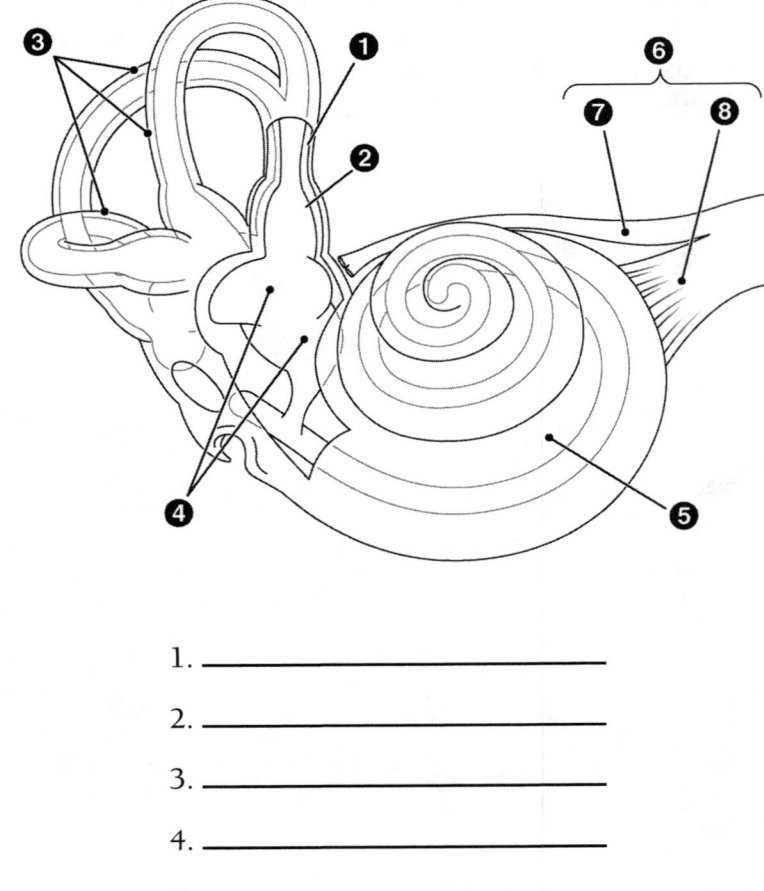

1. _____

2. _____

3. _____

4. _____

5. _____

6. _____

7. _____

8. _____

EXERCISE 10-7: Cochlea and Organ of Corti (text Fig. 10-14)

INSTRUCTIONS

1. Write the name of each labeled part on the numbered lines. Use colors for structures 3–7, 11, and 12. Use black for the other structures.
2. Color structures 3–7, 11, and 12 with the corresponding color.

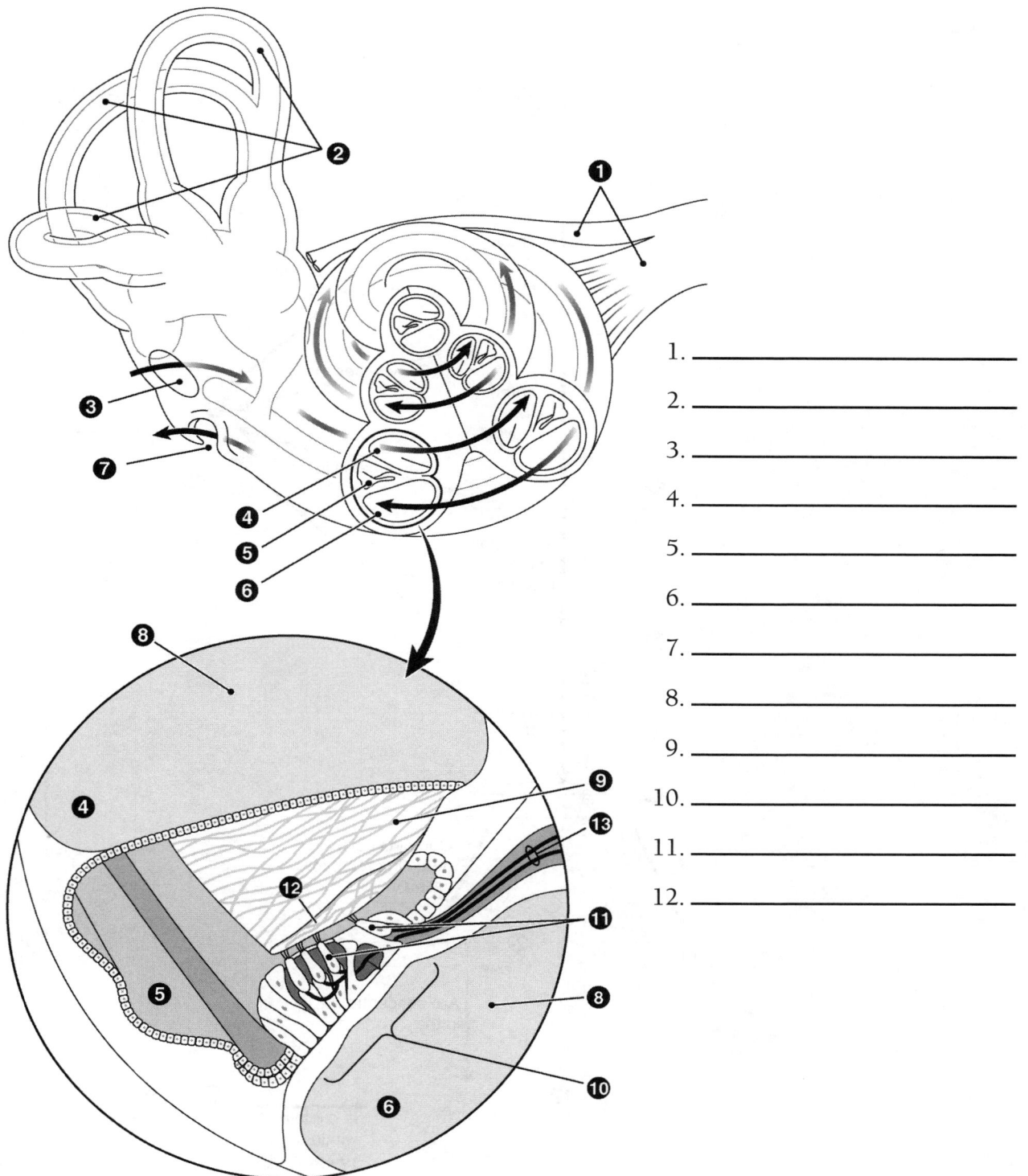

1. _____
2. _____
3. _____
4. _____
5. _____
6. _____
7. _____
8. _____
9. _____
10. _____
11. _____
12. _____

Making the Connections

The following concept map deals with the structure and function of the eye. Each pair of terms is linked together by a connecting phrase into a sentence. The sentence should be read in the direction of the arrow. Complete the concept map by filling in the appropriate term or phrase. There is one right answer for each term. However, there are many correct answers for the connecting phrases (2, 9).

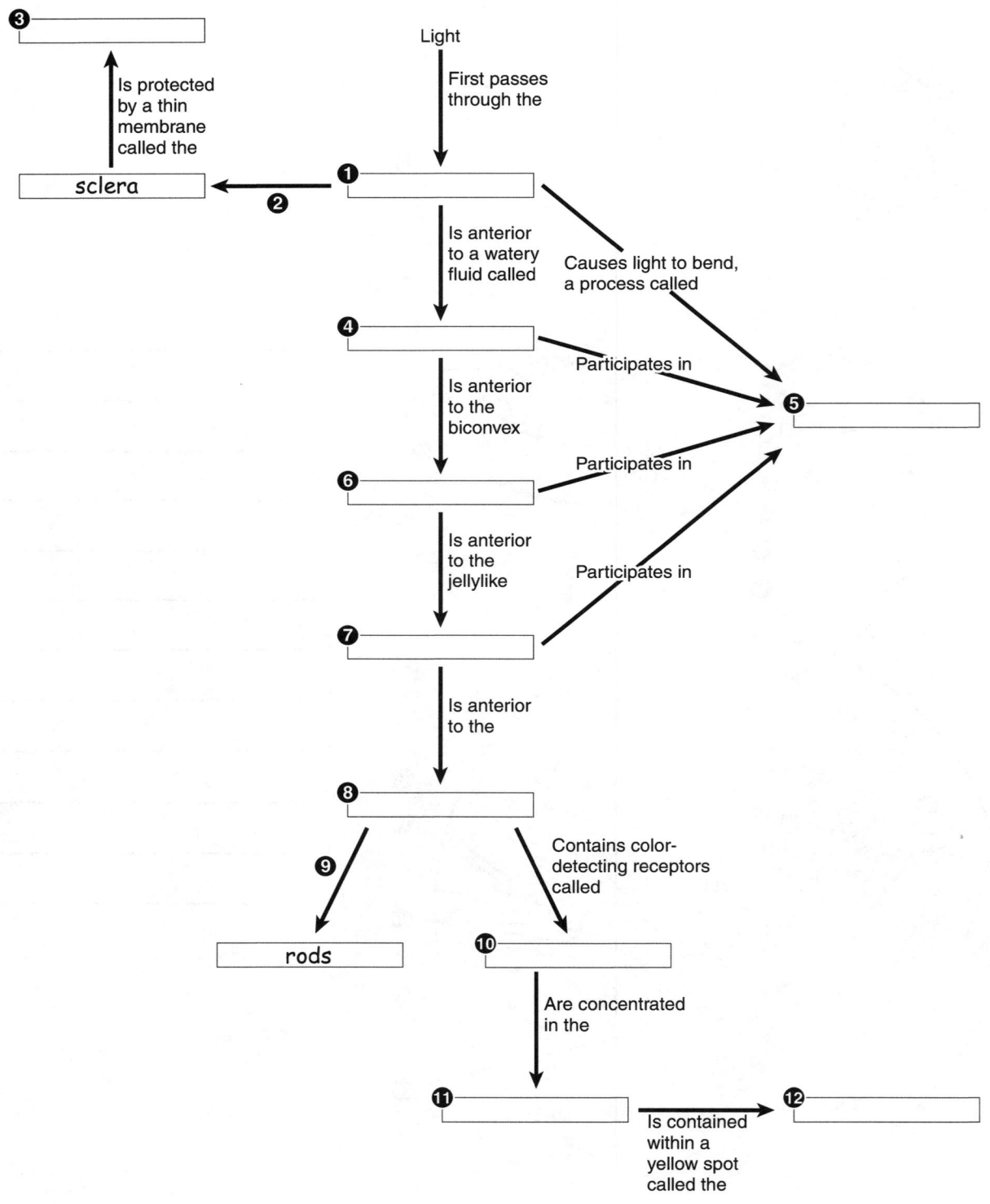

Optional Exercise: Construct a concept map of terms relating to the ear using the following terms and any others you would like to include: tympanic membrane, stapes, malleus, incus, pinna, bony labyrinth, organ of Corti, oval window, round window, cochlear duct, tectorial membrane, cochlear nerve. You may also want to construct concept maps relating to the other special senses (equilibrium, taste, smell) and the general senses (touch, pressure, temperature, proprioception).

Testing Your Knowledge
Building Understanding

I. Matching Exercises

Matching only within each group, write the answers in the spaces provided.

➤ **Group A**

conjunctiva	choroid	cone	cornea
optic disk	retina	rod	sclera

1. The vascular, pigmented middle tunic of the eyeball   _____

2. A vision receptor that is sensitive to color   _____

3. The part of the eye that light rays pass through first as

   they enter the eye   _____

4. The membrane that lines the eyelids   _____

5. Another name for the blind spot, the region where the

   optic nerve connects with the eye   _____

6. The innermost coat of the eyeball, the nervous tissue

   layer that includes the receptors for the sense of vision   _____

7. A vision receptor that functions well in dim light   _____

➤ **Group B**

aqueous humor	vitreous body	lens	ciliary muscle
rhodopsin	pupil	fovea centralis	iris

1. The structure that alters the shape of the lens for

   accommodation   _____

2. The watery fluid that fills much of the eyeball in

   front of the crystalline lens   _____

3. Two sets of muscle fibers that regulate the amount of

   light entering the eye   _____

4. The jelly-like material located behind the crystalline lens

   that maintains the spherical shape of the eyeball   _____

5. A pigment needed for vision   _____

6. The depressed area in the retina that is the point of clearest

   vision   _____

7. The central opening of the iris   _____

➤ Group C

oval window	organ of Corti	malleus
eustachian tube	cochlear duct	endolymph
perilymph	incus	pinna

1. The fluid contained within the membranous labyrinth of

   the inner ear   _____

2. The bone that interacts with the tympanic membrane   _____

3. Another name for the projecting part, or auricle, of the ear _____

4. The channel connecting the middle ear cavity with the

   pharynx   _____

5. The fluid of the inner ear contained within the bony

   labyrinth and surrounding the membranous labyrinth   _____

6. Ciliated receptor cells that detect sound waves   _____

7. The skeleton of the inner ear   _____

➤ Group D

vestibule	dynamic equilibrium	semicircular canals	
cochlear duct	static equilibrium	otoliths	cristae

1. The sense of knowing the position of the head in relation

   to gravity   _____

2. Small crystals that activate maculae   _____

3. The sense organ involved in dynamic equilibrium   _____

4. The receptor cells involved in dynamic equilibrium   _____

5. Two small chambers containing maculae   _____

➤ Group E

kinesthesia	proprioception	tactile corpuscle	cochlear nerve
vestibular nerve	oculomotor nerve	ophthalmic nerve	
optic nerve	free nerve endings	equilibrium	

1. The branch of the vestibulocochlear nerve that carries

   hearing impulses   _____

2. The nerve that carries visual impulses from the retina to

   the brain   _____

3. The branch of the fifth cranial nerve that carries impulses of

   pain, touch, and temperature from the eye to the brain   _____

4. The largest of the three cranial nerves that carry motor fibers

   to the eyeball muscles   _____

5. The sense of knowing the position of one's body and the

   relative positions of different muscles   _____

6. The sense of body movement   _____

7. Receptors that detect changes in temperature   _____

II. Multiple Choice

Select the best answer and write the letter of your choice in the blank.

1. A physician who specializes in eye health and disease is a(n):   1. _____
   a. ophthalmologist
   b. internist
   c. allergist
   d. orthopedic surgeon
2. A term related to the sense of taste is: 2. _____
   a. tactile
   b. gustatory
   c. proprioceptive
   d. thermal
3. Alterations in the lens' shape to allow for near or far vision is called: 3. _____
   a. accommodation
   b. convergence
   c. divergence
   d. dark adaptation
4. The term *lacrimation* refers to the secretion of: 4. _____
   a. mucus
   b. wax
   c. tears
   d. aqueous humor
5. Pain killers that are released from certain regions of the brain are: 5. _____
   a. narcotics
   b. endorphins
   c. anesthetics
   d. nonsteroidal anti-inflammatory drugs

6. A person who lacks cones in the retina will experience: 6. _____
    a. complete blindness
    b. color blindness
    c. night blindness
    d. deafness

7. The organ of Corti is the receptor for: 7. _____
    a. taste
    b. smell
    c. hearing
    d. equilibrium

III. Completion Exercise

1. The transparent portion of the sclera is the   _____
2. The glands that secrete ear wax are called   _____
3. The nerve endings that aid in judging position and changes
   in location of body parts are the   _____
4. The sense of position is partially governed by equilibrium
   receptors in the internal ear, including two small chambers
   in the vestibule and the three   _____
5. The tactile corpuscles are the receptors for the sense of   _____
6. Any drug that relieves pain is called a(n)   _____
7. When you enter a darkened room, it takes a while for the rods
   to begin to function. This interval is known as the period of   _____
8. The receptor tunic (layer) of the eye is the   _____
9. The bending of light rays as they pass through the media of
   the eye is   _____

Understanding Concepts

I. True or False

For each question, write "T" for true or "F" for false in the blank to the left of each number. If a statement is false, correct it by replacing the underlined term and write the correct statement in the blank below the question.

_____ 1. Extrinsic eye muscles control the diameter of the pupil.

_____

_____ 2. There are seven extrinsic muscles connected to each eye.

_____

_____ 3. The iris is an intrinsic muscle of the eye.

_____

_____ 4. The sense of temperature is a <u>general</u> sense.

_____

_____ 5. The <u>rods</u> of the eye function in bright light and detect color.

_____

_____ 6. When the eyes are exposed to a bright light, the pupils <u>constrict</u>.

_____

_____ 7. Sound waves leave the ear through the <u>round window</u>.

_____

_____ 8. The ciliary muscle <u>contracts</u> to thicken the lens.

_____

_____ 9. The sense of smell is also called <u>olfaction</u>.

_____

II. Practical Applications

Study each discussion. Then write the appropriate word or phrase in the space provided.

➤ **Group A**

Baby L was brought in by his mother because he awakened crying and holding the right side of his head. He had been experiencing a cold, but now he seemed to be in pain. Complete the following descriptions relating to his evaluation and treatment.

1. Examination revealed a bulging red eardrum. The eardrum is also called the   _____

2. The cause of baby L's painful bulging eardrum was an infection of the middle ear. The middle ear contains three small bones: the malleus, incus, and   _____

3. Antibiotic treatment of baby L's infection was begun, because this early treatment usually prevents complications. The middle ear is prone to infections, because it is connected to the pharynx by the   _____

4. Baby L was returned to the emergency room the next day because he was falling down repeatedly. The physician suspected a problem with his sense of balance, or   _____

5. Baby L's mother asked how an ear infection could affect balance. The physician explained that two structures were located within the inner ear that are involved with balance, named the semicircular canals and the   _____

6. In particular, the physician feared that the middle ear infection had spread to the fluid within the membranous labyrinth. This fluid is called   _____

➤ Group B

Sixty-year-old Mr. S had ridden his scooter over some broken glass. A fragment of glass bounced up and flew into one eye. Complete the following descriptions relating to his evaluation and treatment.

1. Examination by the eye specialist showed that there was a cut in the transparent window of the eye, the _____

2. On further examination of Mr. S, the colored part of the eye was seen to protrude from the wound. This part of the eye is the _____

3. Mr. S's treatment included antiseptics, anesthetics, and suturing of the wound. Medication was instilled in the sac-like structure at the anterior of the eyeball. This sac is lined with a thin epithelial membrane, the _____

➤ Group C

You are conducting hearing tests at a senior citizens' home. During the course of the afternoon, you encounter the following patients. Complete the following descriptions relating to the evaluation and treatment of hearing loss.

1. Mrs. B reported some hearing loss and a sense of fullness in her outer ear. Examination revealed that her ear canal was plugged with hardened ear wax, which is scientifically called _____

2. Mr. J, age 72, reported gradually worsening hearing loss, although he had no symptoms of pain or other ear problems. Examination revealed that his hearing loss was caused by nerve damage. The cranial nerve that carries hearing impulses to the brain is called the _____

3. Elderly Mr. N had hearing loss (presbycusis) caused by atrophy of the nerve endings located in the spiral-shaped part of the inner ear, a part of the ear that is known as the _____

III. Short Essays

1. Describe several different structural forms of sensory receptors and give examples of each.

_____

_____

_____

2. List three methods to relieve pain that do not involve administration of drugs.

_____

_____

_____

Conceptual Thinking

1. You have probably been sitting in a chair for quite a while, yet you have not been constantly aware of your legs contacting the chair. Why not?

_____

_____

_____

2. Write your name at the bottom of this sheet of paper. Explain the contributions of different sensory receptors that were required to successfully complete that simple task. For instance, proprioceptors are required to indicate where the fingers are each moment of time.

_____

_____

_____

Expanding Your Horizons

1. Imagine if you could taste a triangle, or hear blue. This is reality for individuals with a disorder called synesthesia. Read about some exceptional artists that have this disorder and how synesthesia has helped us understand how the brain processes sensory information, in a Scientific American article (listed below).
2. Here is an exercise you can perform to find your own blind spot. On a separate piece of paper, draw a cross (on the left) and a circle (on the right), separated by a hand-width. Focus on the cross and notice (but do not focus on) the circle. Move the paper closer and further away until the circle disappears. Weird activities to investigate your blind spot can be found at the website http://serendip.brynmawr.edu/bb/blindspot1.html.

Resource List

Ramachandran VS, Hubbard EM. Hearing colors, tasting shapes. Sci Am 2003;288:52–59.

chapter 11

The Endocrine System: Glands and Hormones

Overview

The endocrine system and the nervous system are the main coordinating and controlling systems of the body. Chapter 8 discussed how the nervous system uses chemicals and electrical impulses to control very rapid, short-term responses. This chapter discusses the endocrine system, which uses specific chemicals called **hormones** to induce short-term or long-term changes on the growth, development, and function of specific cells. Hormones travel in the blood to distant sites and exert their effects on any cell (the target cell) that contains a specific **receptor** for the hormone. Hormones are extremely potent, and small variations in hormone concentrations can have significant effects on the body.

Although hormones are produced by many tissues, certain glands, called **endocrine glands**, specialize in hormone production. These endocrine glands include the pituitary (hypophysis), thyroid, parathyroids, adrenals, pancreas, gonads, thymus, and pineal. Together, these glands comprise the endocrine system. The activity of endocrine glands is regulated by negative feedback, other hormones, nervous stimulation, and/or biological rhythms.

One of the most important endocrine glands is the pituitary gland, which comprises the anterior pituitary and the posterior pituitary. The **posterior pituitary gland** is made of nervous tissue—it contains the axons and terminals of neurons that have their cell bodies in a part of the brain called the **hypothalamus**. Hormones are synthesized in the hypothalamus and released from the posterior pituitary. The **anterior pituitary** secretes a number of hormones that act on other endocrine glands. The cells of the anterior pituitary are controlled in part by **releasing hormones** made in the hypothalamus. These releasing hormones pass through the blood vessels of a **portal circulation** to reach the anterior pituitary.

Hormones are also made outside the traditional endocrine glands. Other structures that secrete hormones include the stomach, small intestine, kidney, heart, skin, and placenta.

This chapter contains a lot of details for you to learn. Try to summarize the material using concept maps and summary tables. You should also understand positive and negative feedback (Chapter 1) before you tackle the concepts in this chapter.

Learning the Language: Word Anatomy

Complete the following table by writing the correct word part or meaning in the space provided. For each word part, write a term that contains the word part.

Word Part	Meaning	Example
1. trop/o	_____	_____
2. _____	cortex	_____
3. -poiesis	_____	_____
4. natri-	_____	_____
5. _____	male	_____
6. _____	milk	_____
7. ren/o	_____	_____
8. insul/o-	_____	_____
9. oxy	_____	_____
10. nephr/o	_____	_____

Addressing the Learning Outcomes

I. Writing Exercise

The learning outcomes for Chapter 11 are listed below. These learning outcomes provide an overview of the major topics covered in this chapter. On a separate piece of paper, try to write out an answer to each learning outcome. All of the answers can be found in the pages of the textbook. Learning Outcomes 4 and 6 are also addressed in the Coloring Atlas.

1. Compare the effects of the nervous system and the endocrine system in controlling the body.
2. Describe the functions of hormones.
3. Explain how hormones are regulated.
4. Identify the glands of the endocrine system on a diagram.
5. List the hormones produced by each endocrine gland and describe the effects of each on the body.
6. Describe how the hypothalamus controls the anterior and posterior pituitary.
7. List tissues other than the endocrine glands that produce hormones.
8. List some medical uses of hormones.
9. Explain how the endocrine system responds to stress.
10. Show how word parts are used to build words related to the endocrine system.

II. Labeling and Coloring Atlas

EXERCISE 11-1: The Endocrine Glands (text Fig. 11-2)

INSTRUCTIONS

1. Write the name of each labeled part on the numbered lines in different colors.
2. Color the different structures on the diagram with the corresponding color. Some structures are present in more than one location on the diagram. Try to color all of a particular structure in the appropriate color. For instance, color both adrenal glands, although only one is indicated by a leader line.

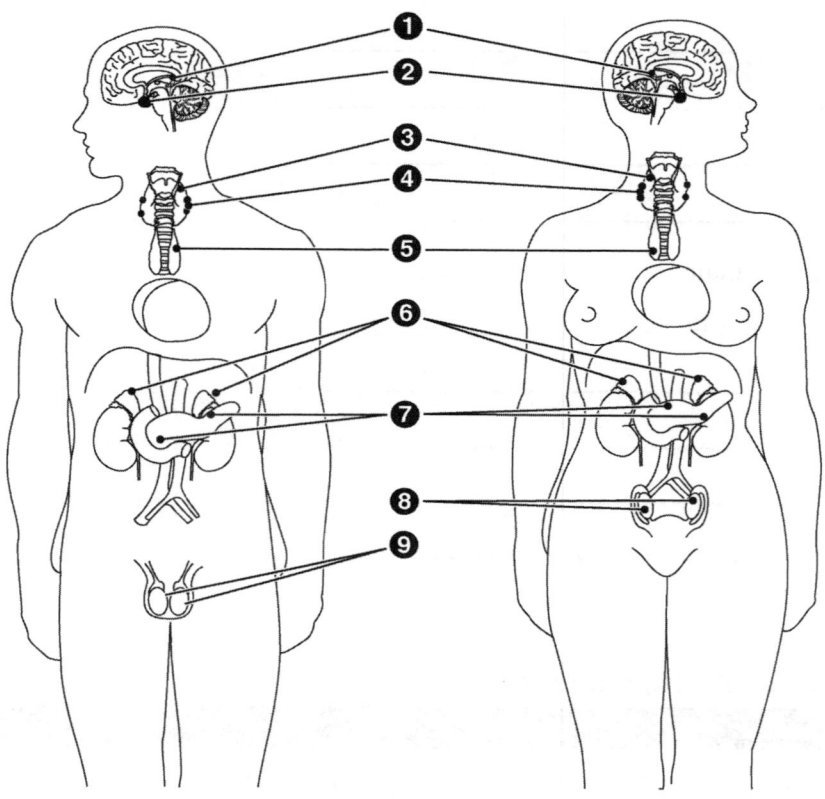

1. _____

2. _____

3. _____

4. _____

5. _____

6. _____

7. _____

8. _____

9. _____

EXERCISE 11-2: The Pituitary Gland (text Fig. 11-3)

INSTRUCTIONS

1. Label the parts of the hypothalamo-pituitary system.
2. Color blood vessels red and nerves yellow.

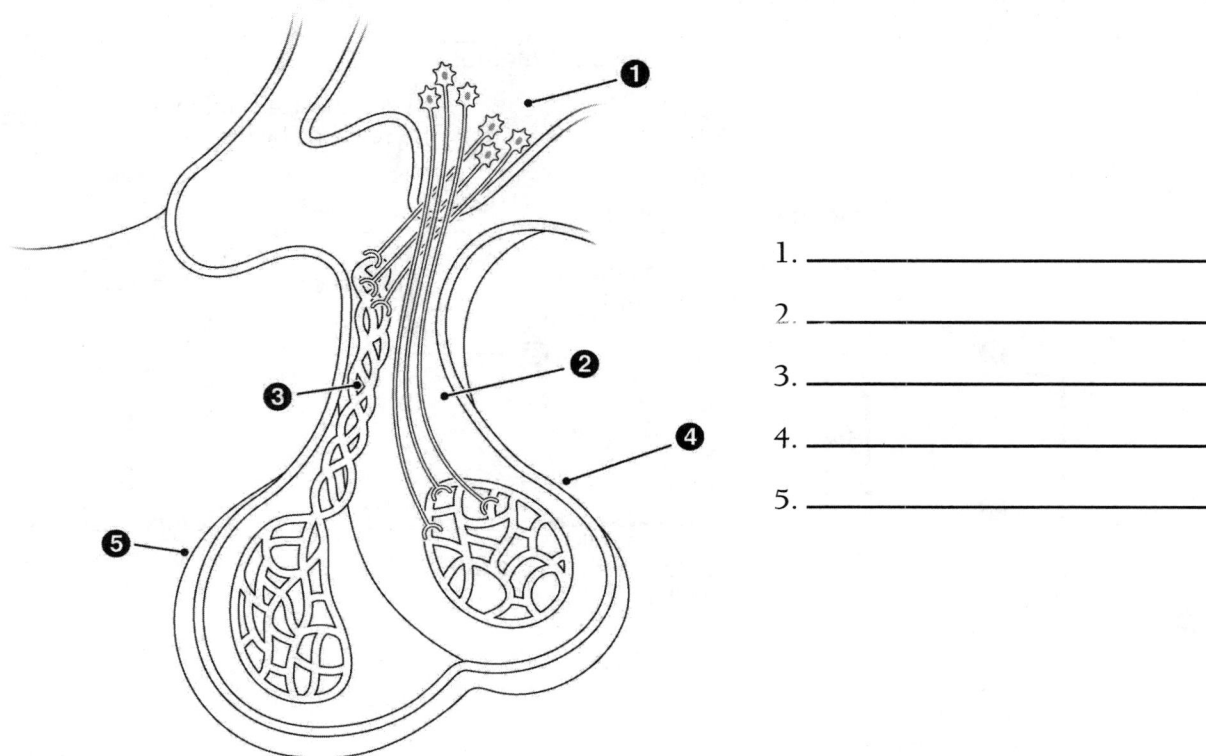

1. _____

2. _____

3. _____

4. _____

5. _____

Making the Connections

The following concept map deals with the relationship between the hypothalamus, pituitary gland, and some target organs. Each pair of terms is linked together by a connecting phrase into a sentence. The sentence should be read in the direction of the arrow. Complete the concept map by filling in the appropriate term or phrase. There is one right answer for each term. However, there are many correct answers for the connecting phrases (1, 4, 5, 9, 12). Write the connecting phrases beside the appropriate number (where space permits) or on a separate piece of paper.

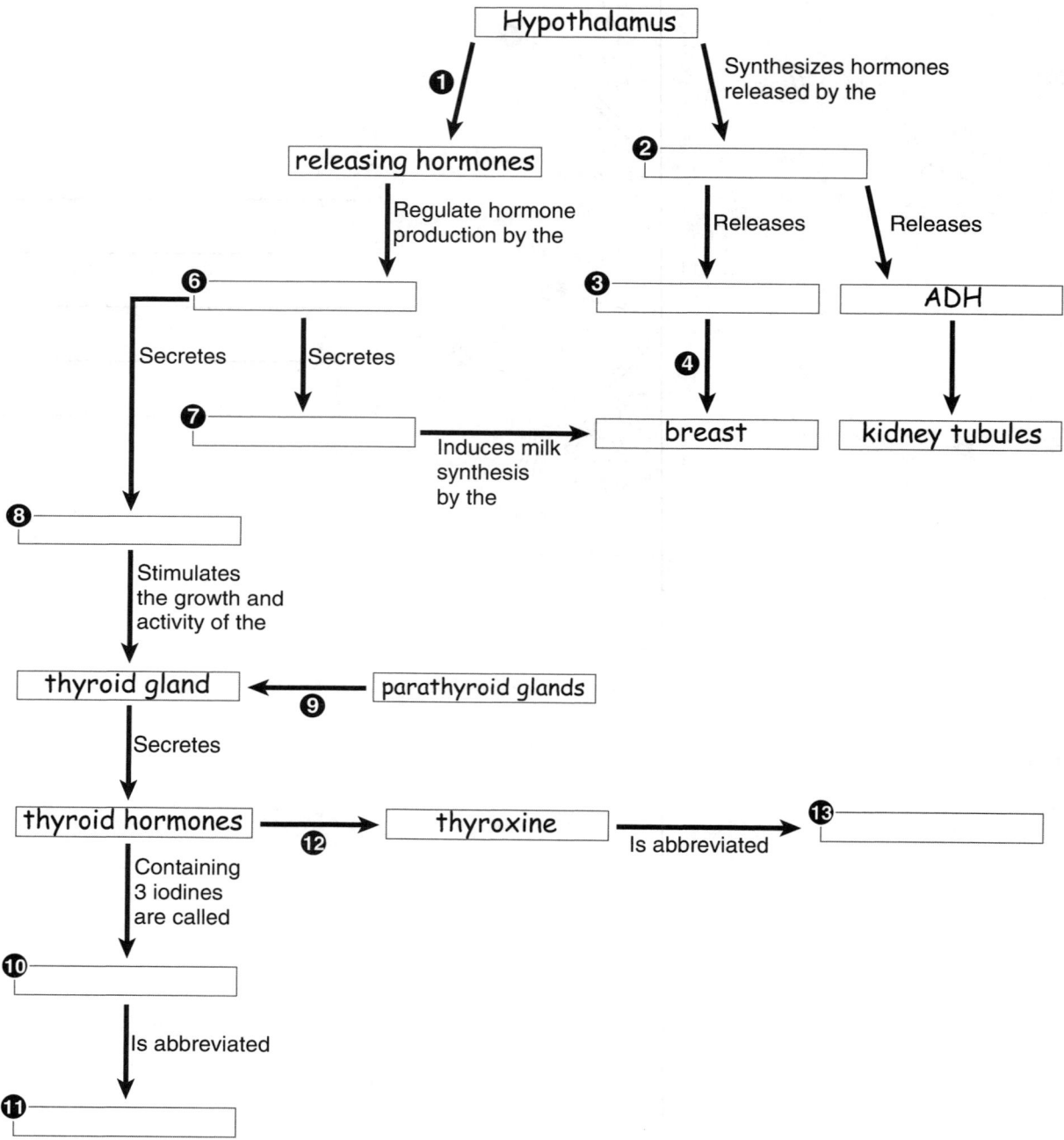

Optional Exercise: Construct your own concept map using the following terms: pancreas, insulin, glucagon, adrenal gland, medulla, cortex, epinephrine, cortisol, aldosterone, raises blood sugar, lowers blood sugar. You can also add other appropriate terms (for instance, target sites or hormone actions).

Testing Your Knowledge

Building Understanding

I. Matching Exercises

Matching only within each group, write the answers in the spaces provided.

➤ Group A

parathyroid	thymus	pineal	hypothalamus
thyroid	adrenal	pancreas	

1. One of the tiny glands located behind the thyroid gland   _____

2. The largest of the endocrine glands, located in the neck   _____

3. The gland in the brain that is regulated by light   _____

4. An organ that contains islets   _____

5. The endocrine gland composed of a cortex and medulla, each
   with specific functions   _____

6. The part of the brain that controls the anterior pituitary   _____

➤ Group B

epinephrine	antidiuretic hormone	ACTH	follicle stimulating hormone
estrogen	calcitonin	aldosterone	prolactin

1. The anterior pituitary hormone that stimulates milk synthesis   _____

2. The main hormone of the adrenal medulla that, among other
   actions, raises blood pressure and increases the heart rate   _____

3. The anterior pituitary hormone that stimulates the adrenal
   cortex   _____

4. A hormone produced by the ovaries   _____

5. The hormone from the adrenal cortex that regulates sodium
   and potassium reabsorption in the kidney tubules   _____

6. A gonadotropic hormone   _____

7. A hormone synthesized in the hypothalamus   _____

➤ Group C

insulin	glucagon	parathyroid hormone	testosterone
thymosin	cortisol	melatonin	atrial natriuretic factor

1. A hormone that raises the blood calcium level   _____

2. A hormone that lowers the blood glucose level   _____

3. A pancreatic hormone that raises the blood glucose level   _____

4. An adrenal hormone that raises the blood glucose level   _____

5. A hormone that aids in the maturation of T lymphocytes   _____

6. The hormone produced by the pineal gland   _____

7. A hormone that lowers blood pressure   _____

➤ **Group D**

steroid hormone   anterior pituitary   posterior pituitary   hypothalamus

cholesterol   amino acid   protein hormone

1. Estrogen is a(n)   _____

2. Steroid hormones are derived from   _____

3. A building block of growth hormone is a(n)   _____

4. Releasing hormones are produced in the   _____

5. Releasing hormones act on the   _____

6. Prolactin is an example of a(n)   _____

II. Multiple Choice

Select the best answer and write the letter of your choice in the blank.

1. An androgen is a(n):   1. _____
   a. female sex hormone
   b. glucocorticoid
   c. male sex hormone
   d. atrial hormone

2. Which of the following hormones is NOT produced by the thyroid gland?   2. _____
   a. calcitonin
   b. thyroxine
   c. triiodothyronine
   d. thymosin

3. The hormone that causes milk ejection from the breasts is: 3. _____
   a. oxytocin
   b. prolactin
   c. progesterone
   d. estrogen

4. Which of the following hormones is derived from cholesterol?   4. _____
   a. progesterone
   b. thyroid hormone
   c. growth hormone
   d. luteinizing hormone

5. The pituitary hormone that regulates the activity of the thyroid
   gland is: 5. _____
   a. TSH
   b. GH
   c. ACTH
   d. MSH

6. Erythropoietin is synthesized in the: 6. _____
   a. kidneys
   b. skin
   c. heart
   d. placenta

III. Completion Exercise

Write the word or phrase that correctly completes each sentence.
1. Releasing hormones are sent from the hypothalamus to the
   anterior pituitary by way of a special circulatory pathway
   called a(n)   _____
2. When the blood glucose level decreases to less than average,
   the islet cells of the pancreas release less insulin. The result is
   an increase in blood glucose. This is an example of the
   regulatory mechanism called   _____
3. The hypothalamus stimulates the anterior pituitary to produce
   ACTH, which, in turn, stimulates hormone production by the   _____
4. The element needed for the production of thyroxine is   _____
5. Local hormones that have a variety of effects, including the
   promotion of inflammation and the production of uterine
   contractions, are the   _____
6. A hormone secreted from the posterior pituitary that is
   involved in water balance is   _____
7. The primary target tissue for prolactin is the   _____

Understanding Concepts

I. True or False

For each question, write "T" for true or "F" for false in the blank to the left of each number. If a statement is false, correct it by replacing the underlined term and write the correct statement in the blanks below the question.

_____ 1. ACTH acts on the adrenal medulla.

_____

_____ 2. Cortisol and the pancreatic hormone insulin both raise blood sugar.

_____

_____ 3. The ovaries and testes produce steroid hormones.

_____

_____ 4. Cortisol is produced by the adrenal cortex.

_____

_____ 5. Islet cells are found in the adrenal gland.

_____

_____ 6. ADH and oxytocin are secreted by the <u>anterior</u> lobe of the pituitary.

_____

_____ 7. Atrial natriuretic peptide (ANP) is produced by the <u>kidneys</u>.

_____

II. Practical Applications

Write the appropriate word or phrase in the space provided.

1. Mr. L, age 42, reported to the hospital emergency room with reports of shortness of breath and heart palpitations. The initial assessment by the nurse included the following findings: rapid heart rate, nervousness with tremor of the hands, skin warm and flushed, sweating, rapid respiration, and protruding eyes. Laboratory tests confirmed the diagnosis of overactivity of the _____

2. After surgery for his endocrine problem, Mr. L had tetany, or contractions of the muscles of the hands and face. This was caused by the incidental surgical removal of the glands that control the release of calcium into the blood. The glands that maintain adequate blood calcium levels are the _____

3. Ms. M has just been stung by a bee. She is extremely allergic to bees. Her sister gave her a life-saving injection of an adrenal hormone. This hormone is called _____

4. Ms. Q was supposed to have her baby 10 days ago. Her relatives are anxiously awaiting the birth of her child, so she asks her obstetrician if he can do something to hasten the birth of her child. The obstetrician agrees to induce labor using a hormone called _____

5. Mr. S is preparing for his final law examinations and is feeling very stressed. His partner is studying for a physiology examination and mentions that he probably has elevated levels of an anterior pituitary hormone that acts on the adrenal cortex. This hormone is called _____

6. Ms. J, age 35, is preparing for a weight-lifting competition. She wants to build muscle tissue very rapidly, so a friend recommends that she tries injections of a male steroid known to stimulate tissue building. This steroid is usually produced by the _____

III. Short Essays

1. Explain why hormones, although they circulate throughout the body, exercise their effects only on specific target cells.

_____

_____

_____

2. List two differences between the endocrine system and the nervous system.

_____

_____

_____

3. Name three organs other than endocrine glands that produce hormones, and name a hormone produced in each organ.

_____

_____

_____

4. Compare the anterior and the posterior lobes of the pituitary.

_____

_____

_____

Conceptual Thinking

1. Young Ms. K has asthma. She uses an inhaler containing epinephrine to treat her attacks. However, lately she has had a very rapid heart beat. Her physician advises her to use her inhaler less frequently. Why?

_____

_____

_____

Expanding Your Horizons

In the past, the only source of protein hormones for therapeutic use was cadavers. Hormone supplies were very limited and only used in severe cases of hormone deficiency. Hormones can now be made in large quantities in the laboratory. Many hormones, including growth hormone and anabolic steroids, are now abused by some athletes. They are also used by the elderly, even though their safety has not been proven. Hormone use and abuse can be investigated using websites (http://www.hormone.org/ and http://www.nlm.nih.gov/medlineplus/). Hormone abuse in athletes is discussed in an article in Scientific American (see below).

Resource List

Zorpette G. The athlete's body: the chemical games. Scientific American Presents: Building the Elite Athlete 2000;11:16–23.

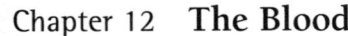

chapter 12

The Blood

Overview

The blood maintains the constancy of the internal environment through its functions of transportation, regulation, and protection. Blood is composed of two elements: the liquid element, or **plasma**, and the formed elements, consisting of the cells and cellular products. The plasma is 91% water and 9% proteins, carbohydrates, lipids, electrolytes, and waste products. The formed elements are composed of the **erythrocytes**, which carry oxygen to the tissues; the **leukocytes**, which defend the body against invaders; and the **platelets**, which are involved in the process of blood coagulation (clotting). The forerunners of the blood cells are called **stem cells**. These are formed in the red bone marrow, where they then develop into the various types of blood cells.

Blood **coagulation** is a protective mechanism that prevents blood loss when a blood vessel is ruptured by an injury. The steps in the prevention of blood loss (**hemostasis**) include constriction of the blood vessels, formation of a platelet plug, and formation of a clot, a complex series of reactions involving many different factors.

If the quantity of blood in the body is severely reduced because of hemorrhage or disease, the cells suffer from lack of oxygen and nutrients. In such instances, a transfusion may be given after typing and matching the blood of the donor with that of the recipient. Donor red cells with different surface antigens (proteins) than the recipient's red cells will react with antibodies in the recipient's blood, causing harmful agglutination reactions and destruction of the donated cells. Blood is most commonly tested for the **ABO system** involving antigens A and B. Blood can be packaged and stored in blood banks for use when transfusions are needed. Whenever possible, blood components such as cells, plasma, plasma fractions, or platelets are used. This practice is more efficient and can reduce the chances of incompatibility and transmission of disease.

The **Rh factor**, another red blood cell protein, also is important in transfusions. If blood containing the Rh factor (Rh positive) is given to a person whose blood lacks that factor (Rh negative), the recipient will produce antibodies to the foreign Rh factor. If an Rh-negative mother is thus sensitized by an Rh-positive fetus, her antibodies may damage fetal red cells in a later pregnancy, resulting in hemolytic disease of the newborn (erythroblastosis fetalis).

Numerous blood studies have been devised to measure the composition of blood. These include the hematocrit, hemoglobin measurements, cell counts, blood chemistry tests, and coagulation studies. These techniques can diagnose blood diseases, some infectious diseases, and some metabolic diseases. Modern laboratories are equipped with automated counters, which rapidly and accurately count blood cells, and with automated analyzers, which measure enzymes, electrolytes, and other constituents of blood serum.

Learning the Language: Word Anatomy

Complete the following table by writing the correct word part or meaning in the space provided. For each word part, write a term that contains the word part.

Word Part	Meaning	Example
1. erythr/o-	_____	_____
2. _____	blood clot	_____
3. pro-	_____	_____
4. morph/o-	_____	_____
5. _____	white, colorless	_____
6. _____	producing, originating	_____
7. hemat/o	_____	_____
8. _____	shape	_____
9. macr/o	_____	_____
10. _____	dissolving	_____

Addressing the Learning Outcomes

I. Writing Exercise

The learning outcomes for Chapter 12 are listed below. These learning outcomes provide an overview of the major topics covered in this chapter. On a separate piece of paper, try to write out an answer to each learning outcome. All of the answers can be found in the pages of the textbook. Learning Outcomes 2, 4, 5, and 8 are also addressed in the Coloring Atlas.

1. List the functions of the blood.
2. List the main ingredients in plasma.
3. Describe the formation of blood cells.
4. Name and describe the three types of formed elements in the blood and give the function of each.
5. Characterize the five types of leukocytes.
6. Define *hemostasis* and cite three steps in hemostasis.
7. Briefly describe the steps in blood clotting.
8. Define *blood type* and explain the relation between blood type and transfusions.
9. List the possible reasons for transfusions of whole blood and blood components.
10. Specify the tests used to study blood.
11. Show how word parts are used to build words related to the blood

II. Labeling and Coloring Atlas

EXERCISE **12-1**: Composition of Whole Blood (text Fig. 12-1)

INSTRUCTIONS

1. Write the names of the different blood components on the appropriate numbered lines in different colors. Use the color red for parts 1, 2, and 3.
2. Color the blood components on the diagram with the appropriate color.

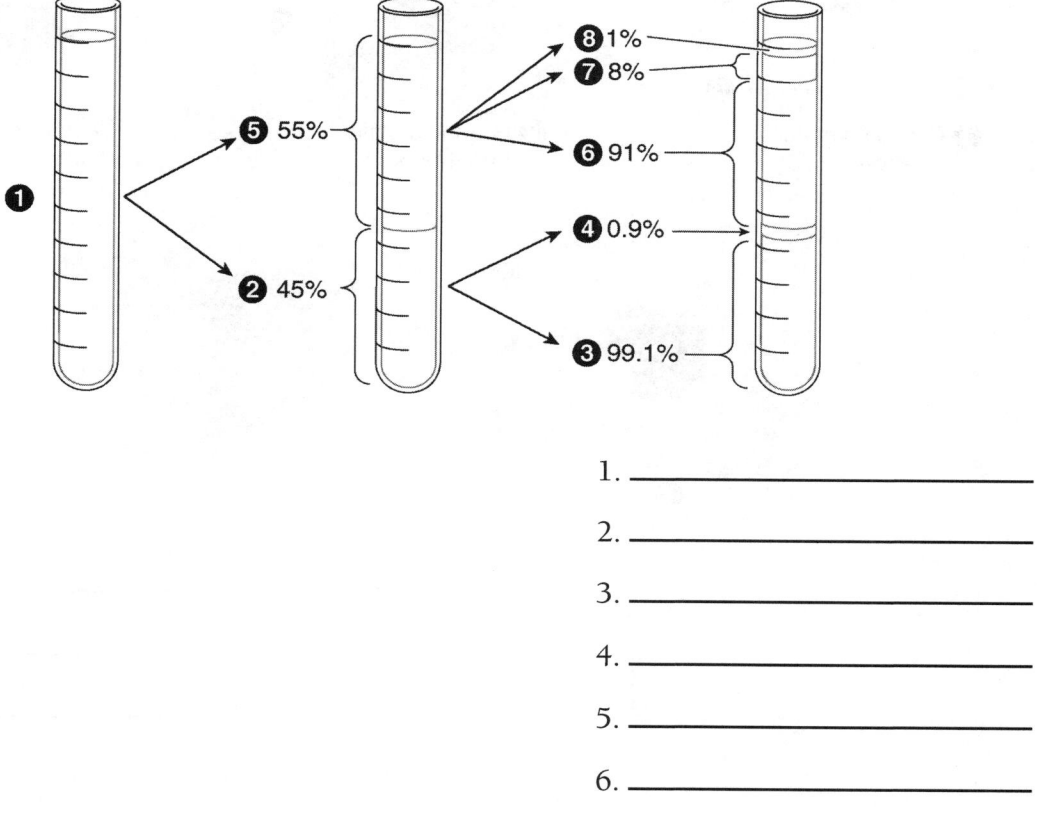

1. _____

2. _____

3. _____

4. _____

5. _____

6. _____

7. _____

8. _____

EXERCISE 12-2: Leukocytes (text Fig. 12-4)

INSTRUCTIONS

1. Write the names of the five types of leukocytes on lines 1–5.
2. Write the names of the labeled cell parts and other blood cells on lines 6–9.

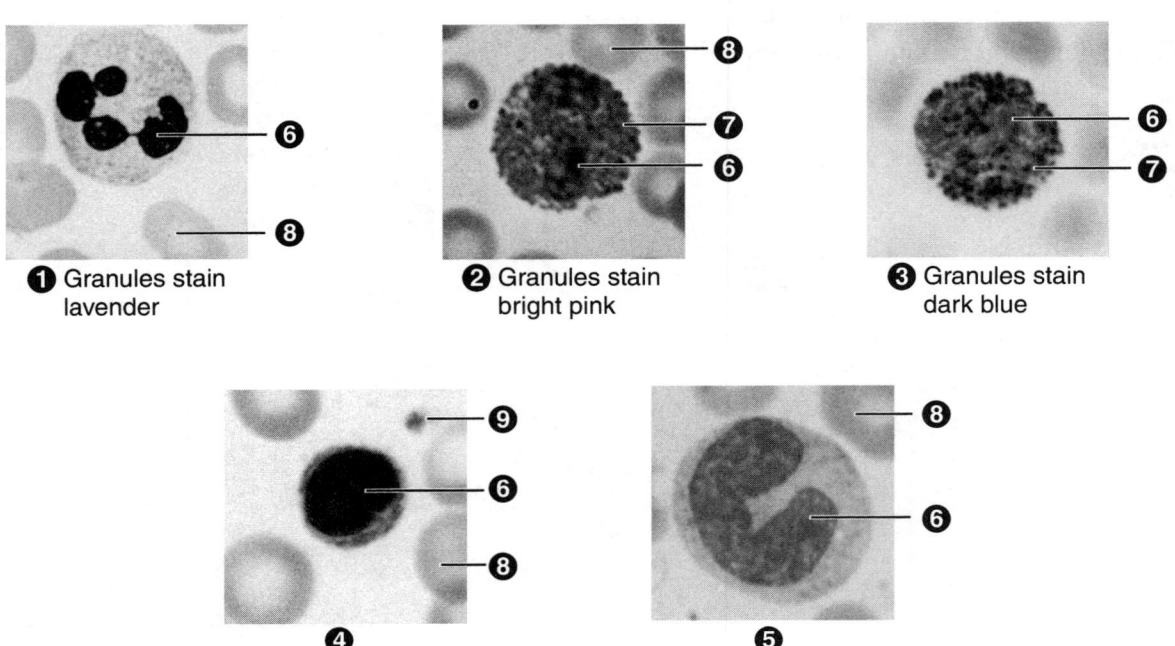

❶ Granules stain
    lavender

❷ Granules stain
    bright pink

❸ Granules stain
    dark blue

❹

❺

1. _____

2. _____

3. _____

4. _____

5. _____

6. _____

7. _____

8. _____

9. _____

EXERCISE 12-3: Formation of a Blood Clot (text Fig. 12-8)
Write the correct term in each of the numbered boxes.

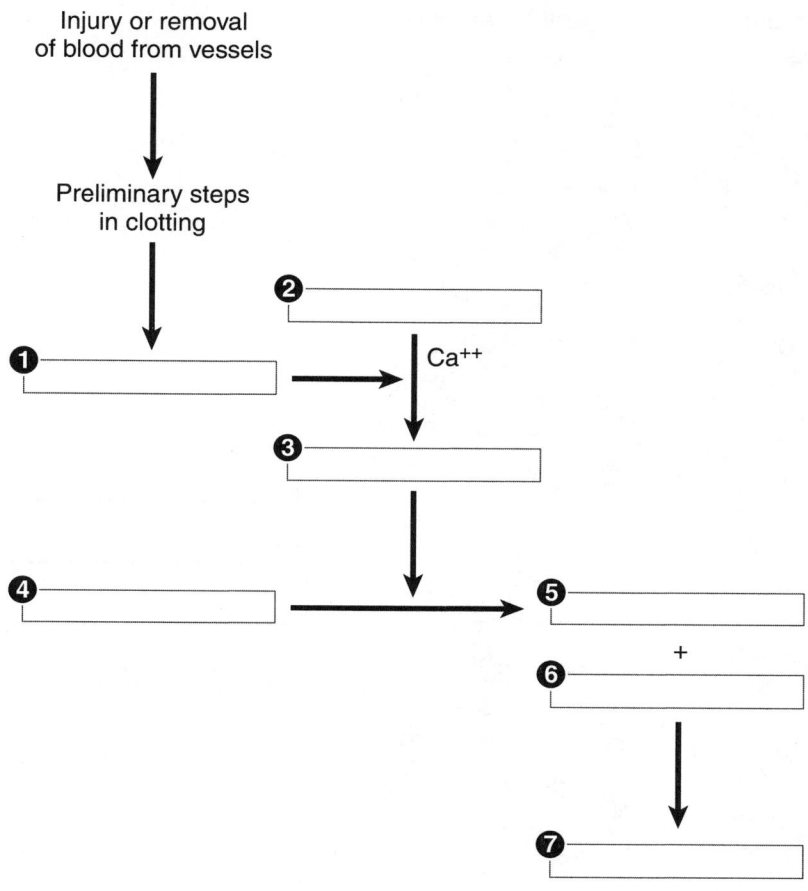

Exercise 12-4: Blood Typing (text Fig. 12-9)

Based on the agglutination reactions, write the name of each blood type on the numbered lines.

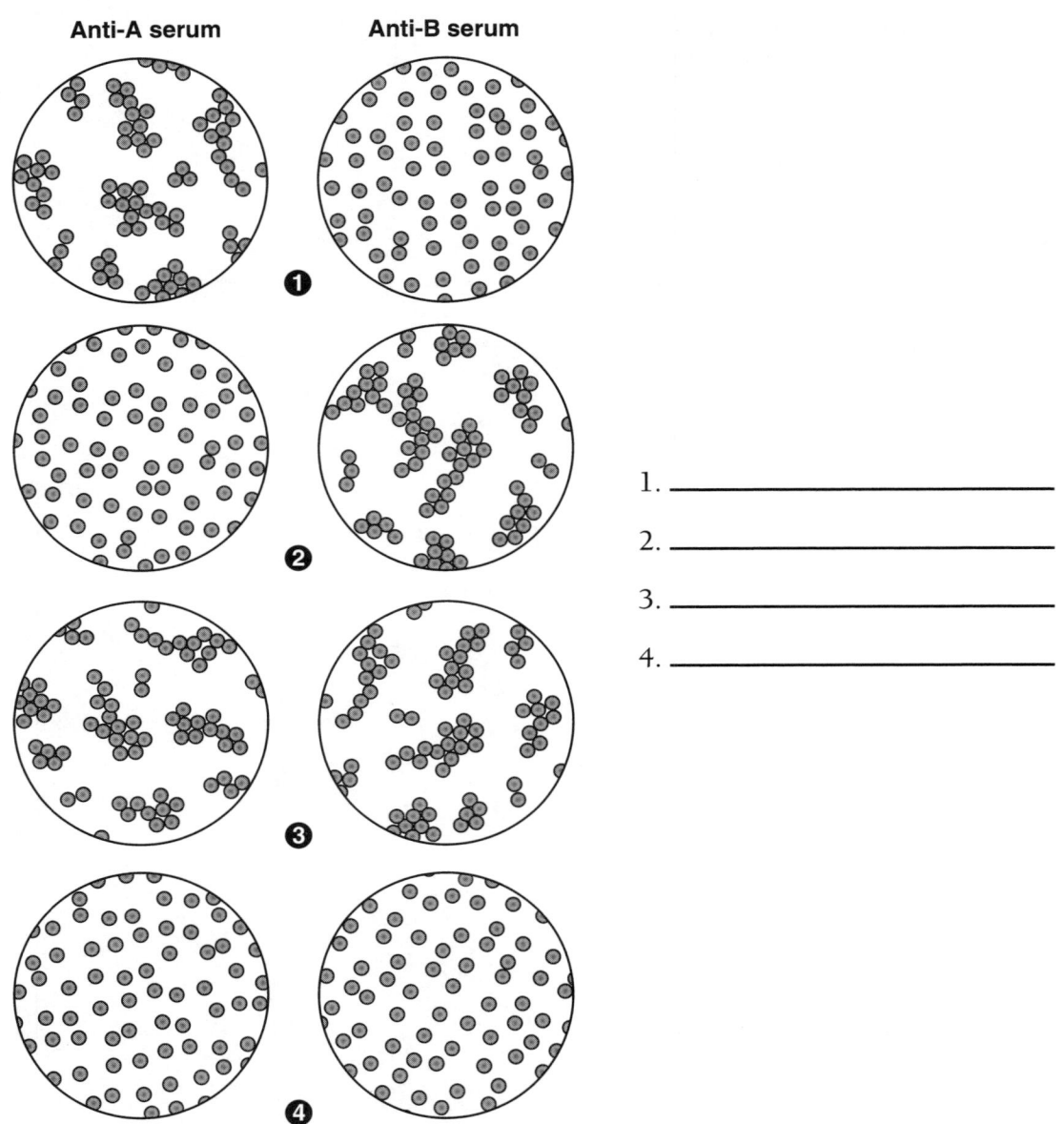

1. _____

2. _____

3. _____

4. _____

Making the Connections

The following concept map deals with the classification of blood cells. Each pair of terms is linked together by a connecting phrase into a sentence. The sentence should be read in the direction of the arrow. Complete the concept map by filling in the appropriate term or phrase. There is one right answer for each term. However, there are many correct answers for the connecting phrases (5, 6, 8, 10, 12, 14, and 16). Write the connecting phrases beside the appropriate number (where space permits) or on a separate piece of paper.

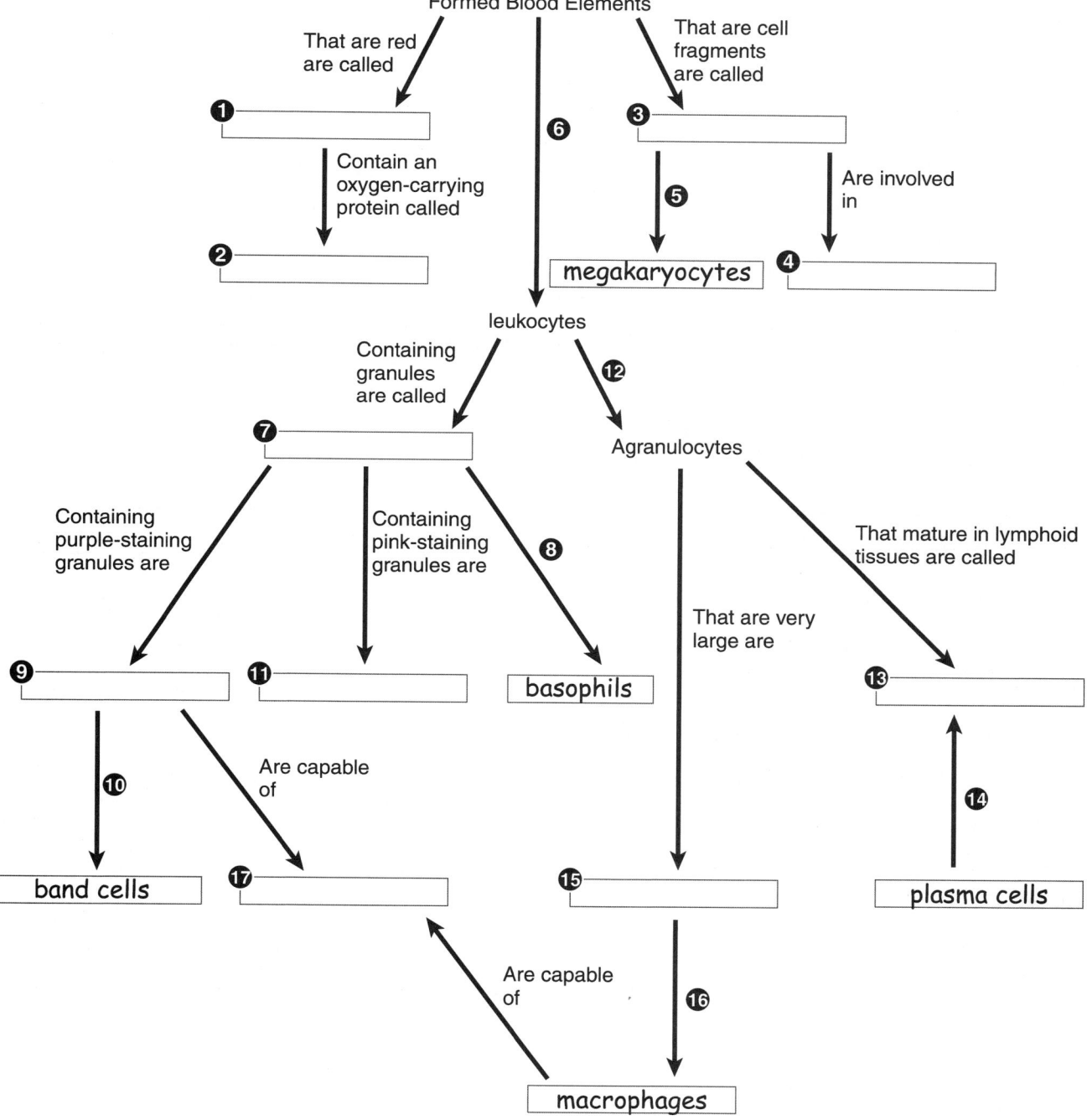

Optional Exercise: Construct your own concept map using the following terms and any others you would like to include: procoagulants, anticoagulants, platelet plug, hemostasis, vasoconstriction, blood clot, fibrinogen, fibrin, prothrombinase, thrombin, serum.

Testing Your Knowledge

Building Understanding

I. Matching Exercises

Matching only within each group, write the answers in the spaces provided.

➤ Group A

erythrocyte	platelet	leukocyte	serum
plasma	albumin	antibodies	complement

1. A red blood cell _____

2. Another name for thrombocyte _____

3. The most abundant protein(s) in blood _____

4. The liquid portion of blood _____

5. A white blood cell _____

6. Enzymes that assist antibodies to battle pathogens _____

7. The watery fluid that remains after a blood clot is removed _____

➤ Group B

neutrophil	macrophage	monocyte	pus
eosinophil	basophil	plasma cell	

1. The most abundant type of white blood cell in whole blood _____

2. A mature monocyte _____

3. A lymphocyte that produces antibodies _____

4. A leukocyte that stains with acidic dyes _____

5. The largest blood leukocyte _____

6. A substance that often accumulates when leukocytes are
   actively destroying bacteria _____

➤ Group C

fibrinogen	vasoconstriction	prothrombinase	coagulation
hemorrhage	antigen	agglutination	

1. A plasma protein that is activated to form a blood clot _____

2. An enzyme that triggers the final clotting mechanism _____

3. The process by which cells become clumped when mixed
   with a specific antiserum _____

4. Contraction of smooth muscles in the blood vessel wall _____

5. Another term for profuse bleeding _____

6. A protein on blood cells that causes incompatibility reactions _____

➤ **Group D**

hematocrit   Rh factor   autologous   AB antigen

hemapheresis   plasmapheresis   transfusion

1. The blood antigen involved in hemolytic disease of the newborn, which results from a blood incompatibility between a mother and fetus _____

2. The procedure for removing plasma and returning formed elements to the donor _____

3. The procedure for removing specific components and returning the remainder of the blood to the donor _____

4. Blood donated by an individual for use by the same individual _____

5. The volume percentage of red cells in whole blood _____

6. The administration of blood or blood components from one person to another person _____

II. Multiple Choice

Select the best answer and write the letter of your choice in the blank.

1. Plasma can be given to anyone without danger of incompatibility because it lacks: 1. _____
   a. serum
   b. red cells
   c. protein
   d. clotting factors

2. Polymorphs, PMNs, and segs are alternate names for: 2. _____
   a. monocytes
   b. neutrophils
   c. basophils
   d. lymphocytes

3. Which of the following is NOT a type of white blood cell?   3. _____
   a. thrombocyte
   b. lymphocyte
   c. eosinophil
   d. monocyte

4. Blood clotting occurs in a complex series of steps. The substance that finally forms the clot is: 4. _____
   a. albumin
   b. anticoagulant
   c. thromboplastin
   d. fibrin

5. Which of the following might result in an Rh incompatibility problem?   5. _____
    a. an Rh-positive mother and an Rh-negative fetus
    b. an Rh-negative mother and an Rh-positive fetus
    c. an Rh-negative mother and a type AB fetus
    d. an Rh-positive mother and an Rh-negative father

6. Intrinsic factor is: 6. _____
    a. the first factor activated in blood clotting
    b. a substance needed for absorption of folic acid
    c. a type of hereditary bleeding disease
    d. a substance needed for absorption of vitamin B_{12}

7. Electrophoresis is the process by which: 7. _____
    a. the volume proportion of red cells is determined
    b. normal and abnormal types of hemoglobin can be separated
    c. red blood cells are counted
    d. white blood cells are counted

8. An immature neutrophil is called a(n):   8. _____
    a. band cell
    b. monocyte
    c. eosinophil
    d. lymphocyte

9. Which of the following cells is NOT a granulocyte?   9. _____
    a. monocyte
    b. eosinophil
    c. neutrophil
    d. polymorph

III. Completion Exercise

Write the word or phrase that correctly completes each sentence.

1. Blood that contains antibodies against the A antigen is termed type _____
2. The conversion of prothrombin into thrombin requires
   the element _____
3. The gas that is necessary for life and that is transported to all
   parts of the body by the blood is _____
4. Some monocytes enter the tissues, mature, and become active
   phagocytes. These cells are called _____
5. One waste product of body metabolism is carried to the lungs
   to be exhaled. This gas is _____
6. The hormone that stimulates red blood cell production is _____
7. Blood cells are formed in the _____
8. The most important function of certain lymphocytes is to
   engulf disease-producing organisms by the process of _____
9. The chemical element that characterizes hemoglobin is _____

Understanding Concepts

I. True or False

For each question, write "T" for true or "F" for false in the blank to the left of each number. If a statement is false, correct it by replacing the underlined term and write the correct statement in the blank below the question.

———— 1. Eosinophils and basophils are underlined granular leukocytes.

————————————————————————

———— 2. Blood cells from a person with type B blood will agglutinate with underlined type A antiserum.

————————————————————————

———— 3. Erythropoietin, a hormone that stimulates production of red blood cells, is produced by the underlined kidneys.

————————————————————————

———— 4. underlined Type AB blood contains antibodies to both A and B antigens.

————————————————————————

———— 5. Monocytes are immature underlined neutrophils.

————————————————————————

———— 6. Substances that induce blood clotting are called underlined procoagulants.

————————————————————————

———— 7. The watery fluid that remains after a blood clot has been removed from the blood is underlined plasma.

————————————————————————

II. Practical Applications

Study each discussion. Then write the appropriate word or phrase in the space provided.

➤ Group A

1. A young girl named AL fell off her bike, sustaining a deep

   gash to her leg that bled copiously from a severed vessel. In

   describing this type of bleeding, the doctor in the Emergency

   Room used the word ————————————

2. While the physician attended to the wound, the technician drew blood for typing and other studies. AL's blood did not agglutinate with either anti-A and anti-B serum. Her blood was classified as group _____

3. Young AL required a blood transfusion. The only type of blood she could receive is _____

4. Further testing of AL's blood revealed that it lacked the Rh factor. She was, therefore, said to be _____

5. If AL were to be given a transfusion of Rh-positive blood, she might become sensitized to the Rh protein. In that event, her blood would produce counteracting substances called _____

6. While they were waiting for the typed blood to arrive, the physician administered the liquid portion of blood to increase AL's blood volume. This liquid is called _____

7. The fluid was obtained by a process in which whole blood is removed from a donor and the formed elements returned. This process is called _____

➤ **Group B**

1. Mr. KK, age 72, had an injury riding his motorized scooter down a steep hill. He sustained only minor scrapes, but he came to the hospital because his scrapes did not stop bleeding. The process by which blood loss is prevented or minimized is called _____

2. The physician discovered that Mr. KK was the great-great-great grandson of Queen Victoria. Like many of her offspring, Mr. KK suffers from hemophilia. Hemophilia results from a deficiency in a substance that regulates blood clotting. These twelve substances, which are designated by Roman numerals, are called _____

3. Mr. KK must be treated with a rich source of clotting factors. The doctor gets a bag of frozen plasma, which has a white powdery substance at the bottom of the bag. The substance is called _____

4. Mr. KK also mentions that he has been very tired and pale lately. His cook recently retired, and he has been surviving on dill pickles and crackers. The physician suspects a deficiency in an element required to synthesize hemoglobin. This element is called _____

5. The physician orders a test to determine the proportion of red blood cells in his blood. The result of this test is called the _____

➤ Group C

1. Ms. J, an elite cyclist, has come to the hospital complaining of a pounding headache. The physician, Dr. L, takes a sample of her blood and notices that it is very thick. He decides to count her red blood cells, but the automatic cell counter is broken. Dr. L calls for a technician to perform a visual count using the microscope and a special slide called a(n) _____

2. The technician comes back with a result of 7.5 million cells per μL. This count is abnormally high. Dr. L is immediately suspicious. He asks Ms. J if she consumes any performance-enhancing drugs. Ms. J admits that she has been taking a hormone to increase blood cell synthesis. This hormone is called _____

3. Dr. L tells Ms. J that she is at risk for blood clot formation. He tells her to stop taking the hormone and to take aspirin for a few days to inhibit blood clotting. Drugs that inhibit clotting are called _____

III. Short Essays

1. What kind of information can be obtained from blood chemistry tests?

_____

_____

_____

_____

_____

2. Briefly describe the final events in blood clot formation, naming the substances involved in each step.

_____

_____

_____

_____

3. Name one reason to transfuse an individual with:
   a. whole blood

   _____

   b. platelets

   _____

   c. plasma

   _____

   d. plasma protein

   _____

Conceptual Thinking

1. A dehydrated individual will have an elevated hematocrit. Explain why.

_____

_____

_____

2. A man named JA has a history of frequent fevers. His skin is pale and his heart rate is rapid. The doctor suspects that he has cancer. His white blood cell count was revealed to be 25,000 per μL of blood.
   a. Is this white blood cell count normal? What is the normal range?

   _____

   _____

b. JA also has a hematocrit of 30%. Is this value normal? What is the normal range?

_____

_____

c. Consider the different functions of blood. Discuss some functions that might be impaired in the case of JA.

_____

_____

_____

3. Mr. R needs a blood transfusion. He has type AB blood. The doctor is considering a transfusion using A blood.
   a. Which antigens are present on his blood cells?

   _____

   b. Which antibodies will be present in his blood?

   _____

   c. Which antigens will be present on donor blood cells?

   _____

   d. Is this blood transfusion safe? Why or why not?

   _____

Expanding Your Horizons

The amount of oxygen carried by the blood is an important determinant of athletic prowess. Some elite athletes are always looking for ways to increase the oxygen in their blood. If you follow competitive cycling, you are probably familiar with the hormone erythropoietin (EPO). EPO came to the public's attention during the 1998 Tour de France, when it was found that EPO use is common among elite athletes. Learn about this and other methods that athletes have used to legally or illegally gain an advantage over their competitors. EPO is discussed in an article in Scientific American (see below), and you can perform a website search for "EPO sport." Information on other methods can be found by performing a website search for "blood doping."

Resource List

Zorpette G. The athlete's body: the chemical games. Scientific American Presents: Building the Elite Athlete 2000;11:16–23.

chapter 13

The Heart

Overview

The ceaseless beat of the heart day and night throughout one's entire lifetime is such an obvious key to the presence of life that it is no surprise that this organ has been the subject of wonderment and poetry. When the heart stops pumping, life ceases. The cells must have oxygen, and it is the heart's pumping action that propels oxygenated blood to them.

In size, the heart is approximately the size of one's fist. It is located between the lungs, more than half to the left of the midline, with the **apex** (point) directed toward the left. Below is the **diaphragm**, the dome-shaped muscle that separates the thoracic cavity from the abdominopelvic cavity.

The heart consists of two sides separated by septa. The septa keeps blood that is higher in oxygen entirely separate from blood that is lower in oxygen. The two sides pump in unison, with the right side pumping blood to the lungs to be oxygenated, and the left side pumping blood to all other parts of the body.

Each side of the heart is divided into two parts or **chambers**. The upper chamber or **atrium** on each side is the receiving chamber for blood returning to the heart. The lower chamber or **ventricle** is the strong pumping chamber. Because the ventricles pump more forcefully, their walls are thicker than the walls of the atria. **Valves** between the chambers keep the blood flowing forward as the heart pumps. The muscle of the heart wall, the **myocardium**, has special features to enhance its pumping efficiency. The coronary circulation supplies blood directly to the myocardium.

The heartbeat originates within the heart at the **sinoatrial (SA) node**, often called the pacemaker. Electrical impulses from the pacemaker spread through special conducting fibers in the wall of the heart to induce contractions, first of the two atria and then of the two ventricles. After contraction, the heart relaxes and fills with blood. The relaxation phase is called **diastole**, and the contraction phase is called **systole**. Together, these two phases make up one **cardiac cycle**. The heart rate is influenced by the nervous system and other circulating factors, such as hormones and drugs.

Learning the Language: Word Anatomy

Complete the following table by writing the correct word part or meaning in the space provided. For each word part, write a term that contains the word part.

Word Part	Meaning	Example
1. _____	chest	_____
2. sin/o	_____	_____
3. cardi/o	_____	_____
4. _____	lung	_____
5. _____	slow	_____
6. _____	rapid	_____

Addressing the Learning Outcomes

I. Writing Exercise

The learning outcomes for Chapter 13 are listed below. These learning outcomes provide an overview of the major topics covered in this chapter. On a separate piece of paper, try to write out an answer to each learning outcome. All of the answers can be found in the pages of the textbook. Learning Outcomes 1–5 and 8 are also addressed in the Coloring Atlas.

1. Describe the three layers of the heart wall.
2. Describe the structure of the pericardium and cite its functions.
3. Compare the functions of the right and left sides of the heart.
4. Name the four chambers of the heart and compare their functions.
5. Name the valves at the entrance and exit of each ventricle and cite the function of the valves.
6. Briefly describe blood circulation through the myocardium.
7. Briefly describe the cardiac cycle.
8. Name and locate the components of the heart's conduction system.
9. Explain the effects of the autonomic nervous system on the heart rate.
10. List and define several terms that describe variations in heart rates.
11. Explain what produces the two main heart sounds.
12. Briefly describe four methods for studying the heart.
13. Show how word parts are used to build words related to the heart.

II. Labeling and Coloring Atlas

EXERCISE 13-1: Layers of the Heart Wall and Pericardium (text Fig. 13-4)

INSTRUCTIONS

1. Write the terms "heart wall" and "serous pericardium" in the appropriate boxes.
2. Write the names of the different structures on the numbered lines in different colors. Use black for structure 6, because it will not be colored.
3. Color the structures on the diagram (except structure 6) with the appropriate colors.

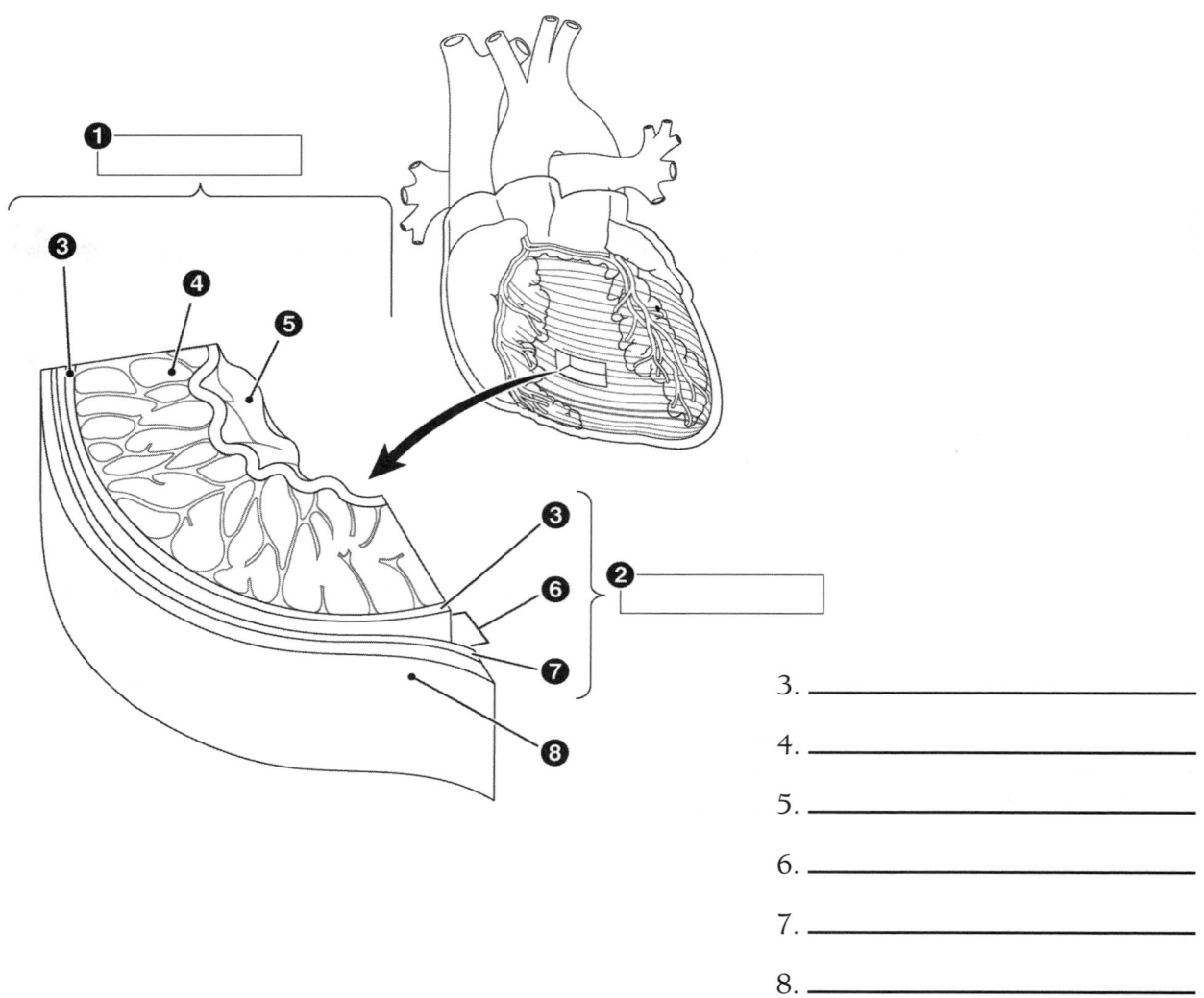

3. _____

4. _____

5. _____

6. _____

7. _____

8. _____

EXERCISE 13-2: The Heart Is a Double Pump (text Fig. 13-4)

INSTRUCTIONS

1. Label the indicated parts.
2. Color the oxygenated blood red and the deoxygenated blood blue.
3. Use arrows to show the direction of blood flow.

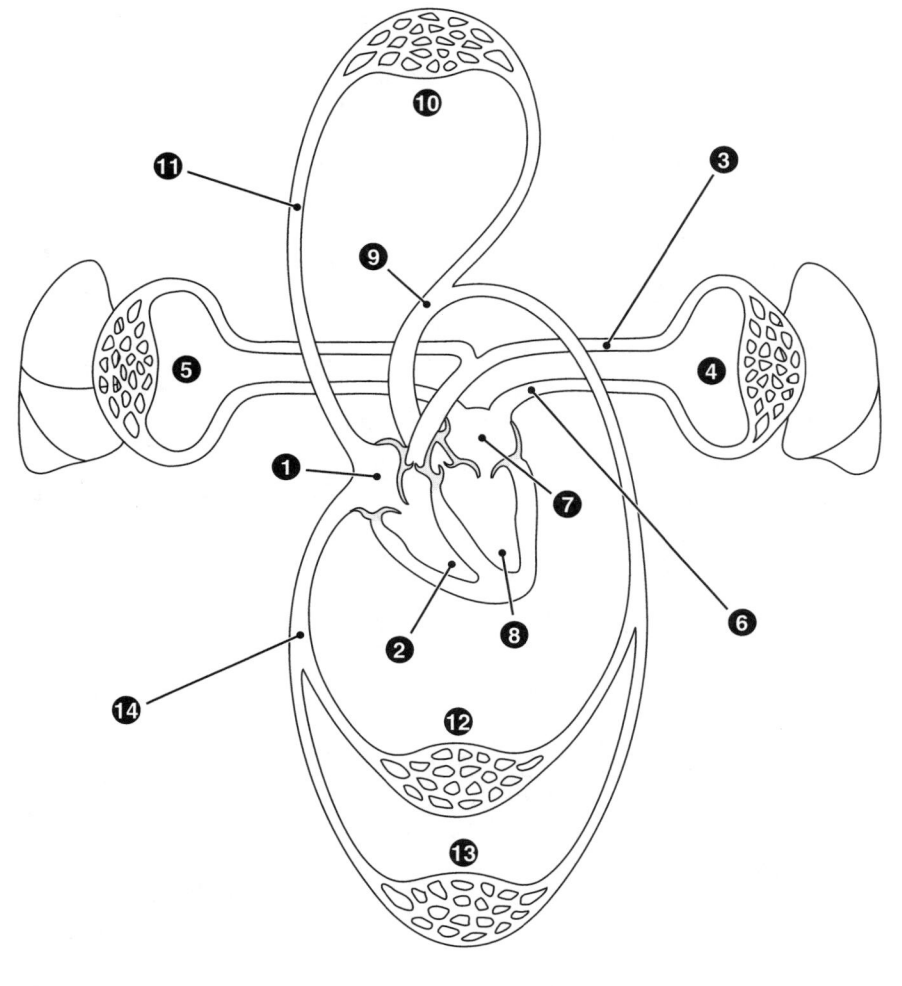

1. _____	8. _____
2. _____	9. _____
3. _____	10. _____
4. _____	11. _____
5. _____	12. _____
6. _____	13. _____
7. _____	14. _____

EXERCISE 13-3: The Heart and Great Vessels (text Fig. 13-5)

INSTRUCTIONS

1. Label the indicated parts.
2. Color the oxygenated blood red and the deoxygenated blood blue.
3. Use arrows to show the direction of blood flow.

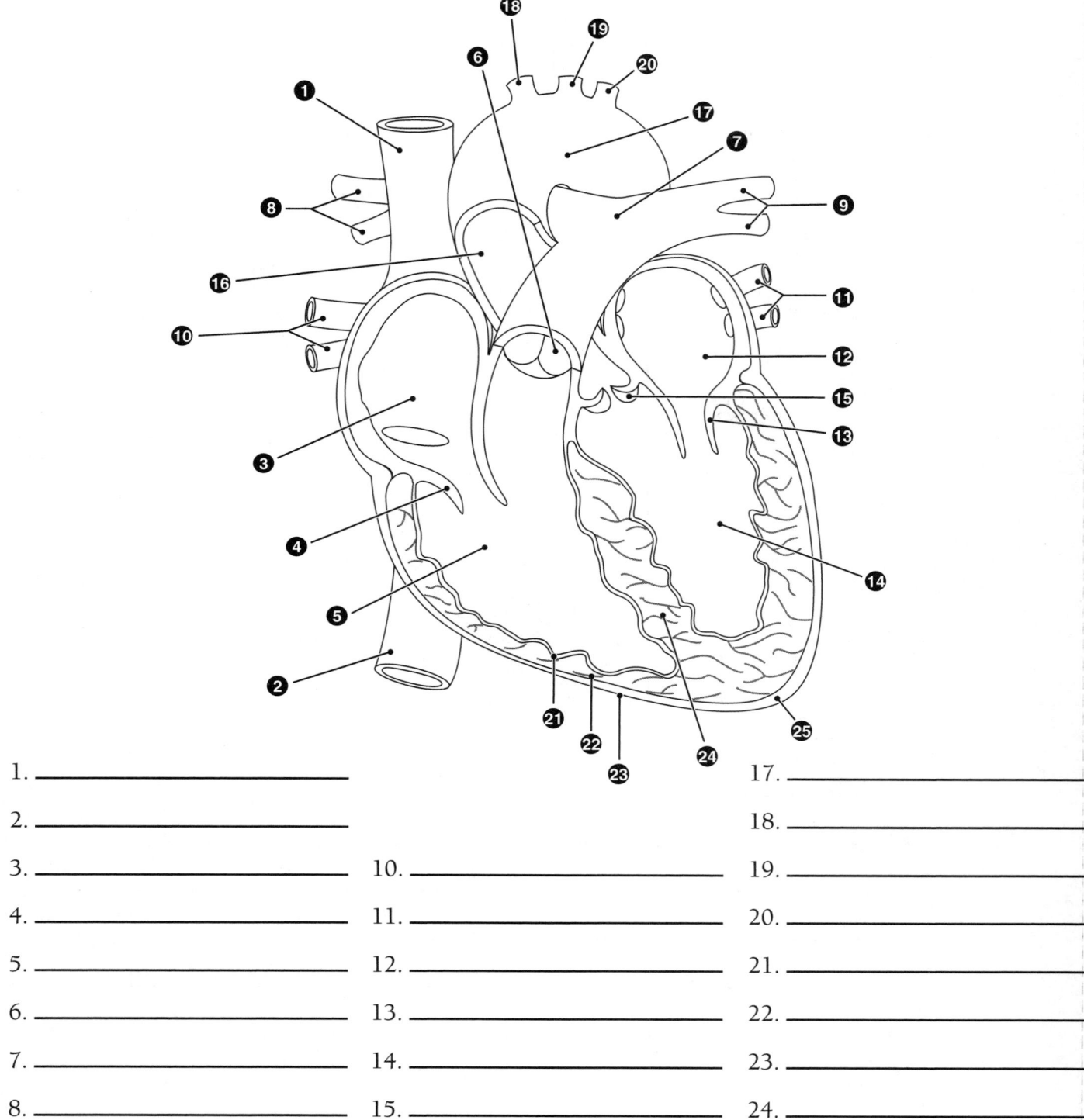

1. _____

2. _____

3. _____ 10. _____

4. _____ 11. _____

5. _____ 12. _____

6. _____ 13. _____

7. _____ 14. _____

8. _____ 15. _____

9. _____ 16. _____

17. _____

18. _____

19. _____

20. _____

21. _____

22. _____

23. _____

24. _____

25. _____

EXERCISE 13-4: The Conducting System of the Heart (text Fig. 13-11)

INSTRUCTIONS

1. Label the indicated parts.
2. Color the oxygenated blood red and the deoxygenated blood blue.
3. Highlight the structures that conduct electrical impulses in yellow. Draw arrows to indicate the direction of impulse conduction.

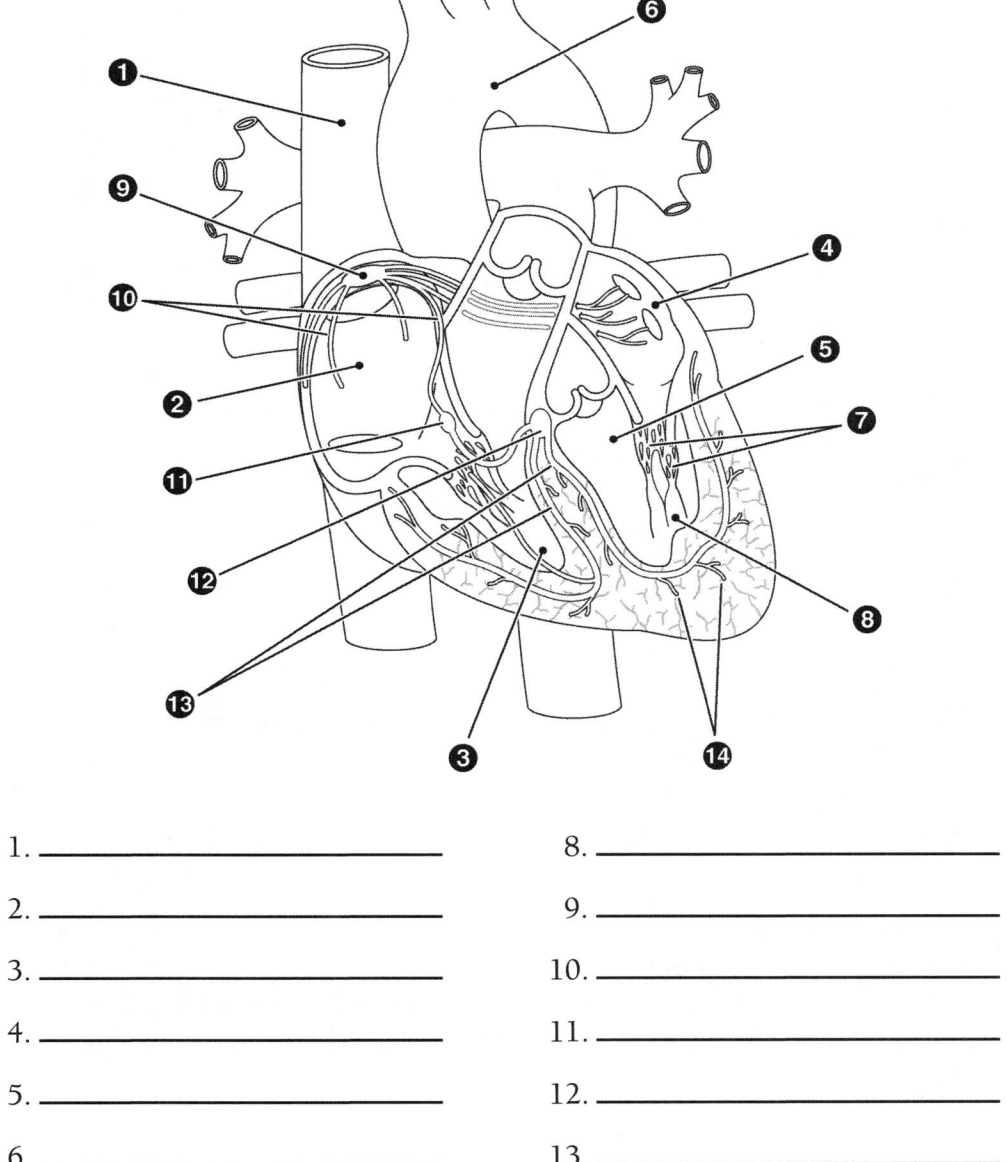

1. _____   8. _____

2. _____   9. _____

3. _____   10. _____

4. _____   11. _____

5. _____   12. _____

6. _____   13. _____

7. _____   14. _____

Making the Connections

The following flow chart deals with the passage of blood through the heart. Beginning with the right atrium, outline the structures a blood cell would pass through in the correct order by filling in the boxes. Use the following terms: left atrium, left ventricle, right ventricle, right AV valve, left AV valve, pulmonary semilunar valve, aortic semilunar valve, superior/inferior vena cava, right lung, left lung, aorta, left pulmonary artery, right pulmonary artery, left pulmonary veins, right pulmonary veins, body. You can write the names of structures that encounter blood high in oxygen in red and the names of structures that encounter blood low in oxygen in blue.

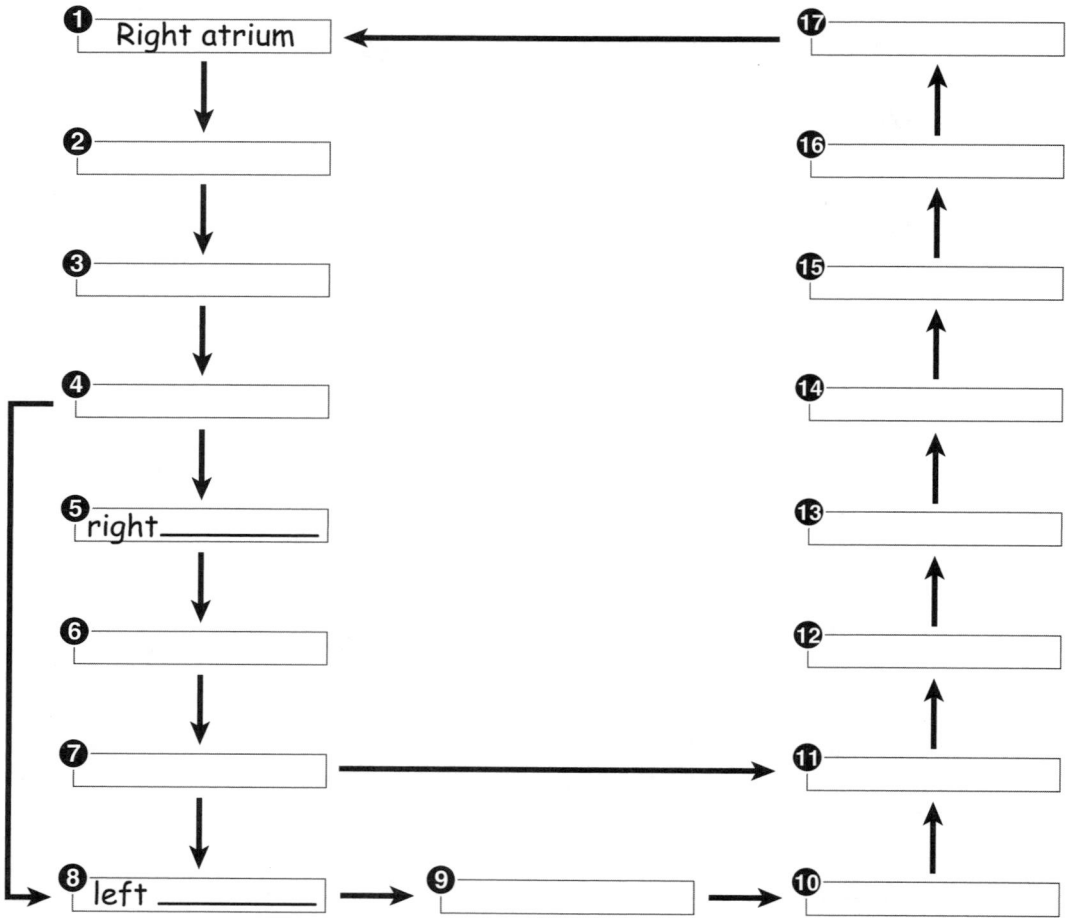

Optional Exercise: Make your own concept map, based on the events of the cardiac cycle. Choose your own terms to incorporate into your map, or use the following list: AV valves open, AV valves closed, blood flow from atria to ventricles, blood flow from ventricles to arteries, atrial diastole, atrial systole, ventricular diastole, ventricular systole. There will be many links between the different terms.

Testing Your Knowledge
Building Understanding

I. Matching Exercises

Matching only within each group, write the answers in the spaces provided.

➤ **Group A**

base	apex	endocardium	epicardium
fibrous pericardium	myocardium	serous pericardium	

1. The pointed, inferior portion of the heart   _____

2. The membrane consisting of a visceral and a parietal layer   _____

3. A layer of epithelial cells in contact with blood within the

   heart   _____

4. The heart layer containing intercalated disks   _____

5. The outermost layer of the sac enclosing the heart   _____

➤ **Group B**

ventricle	atrium	atrioventricular valve	pulmonary valve
aortic valve	coronary artery	interatrial septum	interventricular septum

1. A lower chamber of the heart   _____

2. The valve that prevents blood from returning to the right

   ventricle   _____

3. An upper chamber of the heart   _____

4. The valve that prevents blood from returning to the left

   ventricle   _____

5. The partition that separates the two upper chambers of

   the heart   _____

6. A vessel supplying oxygenated blood to the myocardium   _____

➤ **Group C**

diastole	systole	cardiac output	stroke volume	bundle of His
sinoatrial node	atrioventricular node	Purkinje fibers	sinus rhythm	

1. The group of conduction fibers found in the ventricle walls   _____

2. The mass of conduction tissue located in the septum at the

   bottom of the right atrium   _____

3. The amount of blood ejected from a ventricle with each beat   _____

4. A normal heart beat, originating from the normal heart

   pacemaker   _____

5. The group of conduction fibers carrying the impulse

   from the AV node   _____

6. The contraction phase of the cardiac cycle   _____

7. The resting period that follows the contraction phase of

   the cardiac cycle   _____

8. The pacemaker of the heart, located in the upper wall of

   the right atrium   _____

➤ Group D

echocardiograph	catheterization	bradycardia	fluoroscope
electrocardiograph	tachycardia	stethoscope	

1. Term for a heart rate of greater than 100 beats per minute   _____

2. An instrument used to convey sounds from within the

   patient's body to an examiner's ear   _____

3. An instrument for evaluating heart structure using

   ultrasound waves   _____

4. A procedure required for measuring pressures within the heart

   chambers   _____

5. An instrument for recording the electrical activity of the heart   _____

II. Multiple Choice

Select the best answer and write the letter of your choice in the blank.

1. An average cardiac cycle lasts approximately: 1. _____
   - a. 8 seconds
   - b. 5 seconds
   - c. 0.8 seconds
   - d. 30 seconds
2. The volume of blood pumped by each ventricle in 1 minute is the: 2. _____
   - a. stroke volume
   - b. cardiac output
   - c. heart rate
   - d. ejection rate
3. Which of the following is NOT a part of the conduction system
   of the heart?   3. _____
   - a. bundle of His
   - b. atrioventricular valve

    c. Purkinje fibers

    d. atrioventricular node

4. Activation of the parasympathetic nervous system would: 4. _____

    a. increase heart rate but not myocardial contraction strength

    b. increase heart rate and myocardial contraction strength

    c. decrease heart rate but not myocardial contraction strength

    d. decrease heart rate and myocardial contraction strength

5. The vein that carries blood from the coronary circulation back into

   the right atrium is the: 5. _____

    a. right coronary artery

    b. interatrial septum

    c. pulmonary vein

    d. coronary sinus

III. Completion Exercise

Write the word or phrase that correctly completes each sentence.

1. The autonomic nerve that slows the heart beat is the   _____

2. The fibrous sac that surrounds the heart is the   _____

3. One complete cycle of heart contraction and relaxation
   is called the   _____

4. The fibrous threads connecting the AV valves to muscles
   in the heart wall are called the   _____

5. The right atrioventricular valve is also known as the   _____

6. Normal heart sounds heard while the heart is working
   are called   _____

7. An abnormally slow heart beat is termed   _____

Understanding Concepts

I. True or False

For each question, write "T" for true or "F" for false in the blank to the left of each number. If a statement is false, correct it by replacing the underlined term and write the correct statement in the blank below the question.

_____ 1. The aorta receives blood directly from the left atrium.

_____

_____ 2. Cardiac output equals heart rate divided by stroke volume.

_____

_____ 3. A heart rate of 150 beats/minute is described as tachycardia.

_____

_____ 4. Blood in the heart chambers comes into contact with the epicardium.

_____

_____ 5. The aorta is part of the <u>pulmonary</u> circuit.

_____

_____ 6. Nerve impulses travel down the internodal pathways from the <u>AV node</u>.

_____

_____ 7. A heart rhythm originating at the <u>SA node</u> is termed a sinus rhythm.

_____

II. Practical Applications

Study each discussion. Then write the appropriate word or phrase in the space provided.

➤ **Group A**

1. Ms. J, age 82, was participating in a lawn bowling tournament when she suddenly collapsed with chest pain.
   The paramedics were preparing her for transport to
   the hospital when they noted a sudden onset of pale
   skin and unconsciousness. The heart monitor showed
   a rapid, uncoordinated activity of the lower heart
   chambers, known as the   _____

2. The paramedics administered an electric shock using
   an automated defibrillator with the aim of restoring the
   normal heart rhythm, which is called a(n)   _____

3. In the hospital emergency room, Ms. J was given intravenous medications to dissolve any blood clots in the
   vessels supplying her heart muscle. Together, these
   vessels are called the   _____

4. The drugs were not administered in time to prevent
   damage to the middle layer of the heart wall, which
   is known as the   _____

5. The electrical activity of Ms. J's heart was analyzed
   using a(n)   _____

6. The analysis showed that the conduction system was
   damaged. The electrical impulse generated by her
   sinoatrial node was not reaching the conducting
   fibers that pass down the interventricular septum.
   These fibers are collectively known as the   _____

➤ **Group B**

1. Baby L has just been born. To her parents' dismay, her
   skin and mucous membranes are tinged with blue.
   The obstetrician listens to her heartbeat using an
   instrument called a(n)   _____

2. The doctor notices an abnormality in the second heart
   sound (or "dupp"), which is largely caused by the closure
   of the two   _____

3. This abnormal sound probably reflects a structural problem
   with baby L's heart, and is thus termed a(n)   _____

4. The baby is sent for a test that uses ultrasound waves to
   examine her heart structure. This technique is known as   _____

III. Short Essays

1. Although the heartbeat originates within the heart itself, it is influenced by factors in the internal environment. Describe some of the factors that can affect the heart.

   _____

   _____

   _____

2. Describe the pathway followed by an electrical impulse that originates in the sinotrial node and excites a ventricular myocardial cell.

   _____

   _____

   _____

Conceptual Thinking

1. Atropine is a drug that inhibits activity of the parasympathetic nervous system. Discuss the effects of atropine on the heart. How does the parasympathetic nervous system affect the heart, and which aspects of heart function will be affected and which will be unaffected?

   _____

   _____

   _____

2. Mr. J is undertaking a gentle exercise program, primarily involving walking, to lose weight. His heart rate is 100 beats/minute and his stroke volume is 75 mL. What is his cardiac output, and what does cardiac output mean?

   _____

   _____

   _____

Expanding Your Horizons

How low can you go? You may have heard of the exploits of free divers, who dive to tremendous depths without the aid of SCUBA equipment. The world record for assisted free diving is held by Pipin Ferreras, who dove to 170 m (558 feet) with the aid of a sled. Free diving is not without its dangers. Pipin's wife (Audrey) died during a world record attempt. Free diving is facilitated by the mammalian dive reflex, which allows mammals to hold their breath for long periods of time underwater. Immersing one's face in cold water induces bradycardia and diverts blood away from the periphery. How would these modifications increase the ability to free dive? You can learn more about the underlying mechanisms, rationale, and dangers of the dive reflex by performing a Google search for "dive reflex." Information is also available in an article in the journal Physiology and Behaviour (see below).

Resource List

Hurwitz BE, Furedy JJ. The human dive reflex: an experimental, topographical, and physiological analysis. Physiol Behav 1986;36:287–294.

chapter 14

Blood Vessels and Blood Circulation

Overview

The blood vessels are classified as arteries, veins, or capillaries according to their function. **Arteries** carry blood away from the heart, **veins** return blood to the heart, and **capillaries** are the site of gas, nutrient, and waste exchange between the blood and tissues. Small arteries are called **arterioles**, and small veins are called **venules**. The walls of the arteries are thicker and more elastic than the walls of the veins to withstand higher pressure. All vessels are lined with a single layer of simple epithelium called **endothelium**. The smallest vessels, the capillaries, are made only of this single layer of cells. The exchange of fluid between the blood and interstitial spaces is influenced by **blood pressure**, which pushes fluid out of the capillary, and **osmotic pressure**, which draws fluid back in. Blood pressure is determined by the **cardiac output** and the **total peripheral resistance**.

The vessels carry blood through two circuits. The **pulmonary circuit** transports blood between the heart and the lungs for gas exchange. The **systemic circuit** distributes blood high in oxygen to all other body tissues and returns deoxygenated blood to the heart.

The walls of the vessels, especially the small arteries, contain smooth muscle that is under the control of the involuntary nervous system. The diameters of the vessels can be increased (**vasodilation**) or decreased (**vasoconstriction**) by the nervous system to alter blood pressure and blood distribution.

Several forces work together to drive blood back to the heart in the venous system. Contraction of skeletal muscles compresses the veins and pushes blood forward, **valves** in the veins keep blood from flowing backward, and changes in pressure that occur during breathing help to drive blood back to the heart. The **pulse rate** and **blood pressure** can provide information about the cardiovascular health of an individual.

Learning the Language: Word Anatomy

Complete the following table by writing the correct word part or meaning in the space provided. For each word part, write a term that contains the word part.

Word Part	Meaning	Example
1. _____	foot	_____
2. man/o-	_____	_____
3. _____	mouth	_____
4. hepat/o	_____	_____
5. phren/o	_____	_____
6. _____	stomach	_____
7. _____	arm	_____
8. _____	intestine	_____
9. sphygm/o	_____	_____
10. celi/o	_____	_____

Addressing the Learning Outcomes

I. Writing Exercise

The learning outcomes for Chapter 14 are listed below. These learning outcomes provide an overview of the major topics covered in this chapter. On a separate piece of paper, try to write out an answer to each learning outcome. All of the answers can be found in the pages of the textbook. Learning Outcomes 1, 3, 5, 6, 7, and 8 are also addressed in the Coloring Atlas.

1. Differentiate among the five types of blood vessels with regard to structure and function.
2. Compare the pulmonary and systemic circuits relative to location and function.
3. Name the four sections of the aorta and list the main branches of each section.
4. Define *anastomosis*. Cite the function of anastomoses and give several examples.
5. Compare superficial and deep veins and give examples of each type.
6. Name the main vessels that drain into the superior and inferior venae cavae.
7. Define *venous sinus* and give several examples of venous sinuses.
8. Describe the structure and function of the hepatic portal system.
9. Explain the forces that affect exchange across the capillary wall.
10. Describe the factors that regulate blood flow.
11. Define *pulse* and list factors that affect pulse rate.
12. List the factors that affect blood pressure.
13. Explain how blood pressure is commonly measured.
14. Show how word parts are used to build words related to the blood vessels and circulation.

II. Labeling and Coloring Atlas

EXERCISE 14-1: Sections of Small Blood Vessels (text Fig. 14-2)

INSTRUCTIONS

1. Write the names of the different vessel types on lines 1–5.
2. Write the names of the different vascular layers on the appropriate numbered lines (6–10) in different colors. Use black for structure 10, because it will not be colored.
3. Color the structures on the diagram with the appropriate color (except for structure 10).
4. Draw an arrow in the box to indicate the direction of blood flow.

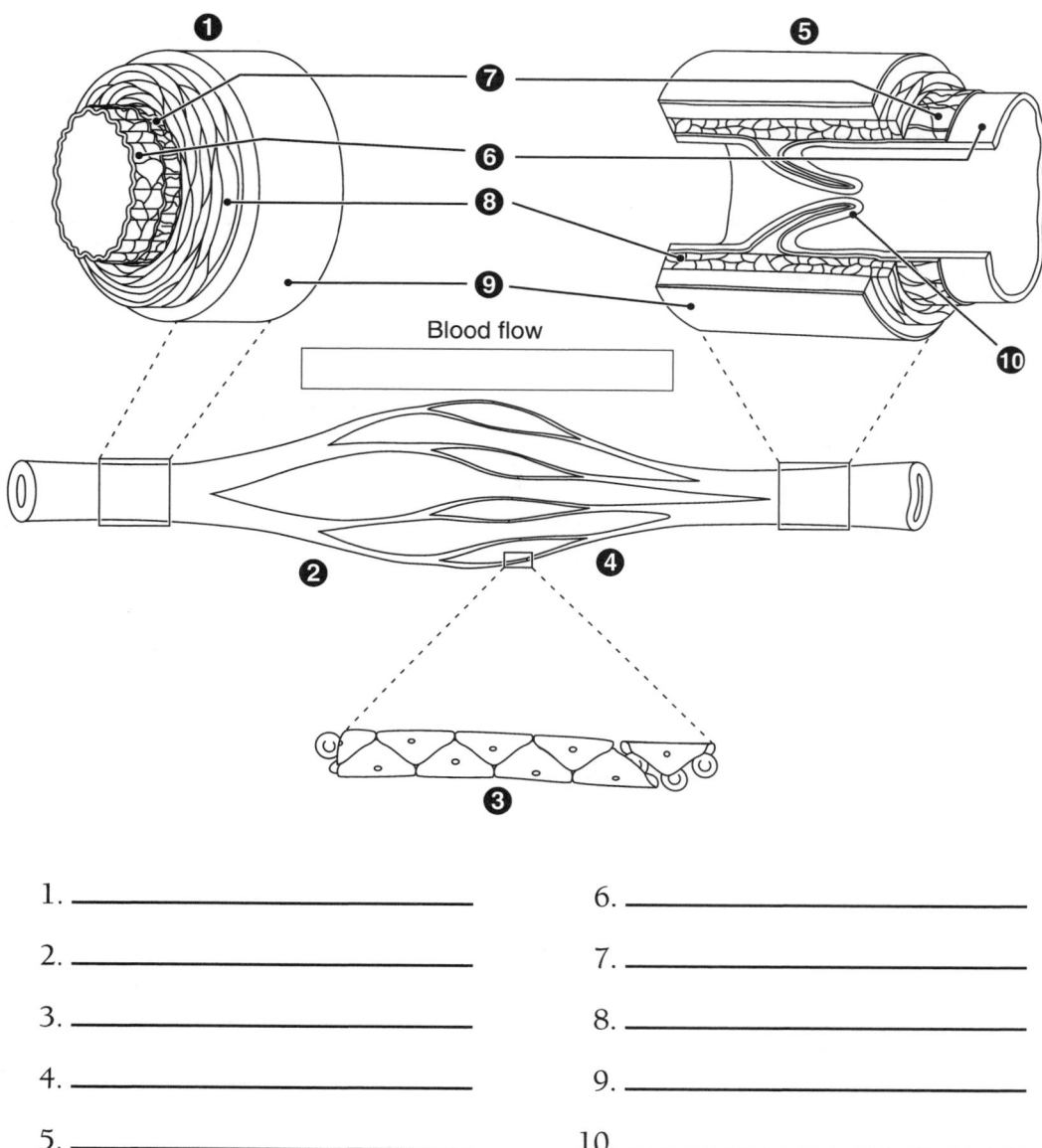

Blood flow

1. _____	6. _____
2. _____	7. _____
3. _____	8. _____
4. _____	9. _____
5. _____	10. _____

Exercise 14-2: The Aorta and Its Branches (text Fig. 14-4)

Instructions

1. Write the names of the aortic sections on lines 1–4 in different colors, and color the sections on the diagram. Although the aorta is continuous, lines have been added to the diagram to indicate the boundaries of the different sections.
2. Write the names of the aortic branches on the appropriate lines 5–22 in different colors, and color the corresponding artery on the diagram. Use the same color for structures 8 and 9 and for structures 7 and 10. Use black for structure 15, because it will not be colored.

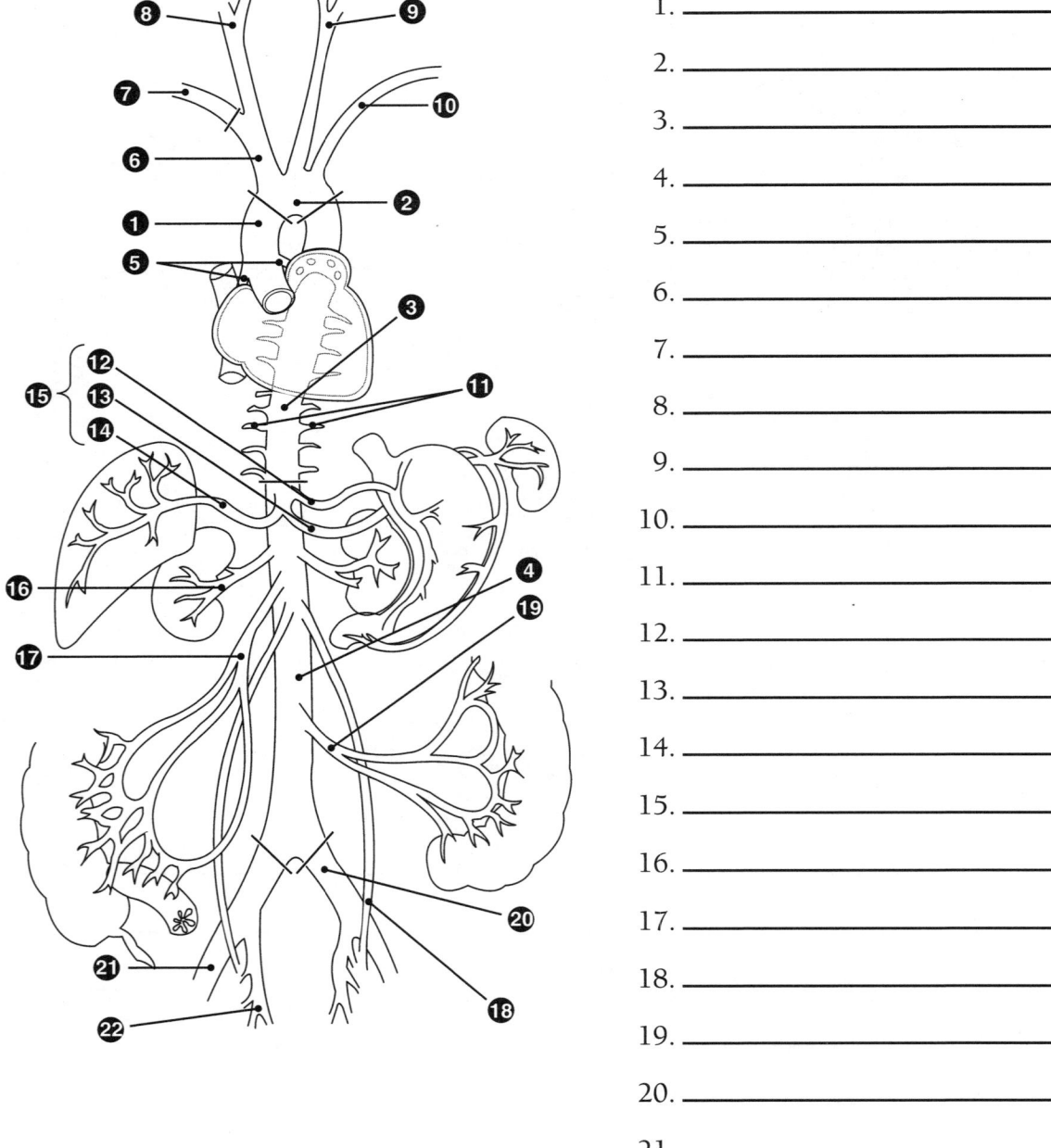

1. _____

2. _____

3. _____

4. _____

5. _____

6. _____

7. _____

8. _____

9. _____

10. _____

11. _____

12. _____

13. _____

14. _____

15. _____

16. _____

17. _____

18. _____

19. _____

20. _____

21. _____

22. _____

EXERCISE 14-3: Principal Systemic Arteries (text Fig. 14-5)

INSTRUCTIONS

1. Write the names of the aortic segments and the principal systemic arteries on the appropriate lines in different, preferably darker, colors. Felt tip pens would work well for this exercise. Some structures were also labeled in Exercise 14-2 (for instance, the thoracic aorta); you may want to use the same color scheme for both exercises. Use black for structure 15, because it will not be colored.
2. Outline the arteries on the diagram with the appropriate color. If appropriate, color the left and right versions of each artery (for instance, you can color the right and left anterior tibial arteries). Some arteries change names along their length (for instance, the brachiocephalic artery). The boundary between different artery names is indicated by a perpendicular line.

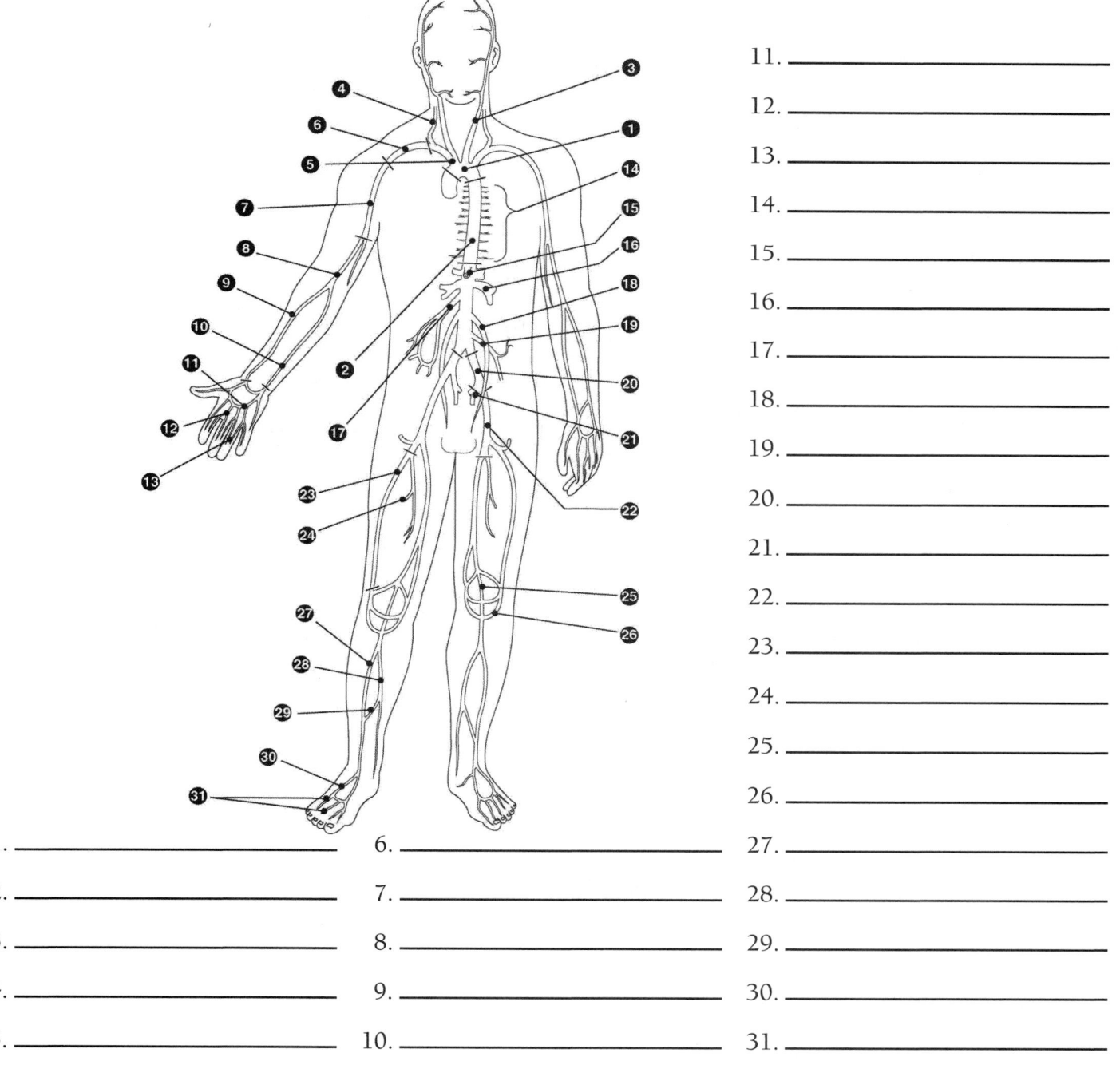

11. _____

12. _____

13. _____

14. _____

15. _____

16. _____

17. _____

18. _____

19. _____

20. _____

21. _____

22. _____

23. _____

24. _____

25. _____

26. _____

27. _____

28. _____

29. _____

30. _____

31. _____

1. _____ 6. _____

2. _____ 7. _____

3. _____ 8. _____

4. _____ 9. _____

5. _____ 10. _____

Exercise 14-4: Principal Systemic Arteries of the Head (text Fig. 14-5)

Instructions

1. Write the names of cranial arteries on the appropriate lines in different, preferably darker, colors. Felt tip pens would work well for this exercise.
2. Outline the arteries on the diagram with the appropriate color.

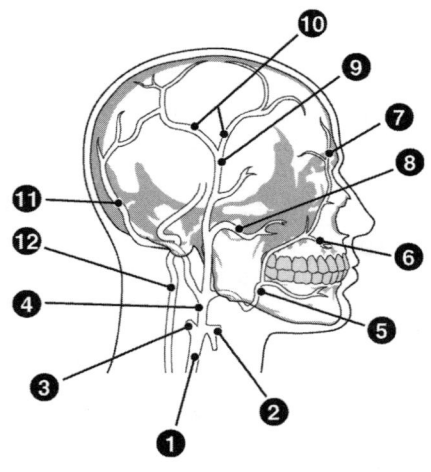

1. _____

2. _____

3. _____

4. _____

5. _____

6. _____

7. _____

8. _____

9. _____

10. _____

11. _____

12. _____

EXERCISE 14-5: Principal Systemic Veins (text Fig. 14-8)
Label each of the indicated veins.

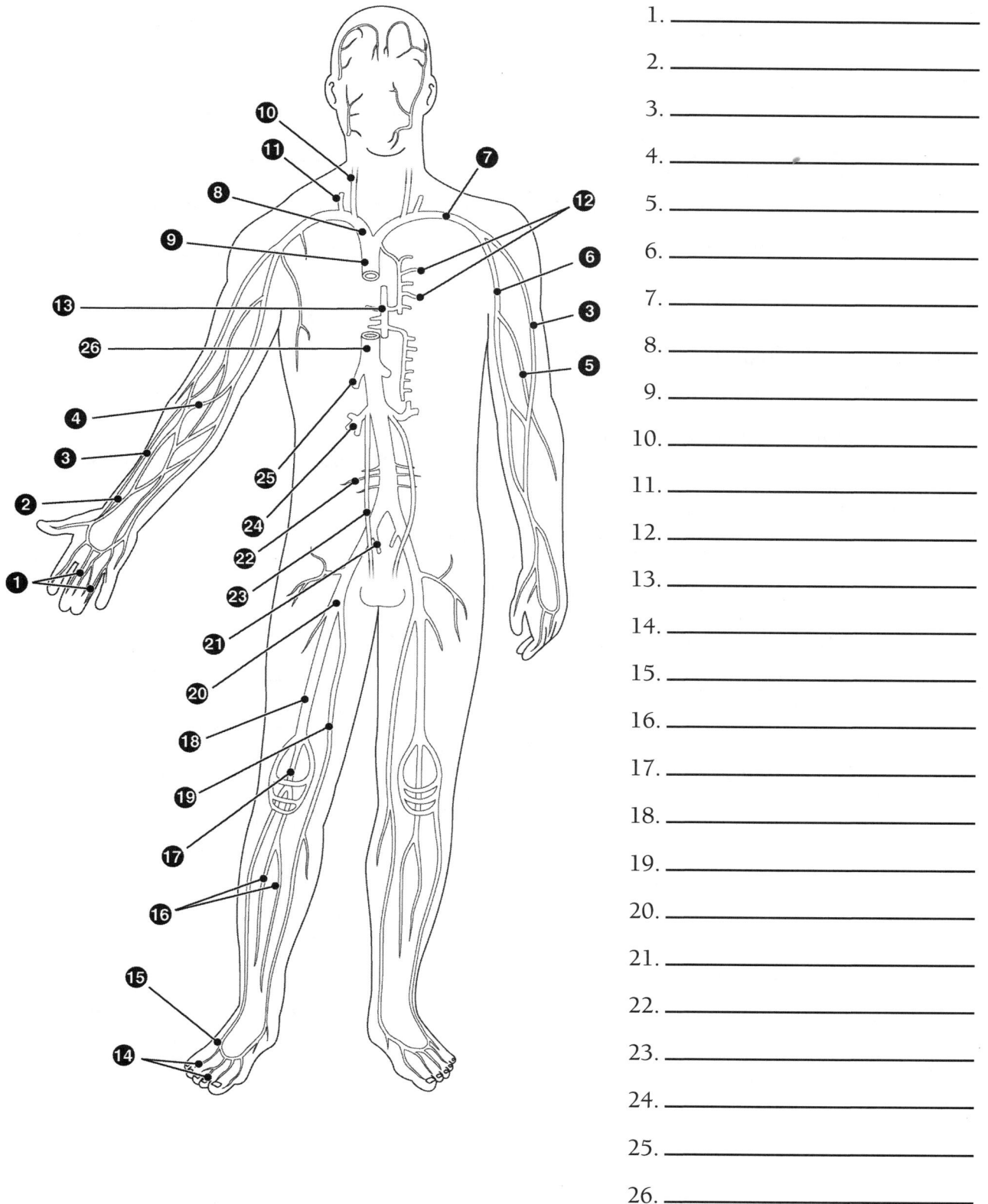

1. _____

2. _____

3. _____

4. _____

5. _____

6. _____

7. _____

8. _____

9. _____

10. _____

11. _____

12. _____

13. _____

14. _____

15. _____

16. _____

17. _____

18. _____

19. _____

20. _____

21. _____

22. _____

23. _____

24. _____

25. _____

26. _____

EXERCISE 14-6: Principal Systemic Veins of the Head (text Fig. 14-8)

Label each of the indicated veins.

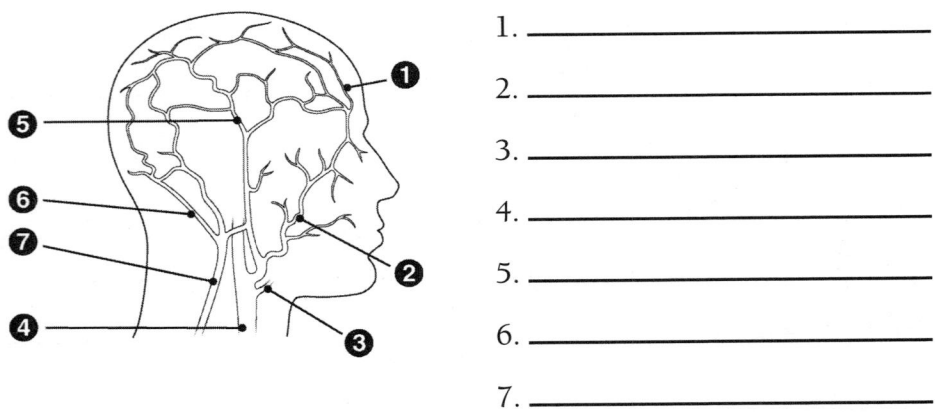

1. _____
2. _____
3. _____
4. _____
5. _____
6. _____
7. _____

EXERCISE 14-7: Cranial Venous Sinuses (text Fig. 14-9)

INSTRUCTIONS

1. Label each of the indicated veins and sinuses.
2. Draw arrows to indicate the direction of blood flow through the sinuses into the internal jugular vein.

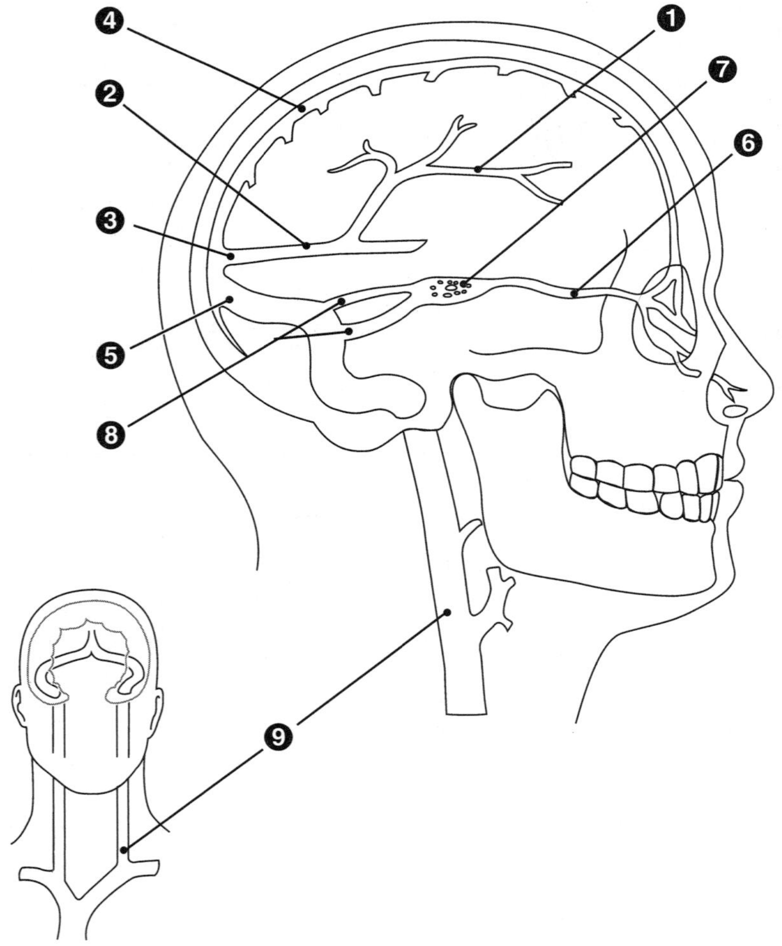

1. _____
2. _____
3. _____
4. _____
5. _____
6. _____
7. _____
8. _____
9. _____

EXERCISE 14-8: Hepatic Portal Circulation (text Fig. 14-10)
Label each of the indicated parts.

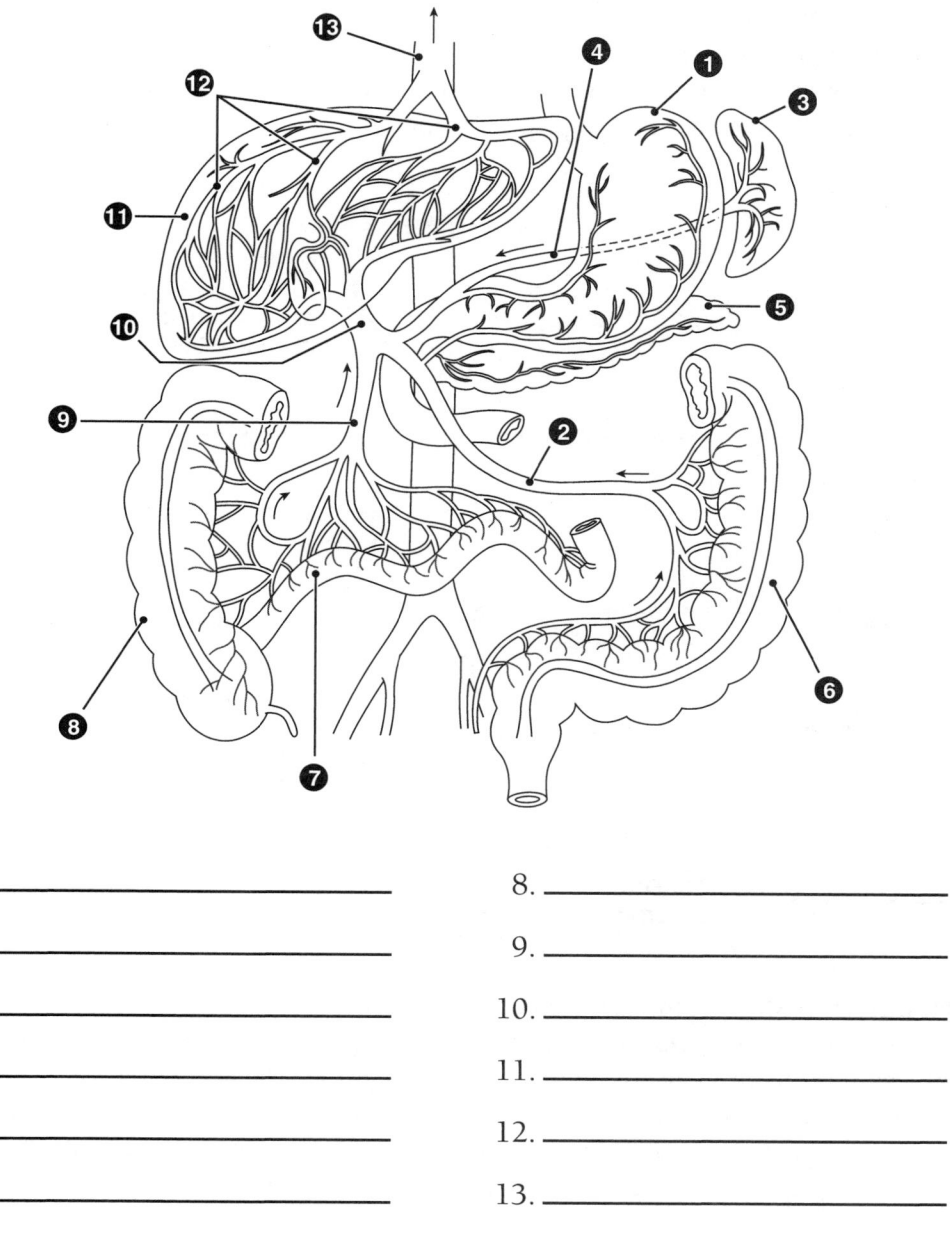

1. _____   8. _____

2. _____   9. _____

3. _____   10. _____

4. _____   11. _____

5. _____   12. _____

6. _____   13. _____

7. _____

Making the Connections

The following concept map deals with the measurement and regulation of blood pressure. Each pair of terms is linked together by a connecting phrase into a sentence. The sentence should be read in the direction of the arrow. Complete the concept map by filling in the appropriate term or phrase. There is one right answer for each term. However, there are many correct answers for the connecting phrases (3, 6, 8, and 11). Write the connecting phrases beside the appropriate number (where space permits) or on a separate piece of paper.

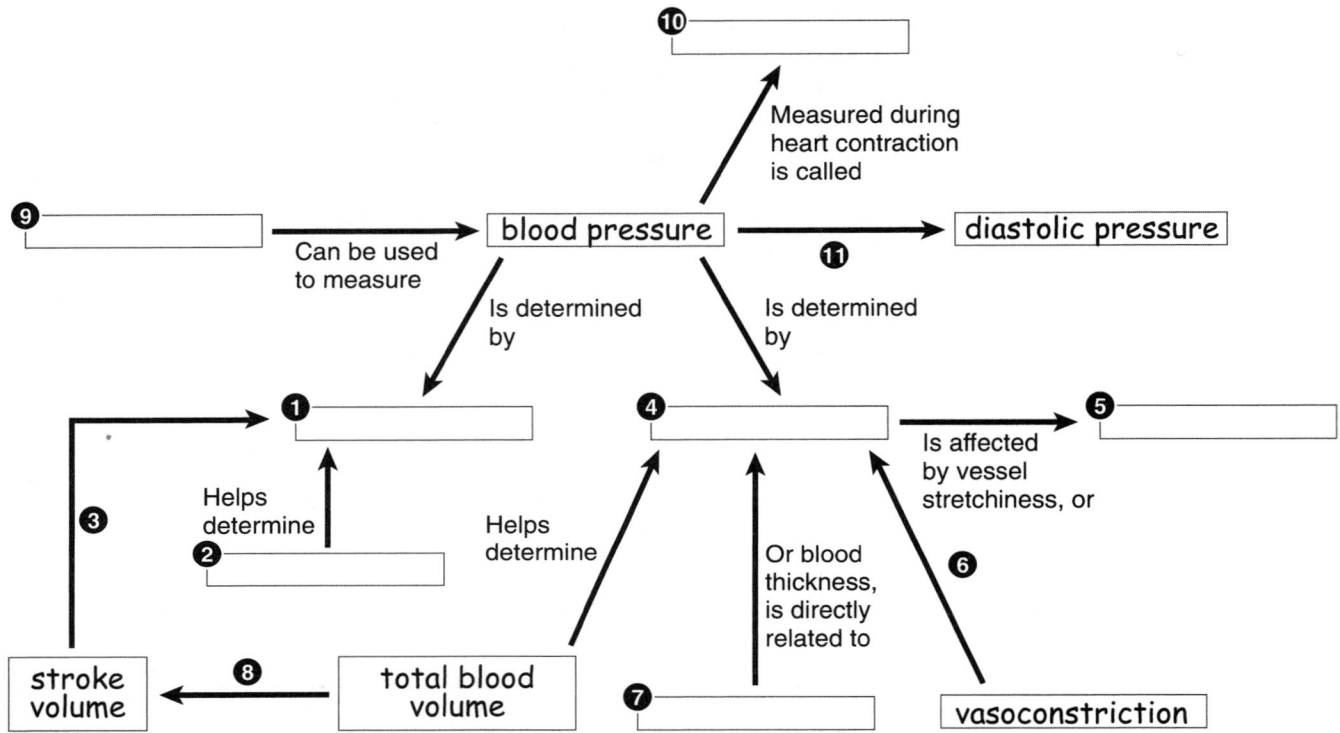

Optional Exercise: Make your own concept map/flow chart, based on the flow of blood from the left ventricle to the foot. It is not necessary to include connecting statements between the terms. Choose your own terms to incorporate into your map, or use the following list: left ventricle, dorsalis pedis, femoral, anterior tibial, aortic arch, abdominal aorta, descending aorta, ascending aorta, popliteal, common iliac, external iliac. You can also make flow charts based on the flow of blood from the leg to the heart, or to and from the arm and/or head.

Testing Your Knowledge

Building Understanding

I. Matching Exercises

Matching only within each group, write the answers in the spaces provided.

➤ Group A

artery	capillary	vein	pulmonary circuit	systemic circuit
venule	anastomosis	portal system	arteriole	sinus

1. A small vessel through which exchanges between the blood and the cells take place   _____

2. A vessel that receives blood from the capillaries   _____

3. A communication between two blood vessels   _____

4. The group of vessels that carries nutrients and oxygen to all tissues of the body except the lungs   _____

5. The term for a circuit that carries venous blood to a second capillary bed before it returns to the heart   _____

6. A vessel that branches off the aorta   _____

7. A small vessel that delivers blood to the capillaries   _____

8. The group of vessels that carries blood to and from the lungs for gas exchange   _____

➤ Group B

coronary arteries	carotid arteries	lumbar arteries	common iliac arteries
phrenic arteries	intercostal arteries	ovarian arteries	renal arteries
suprarenal arteries	brachial arteries		

1. Paired branches of the abdominal aorta that supply the diaphragm   _____

2. The vessels that branch off the ascending aorta and supply the heart muscle   _____

3. The large, paired branches of the abdominal aorta that supply blood to the kidneys   _____

4. The vessels formed by final division of the abdominal aorta   _____

5. The vessels that supply blood to the head and neck on each side   _____

6. The paired arteries that branch into the radial and ulnar
   arteries   _____

7. A group of paired vessels that extend between the ribs   _____

8. Paired branches of the abdominal aorta that extend
   into the abdominal wall musculature   _____

➤ **Group C**

| ascending aorta | aortic arch | thoracic aorta | abdominal aorta | basilar artery |
| brachiocephalic artery | celiac trunk | volar arch | hepatic artery | circle of Willis |

1. The short artery that branches into the left gastric artery,
   the splenic artery, and the hepatic artery   _____

2. A large vessel found within the pericardial sac   _____

3. An anastomosis under the center of the brain formed
   by two internal carotid arteries and the basilar artery   _____

4. The portion of the aorta supplying the upper extremities,
   neck, and head   _____

5. The large vessel that branches into the right subclavian
   artery and the right common carotid artery   _____

6. The most inferior portion of the aorta   _____

7. The vessel supplying oxygenated blood to the liver   _____

8. The vessel formed by union of the two vertebral arteries   _____

➤ **Group D**

| mesenteric arch | arterial arch | saphenous vein | jugular vein | cephalic vein |
| femoral vein | lumbar vein | hepatic portal vein | common iliac vein | |

1. The vein that drains the area supplied by the carotid artery _____

2. The longest vein   _____

3. An anastomosis between vessels supplying the intestines   _____

4. A vessel that drains into the subclavian vein   _____

5. A deep vein of the thigh   _____

6. One of four pairs of veins that drain the dorsal part of the
   trunk   _____

7. A vein that sends blood to hepatic capillaries   _____

➤ **Group E**

coronary sinus	azygos vein	superior vena cava
inferior vena cava	transverse sinus	superior sagittal sinus
gastric vein	median cubital vein	cavernous sinus

1. A vessel that drains blood from the chest wall and empties
   into the superior vena cava   _____

2. The vein that receives blood draining from the head,
   the neck, the upper extremities, and the chest   _____

3. A vein frequently used for removing blood for testing
   because of its location near the surface at the front of
   the elbow   _____

4. The large vein that drains blood from the parts of the
   body below the diaphragm   _____

5. The channel that drains blood from the ophthalmic vein
   of the eye   _____

6. A vein that drains the stomach and empties into the
   hepatic portal vein   _____

7. The channel that receives blood from most of the veins
   of the heart wall   _____

➤ **Group F**

vasomotor center	vasodilation	vasoconstriction	precapillary sphincter	pulse
valve	viscosity	sphygmomanometer	systolic	diastolic

1. Term for the blood pressure reading taken during
   ventricular relaxation   _____

2. An instrument that is used to measure blood pressure   _____

3. Term for blood pressure measured during heart muscle
   contraction   _____

4. A wave of increased pressure that begins at the heart
   when the ventricles contract and travels along the arteries   _____

5. A term that describes the thickness of a solution   _____

6. Structure that prevents blood from moving backward in

   the veins   _____

7. The change in blood vessel diameter caused by smooth

   muscle contraction   _____

8. A region of the medulla oblongata that controls blood

   vessel diameter   _____

II. Multiple Choice

Select the best answer and write the letter of your choice in the blank.

1. Which of the following arteries is unpaired?   1. _____
    a. renal
    b. brachial
    c. brachiocephalic
    d. common carotid
2. The precapillary sphincter is a: 2. _____
    a. ring of smooth muscle that regulates blood flow
    b. dilated vein in the liver
    c. tissue flap that prevents blood backflow in veins
    d. valve at the entrance to the iliac artery
3. Which of the following arteries carries blood low in oxygen?   3. _____
    a. pulmonary artery
    b. hepatic portal artery
    c. brachiocephalic artery
    d. superior vena cava
4. The cavernous sinus is found in the: 4. _____
    a. lung
    b. liver
    c. heart
    d. head
5. As blood flows through the tissues, a force that draws fluid
   back into the capillaries is: 5. _____
    a. blood pressure
    b. osmotic pressure
    c. hypertension
    d. vasoconstriction
6. Which of the following veins is found in the lower extremity?   6. _____
    a. jugular
    b. brachial
    c. basilic
7. Which of the following arteries is NOT found in the circle of Willis?   7. _____
    a. anterior cerebral
    b. posterior communicating
    c. vertebral
    d. middle cerebral

8. Which of the following layers is found in arteries AND capillaries? 8. _____
    a. smooth muscle
    b. inner tunic
    c. outer tunic
    d. middle tunic

9. Blood pressure would be increased by: 9. _____
    a. narrowing the blood vessels
    b. reducing the pulse rate
    c. increasing vasodilation
    d. decreasing blood viscosity

10. Which of the following is NOT a subdivision of the aorta? 10. _____
    a. thoracic aorta
    b. descending aorta
    c. pulmonary aorta
    d. abdominal aorta

11. Which of the following changes would increase blood pressure? 11. _____
    a. activation of the vagus nerve
    b. vasodilation
    c. increased stroke volume
    d. decreased heart rate

12. The two veins that unite to form the inferior vena cava are the: 12. _____
    a. gastric veins
    b. common iliac veins
    c. jugular veins
    d. mesenteric veins

III. Completion Exercise

Write the word or phrase that correctly completes each sentence.

1. One example of a portal system is the system that carries blood from the abdominal organs to the _____

2. The inner, epithelial layer of blood vessels is called the _____

3. The force that draws fluid and dissolved substances into capillaries is called _____

4. The longest veins of the body, extending from the feet to the groin, are called the _____

5. The aorta is part of the group, or circuit, of blood vessels called the _____

6. A large channel that drains deoxygenated blood is called a(n) _____

7. The smallest subdivisions of arteries have thin walls in which there is little connective tissue and relatively more muscle. These vessels are _____

8. A decrease in a blood vessel's diameter is called _____

9. The circle of Willis is formed by a union of the internal carotid arteries and the basilar artery. Such a union of vessels is called a(n) _____

Understanding Concepts

I. True or False

For each question, write "T" for true or "F" for false in the blank to the left of each number. If a statement is false, correct it by replacing the underlined term and write the correct statement in the blank below the question.

_____ 1. The anterior and posterior communicating arteries are part of the anastomosis supplying the brain.

_____

_____ 2. Contraction of the smooth muscle in arterioles would decrease blood pressure.

_____

_____ 3. Increased blood pressure would decrease the amount of fluid leaving the capillaries.

_____

_____ 4. The external iliac artery continues in the thigh as the femoral artery.

_____

_____ 5. The transverse sinuses receive most of the blood leaving the heart.

_____

_____ 6. Sinusoids are found in the kidney.

_____

_____ 7. Blood flow into individual capillaries is regulated by precapillary sphincters.

_____

_____ 8. Blood pressure is equal to the pulse rate × peripheral resistance.

_____

II. Practical Applications

Study each discussion. Then write the appropriate word or phrase in the space provided.

➤ **Group A**

Ms S, aged 68, was admitted to the hospital suffering from lightheadedness and mental confusion.

1. Physical examination showed a narrowing of the large artery on the side of the neck that carries blood to the brain. This artery is the _____

2. Small amounts of blood could still reach Ms S's brain through the two vertebral arteries. These join at the base of the brain to form a single artery called the _____

3. Despite the impaired blood supply, blood could still access all
   parts of Ms S's brain because blood could pass through the
   Circle of Willis. This connecting vessel is an example of a(n)   _____
4. Connecting vessels also link the arteries supplying the
   intestinal tract. These connecting vessels are collectively
   called the   _____

➤ **Group B**

1. Ms. L, age 42, had her blood pressure examined during a
   routine physical. Her pressure reading was 165/120.
   Her diastolic pressure is thus   _____
2. The physician was very alarmed by the finding and immediately prescribed a drug to reduce the production of an
   enzyme produced in the kidneys that causes blood pressure
   to increase. This enzyme is called   _____
3. Further tests showed evidence of artery disease in several
   of the larger vessels. One area involved was the first
   portion of the aorta called the   _____
4. Another vessel that was seriously damaged was the short one
   that is the first branch of the aortic arch. This artery is called the   _____
5. The damage reflects the accumulation of fatty material in the
   vessel walls. The lining of the arteries was roughened, which
   could lead to the fatal formation of a blood clot. The innermost
   damaged layer of the arteries is known as the   _____

III. Short Essays

1. Explain the purpose of vascular anastomoses.

   _____

   _____

   _____

2. What is the function of the hepatic portal system, and what vessels contribute to this system?

   _____

   _____

   _____

3. List the vessels a drop of blood will encounter traveling from deep within the left thigh to the
   right atrium.

   _____

   _____

   _____

Conceptual Thinking

1. Mr. B, age 54, is losing substantial amounts of blood because of a bleeding ulcer. What will be the effect on his blood pressure? What are some physiological changes that could be made to correct this effect?

_____

_____

_____

Expanding Your Horizons

Eat, drink, and have happy arteries. Eat more fish. Eat less fish. Drink wine. Do not drink wine. We receive conflicting messages about the effect of different foodstuffs on arterial health. The following two articles discuss some of these claims.

Resource List

Klatsky AL. Drink to your health? Sci Am 2003;288:74–81.
Covington MB. Omega-3 fatty acids. Am Fam Physician 2004;70:133–140.

chapter 15

The Lymphatic System and Body Defenses

Overview

Lymph is the watery fluid that flows within the lymphatic system. It originates from the blood plasma and from the tissue fluid that is found in the minute spaces around and between the body cells. The fluid moves from the **lymphatic capillaries** through the **lymphatic vessels** and then to the **right lymphatic duct** and the **thoracic duct**. These large terminal ducts drain into the subclavian veins, adding the lymph to blood that is returning to the heart. Lymphatic capillaries resemble blood capillaries, but they begin blindly and larger gaps between the cells make them more permeable than blood capillaries. The larger lymphatic vessels are thin-walled and delicate; like some veins, they have valves that prevent backflow of lymph.

The **lymph nodes**, which are the lymphatic system's filters, are composed of lymphoid tissue. These nodes remove impurities and process **lymphocytes**, cells active in immunity. Chief among them are the cervical nodes in the neck, the axillary nodes in the armpit, the tracheobronchial nodes near the trachea and bronchial tubes, the mesenteric nodes between the peritoneal layers, and the inguinal nodes in the groin.

In addition to the nodes, there are several organs of lymphoid tissue with somewhat different functions. The **tonsils** filter tissue fluid; the **thymus** is essential for development of the immune system during early life. The **spleen** has numerous functions, including destruction of worn out red blood cells, serving as a reservoir for blood, and producing red blood cells before birth.

The **reticuloendothelial system** consists of cells such as macrophages and natural killer cells involved in the destruction of bacteria, cancer cells, and other possibly harmful substances. Other nonspecific defenses include the intact **skin** and **mucous membranes**, which serve as mechanical barriers. Body secretions wash away impurities and may kill bacteria as well. By the process of **inflamma-**

tion, the body tries to get rid of an irritant or to minimize its harmful effects. **Fever** boosts the immune system and inhibits the growth of some organisms.

The ultimate defense against disease is **immunity,** the means by which the body resists or overcomes the effects of a particular disease or other harmful agent. There are two basic types of immunity: inborn and acquired. **Inborn immunity** is inherited; it may exist on the basis of **species, population,** or **individual** characteristics. **Acquired immunity** is gained during a person's lifetime. It involves reactions between foreign substances or **antigens** and the white blood cells known as **lymphocytes.** The **T cells** (T lymphocytes) respond to the antigen directly and produce **cell-mediated immunity.** There are different types of T cells involved in immune reactions, some acting to control the response. **Macrophages** participate by presenting the foreign antigen to the T cells. **B cells** (B lymphocytes), when stimulated by an antigen, multiply into **plasma cells.** These cells produce specific **antibodies,** which react with the antigen. Circulating antibodies make up the form of immunity termed **humoral immunity.**

Acquired immunity may be **natural** (acquired by transfer of maternal antibodies or by contact with the disease) or **artificial** (provided by a vaccine or an immune serum). Immunity that involves production of antibodies by the individual is termed **active immunity;** immunity acquired as a result of the transfer of antibodies to an individual from some outside source is described as **passive immunity.**

Learning the Language: Word Anatomy

Complete the following table by writing the correct word part or meaning in the space provided. For each word part, write a term that contains the word part.

Word Part	Meaning	Example
1. _____	gland	_____
2. lingu/o	_____	_____
3. -oid	_____	_____

Addressing the Learning Outcomes

The learning outcomes for Chapter 15 are listed below. These learning outcomes provide an overview of the major topics covered in this chapter. On a separate piece of paper, try to write out an answer to each learning outcome. All of the answers can be found in the pages of the textbook. Learning Outcomes 3 and 4 are also addressed in the Coloring Atlas.

1. List the functions of the lymphatic system.
2. Explain how lymphatic capillaries differ from blood capillaries.
3. Name the two main lymphatic ducts and describe the area drained by each.
4. List the major structures of the lymphatic system and give the locations and functions of each.
5. Describe the composition and function of the reticuloendothelial system.
6. Differentiate between nonspecific and specific body defenses and give examples of each.
7. Briefly describe the inflammatory reaction.
8. List several types of inborn immunity.
9. Define *antigen* and *antibody*.
10. Compare T cells and B cells with respect to development and type of activity.
11. Explain the role of macrophages in immunity.
12. Describe some protective effects of an antigen–antibody reaction.
13. Differentiate between naturally acquired and artificially acquired immunity.
14. Differentiate between active and passive immunity.
15. Define the terms *vaccine* and *immune serum*.
16. Show how word parts are used to build words related to the lymphatic system.

II. Labeling and Coloring Atlas

EXERCISE 15-1: Lymphatic System in Relation to the Cardiovascular System (text Fig. 15-1)

INSTRUCTIONS

1. Label the indicated parts.
2. Color the oxygenated blood red, the deoxygenated blood blue, and the lymph yellow.

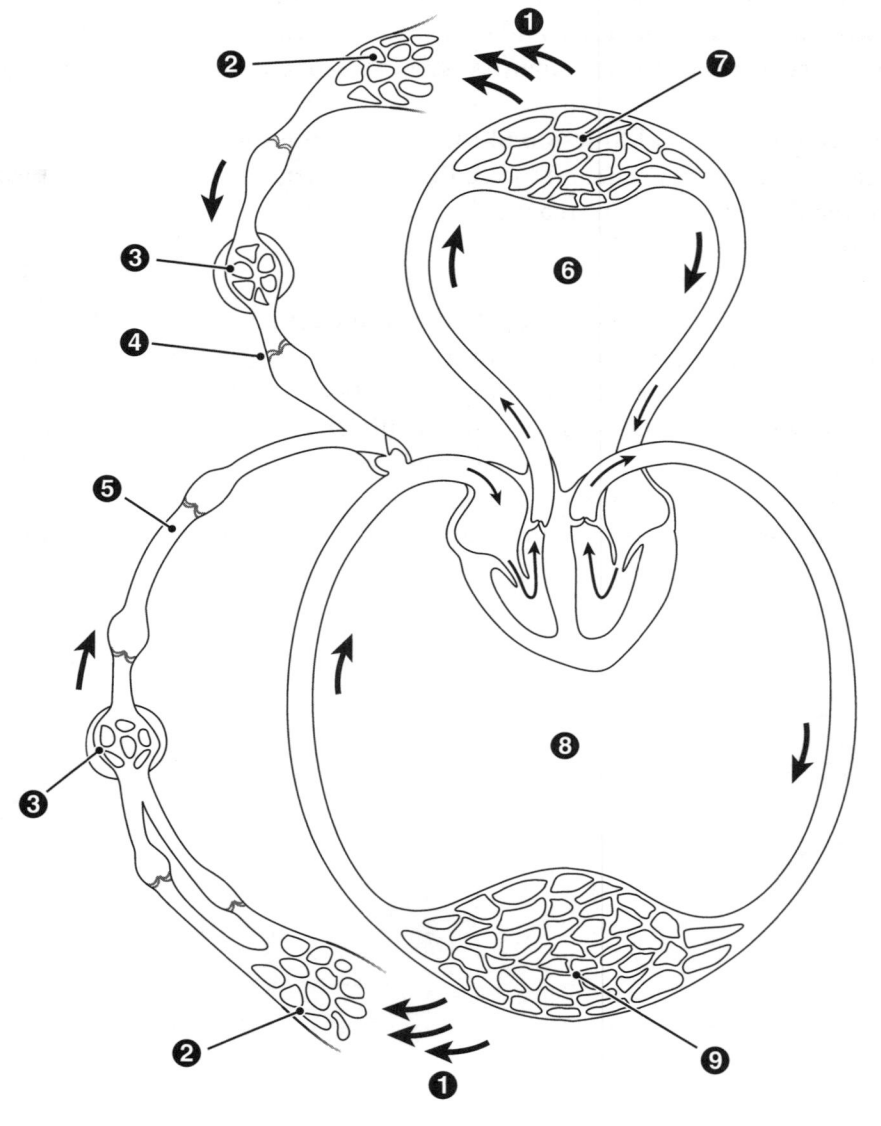

1. _____   6. _____

2. _____   7. _____

3. _____   8. _____

4. _____   9. _____

5. _____

EXERCISE 15-2: Lymphatic System (text Fig. 15-4)
Label the indicated parts.

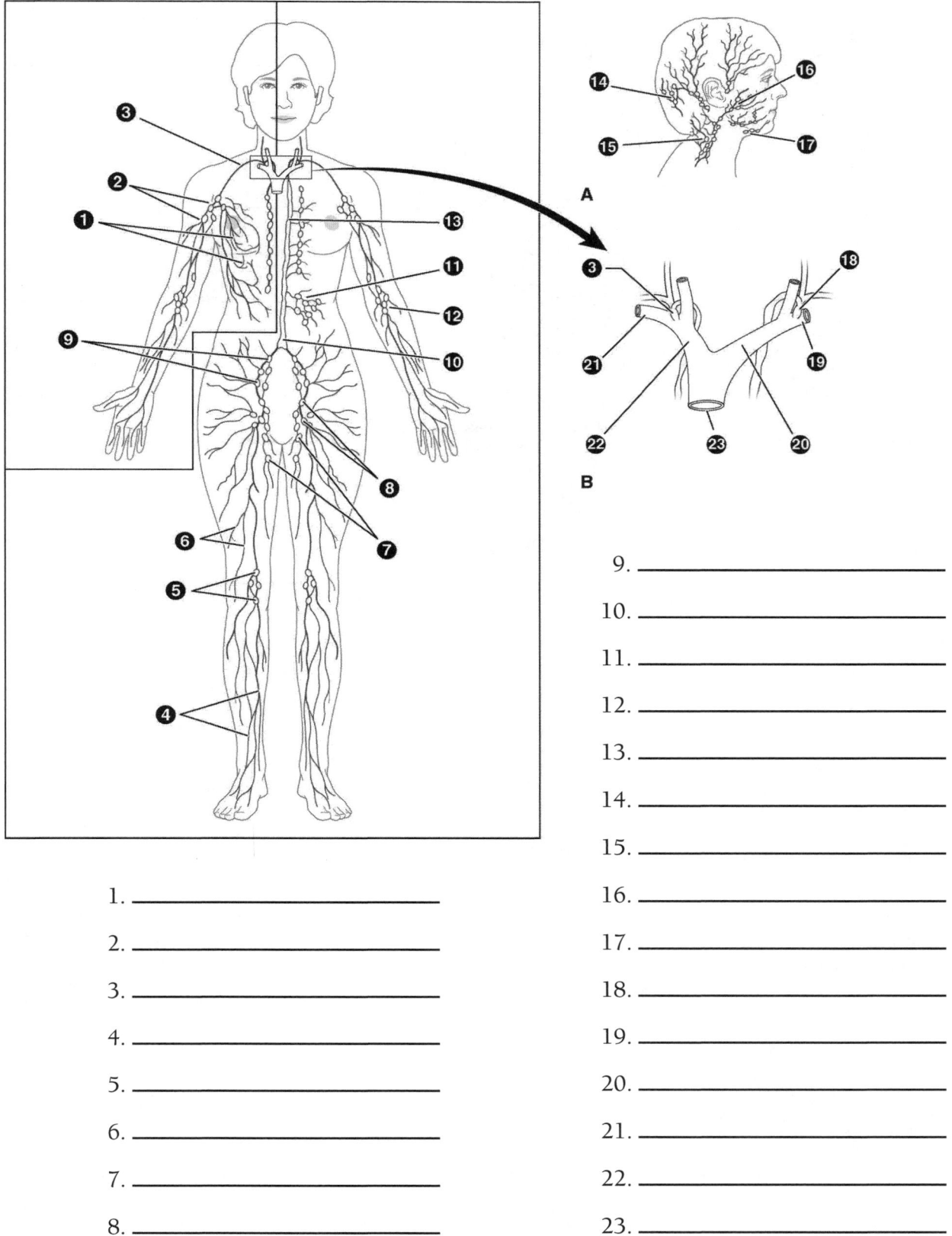

A

B

1. _____

2. _____

3. _____

4. _____

5. _____

6. _____

7. _____

8. _____

9. _____

10. _____

11. _____

12. _____

13. _____

14. _____

15. _____

16. _____

17. _____

18. _____

19. _____

20. _____

21. _____

22. _____

23. _____

EXERCISE 15-3: Lymph Node (text Fig. 15-5)
Label the indicated parts.

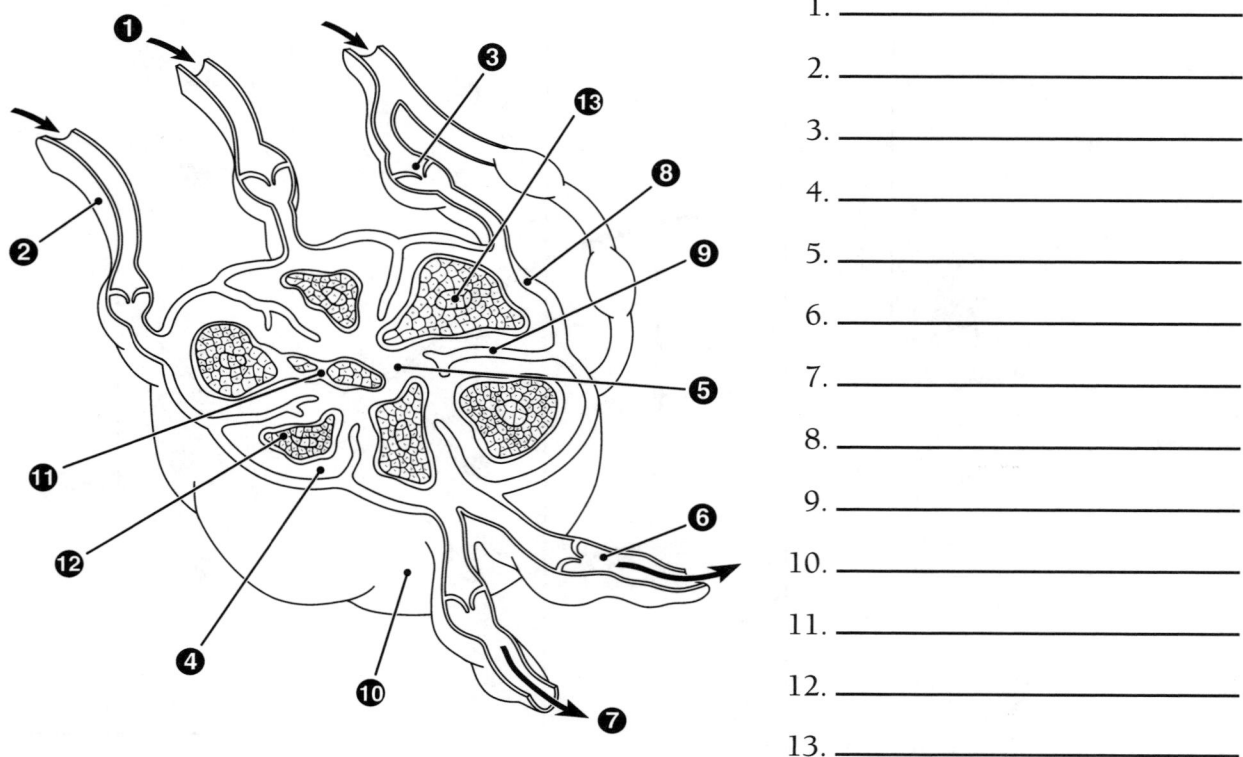

1. _____

2. _____

3. _____

4. _____

5. _____

6. _____

7. _____

8. _____

9. _____

10. _____

11. _____

12. _____

13. _____

EXERCISE 15-4: Location of Lymphoid Tissue (text Fig. 15-6)

INSTRUCTIONS

1. Write the names of the different lymphoid organs on the numbered lines in different colors.
2. Color the structures on the diagram with the appropriate colors.

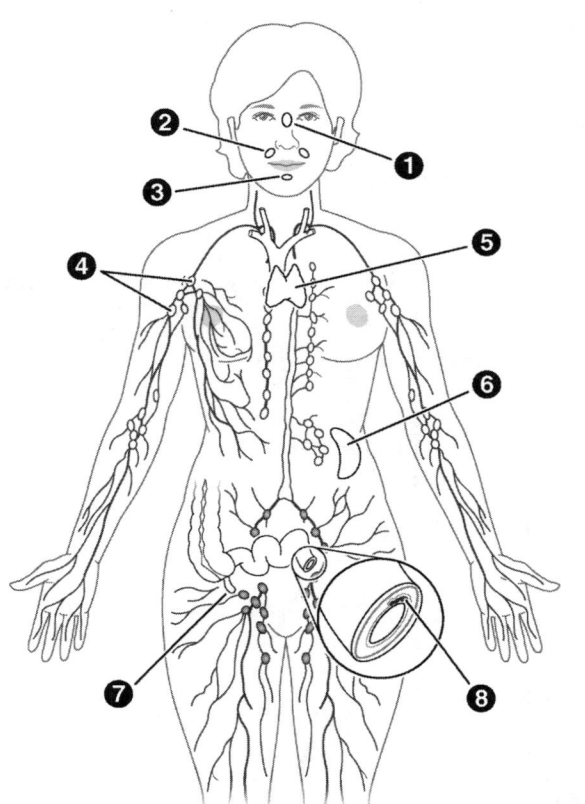

1. _____

2. _____

3. _____

4. _____

5. _____

6. _____

7. _____

8. _____

Making the Connections

The following concept maps deal with the structure and function of the lymphatic system (Map A) and the processes of immunity (Map B). Each pair of terms is linked together by a connecting phrase into a sentence. The sentence should be read in the direction of the arrow. Complete the concept maps by filling in the appropriate term or phrase. There is one right answer for each term. However, there are many correct answers for the connecting phrases. Write the connecting phrases beside the appropriate number (where space permits) or on a separate piece of paper.

MAP A

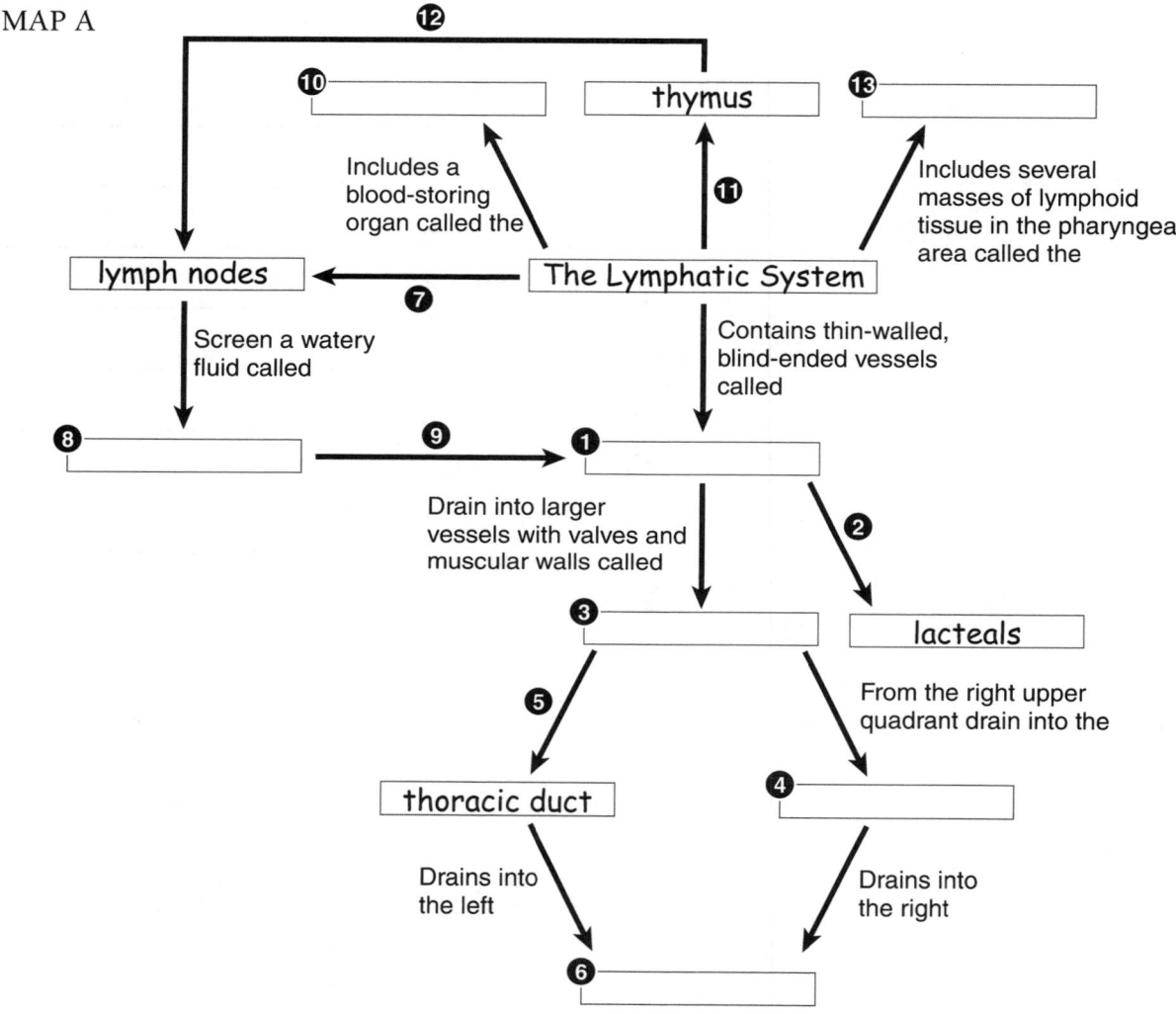

MAP B

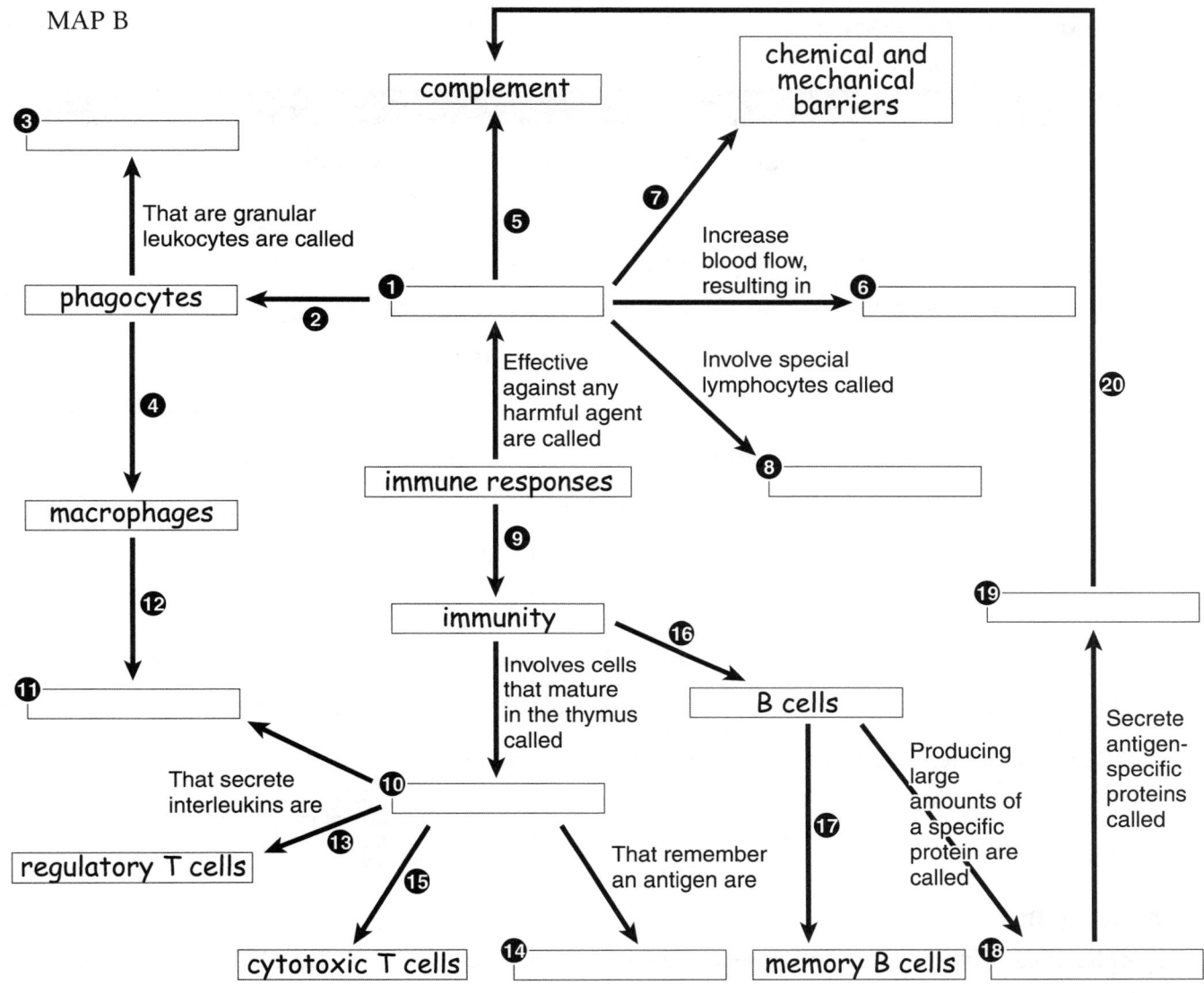

Optional Exercise: Make your own concept map/flow chart, based on the flow of lymph from a body part to the left atrium. It is not necessary to include connecting statements between the terms. For instance, you could map the flow of lymph from the right breast to the right atrium by linking the following terms: superior vena cava, right subclavian vein, right brachiocephalic vein, mammary vessels, axillary nodes, right lymphatic duct.

Testing Your Knowledge
Building Understanding

I. Matching Exercises

Matching only within each group, write the answers in the spaces provided.

➤ Group A

lacteal	endothelium	superficial	mesothelium
deep	inguinal nodes	axillary nodes	cervical nodes

1. The nodes that filter lymph from the lower extremities and
   the external genitalia   _____

2. The lymph nodes located in the armpits   _____

3. Term for lymphatic vessels located under the skin   _____

4. The single layer of cells that makes up the walls of lymphatic
   capillaries   _____

5. A specialized vessel in the small intestine wall that absorbs
   digested fats   _____

6. The lymph nodes located in the neck that drain certain parts
   of the head and neck   _____

➤ Group B

lymphatic capillary	right lymphatic duct	chyle	lymph
valve	subclavian vein	thoracic duct	cisterna chyli

1. The temporary storage area formed by an enlargement of
   the first part of the thoracic duct   _____

2. The fluid formed when tissue fluid passes from the
   intercellular spaces into the lymphatic vessels   _____

3. The large lymphatic vessel that drains lymph from below the
   diaphragm and from the left side above the diaphragm   _____

4. The milky-appearing fluid that is a combination of fat
   globules and lymph   _____

5. Structure that prevents backflow of fluid in lymphatic vessels   _____

6. Blind-ended, thin-walled vessel that absorbs excess tissue
   fluid and proteins   _____

➤ **Group C**

hilum	germinal center	trabeculae	spleen
palatine tonsil	lingual tonsil	pharyngeal tonsil	thymus

1. An oval lymphoid body located at the side of the soft palate   _____

2. The organ that filters blood and is located in the upper left
   quadrant (left hypochondriac region) of the abdomen   _____

3. A mass of lymphoid tissue at the back of the tongue   _____

4. The mass of lymphoid tissue located in the pharynx behind
   the nose and commonly called adenoids   _____

5. The organ in which T cells mature   _____

6. The indented area of a lymph node where efferent
   lymphatic vessels exit the node   _____

➤ **Group D**

Peyer patch	MALT	GALT	monocyte
Kupffer cell	macrophage	reticuloendothelial system	immune system

1. A different name for the tissue macrophage system   _____

2. Areas of lymphoid tissue found in mucous membranes   _____

3. Areas of lymphoid tissue specifically found throughout the
   gastrointestinal system   _____

4. The name given to a phagocyte found in the liver   _____

5. An area of lymphoid tissue specifically found in the small
   intestine wall   _____

6. A large white blood cell circulating in the blood   _____

➤ **Group E**

nonspecific defenses	specific defenses	inflammatory exudate	histamine
toxin	species immunity	natural killer cell	neutrophil

1. The type of protection that prevents humans from contracting
   certain animal diseases   _____

2. A lymphocyte that nonspecifically destroys abnormal cells   _____

3. A mixture of lymphocytes and fluid   _____

4. A poison produced by a pathogen   _____

5. Immune responses effective against any pathogen   _____

6. Immune responses directed against an individual pathogen _____

7. A phagocyte that participates in nonspecific defenses _____

➤ **Group F**

active immunity	passive immunity	antigen	antibody	interferon
complement	plasma cell	T_h cell	T_{reg} cell	T_c cell

1. A substance that prevents multiplication of viruses _____

2. The type of immunity that results from transfer of antibodies from mother to fetus through the placenta _____

3. A cell that matures in the thymus that directly destroys a foreign cell _____

4. The type of long-term immunity produced by infection or exposure to a microbial toxin _____

5. Any foreign substance introduced into the body that provokes an immune response _____

6. An antibody-producing cell derived from a B cell _____

7. A cell that reduces an immune response by inhibiting or destroying activated lymphocytes _____

8. A circulating protein also known as an immunoglobulin _____

➤ **Group G**

toxoid	attenuation	immunization	complement	memory cell
antitoxin	gamma globulin	antivenin	rubella	toxin

1. The process of reducing the virulence of a pathogen to prepare a vaccine _____

2. A toxin treated with heat or chemicals to reduce its harmfulness so that it may be used as a vaccine _____

3. A group of blood proteins that may be needed to help an antibody destroy a foreign antigen _____

4. The fraction of the blood plasma that contains antibodies _____

5. A process designed to induce an immune response against a particular pathogen, resulting in the acquisition of active artificially acquired immunity _____

6. A B cell or T cell that can rapidly activate an immune response when the pathogen is encountered for a second time _____

7. The type of immune serum used to provide passive immunity

   to botulism   _____

8. An immune serum administered to a snake bite victim   _____

II. Multiple Choice

Select the best answer and write the letter of your choice in the blank.

1. Which of the following is NOT a type of cell associated with the
   reticuloendothelial system?   1. _____
       a. monocytes
       b. macrophages
       c. dust cells
       d. red blood cells
2. Which of the following is NOT a function of the spleen? 2. _____
       a. destruction of old red blood cells
       b. blood filtration
       c. blood storage
       d. chyle drainage
3. The mesenteric nodes are found: 3. _____
       a. in the groin region
       b. near the trachea
       c. between the two peritoneal layers
       d. in the armpits
4. An organ that shrinks in size after puberty is the: 4. _____
       a. cisternal chyli
       b. thymus
       c. spleen
       d. liver
5. Unlike blood capillaries, lymphatic capillaries: 5. _____
       a. contain a thin muscular layer
       b. are virtually impermeable to water and solutes
       c. are blind-ended
       d. do not contain any cells
6. The enlarged portion of the thoracic duct is called the: 6. _____
       a. cisterna chyli
       b. right lymphatic duct
       c. hilum
       d. lacteal
7. The type of lymphocyte involved in nonspecific immunity is the: 7. _____
       a. B cells
       b. natural killer cells
       c. macrophages
       d. cytotoxic T cells
8. Which of the following describes an activity of B cells? 8. _____
       a. suppression of the immune response
       b. manufacture of antibodies

     c. direct destruction of foreign cells

     d. phagocytosis

9. Which of the following is a specific defense against infection?   9. _____

     a. skin

     b. mucus

     c. antibodies

     d. cilia

10. Cells that combine with foreign antigens and present them to T cells

    are the: 10. _____

     a. macrophages

     b. B cells

     c. interferons

     d. viruses

11. Complement proteins: 11. _____

     a. promote inflammation

     b. attract phagocytes

     c. destroy cells

     d. all of the above

12. Interleukins are: 12. _____

     a. substances in the blood that react with antigens

     b. the antibody fraction of the blood

     c. a group of nonspecific proteins needed for agglutination

     d. substances released from T_h cells that stimulate other leukocytes

13. MHC antigens are: 13. _____

     a. bacterial proteins

     b. foreign proteins

     c. one's own proteins

     d. antibodies

14. Which of the following will result in active immunity?   14. _____

     a. vaccination

     b. antiserum administration

     c. breast feeding

     d. none of the above

III. Completion Exercise

Write the word or phrase that correctly completes each sentence.

1. Thymosin is synthesized by the   _____

2. The milky-appearing lymph that drains from the small
   intestine is called   _____

3. The fluid that moves from tissue spaces into special collecting
   vessels for return to the blood is called   _____

4. Lymph from the right side of the body above the diaphragm
   joins the bloodstream when the right lymphatic duct empties
   into the   _____

5. The lymph nodes surrounding the breathing passageways may
   become black in individuals living in highly polluted areas.
   The nodes involved are the   _____

6. Nearly all of the lymph from the arm, shoulder, and breast passes through the lymph node known as the _____

7. The spleen contains many cells that can engulf harmful bacteria and other foreign cells by a process called _____

8. Circulating antibodies are responsible for the type of immunity termed _____

9. Heat, redness, swelling, and pain are considered the classic symptoms of _____

10. Antibodies that neutralize toxins but do not affect the organism producing the toxin are called _____

11. Antibodies transmitted from a mother's blood to a fetus provide a type of short-term borrowed immunity called _____

12. The administration of vaccine, however, stimulates the body to produce a longer-lasting type of immunity called _____

13. The action of leukocytes in which they engulf and digest invading pathogens is known as _____

Understanding Concepts

I. True or False

For each question, write "T" for true or "F" for false in the blank to the left of each number. If a statement is false, correct it by replacing the underlined term and write the correct statement in the blank below the question.

_____ 1. Lymph filtered through the mesenteric nodes will drain into the <u>thoracic duct</u>.

_____

_____ 2. Thymosin is produced by the <u>spleen</u>.

_____

_____ 3. Kupffer cells are part of the <u>GALT system</u>.

_____

_____ 4. Lacteals are a type of <u>blood capillary</u>.

_____

_____ 5. <u>Complement</u> is a substance that participates in non-specific body defenses directed against viruses.

_____

_____ 6. Cytoxotic T-cells participate in <u>humoral</u> immunity.

_____

_____ 7. Any process in which an individual produces his or her own antibodies is called <u>active</u> immunity.

_____

_____ 8. The action of histamine in the inflammatory reaction is an example of a <u>nonspecific</u> defense.

_____

_____ 9. Immunoglobulin is another name for <u>antigens</u>.

_____

_____ 10. <u>Interferons</u> are released by helper T cells to stimulate the activity of other leukocytes.

_____

_____ 11. Administration of an antiserum is an example of <u>artificially acquired, passive</u> immunity.

_____

II. Practical Applications

Study each discussion. Then write the appropriate word or phrase in the space provided.

➤ **Group A**

1. Ms. L traveled in Asia for 2 years before starting nursing school. During the first week of classes, she noticed swelling in one of her legs. She looked through her pathophysiology textbook to try to identify the cause. She read that excess fluid from tissues drains into small blunt-ended vessels called _____

2. To her alarm, she discovered that small worms can obstruct these vessels, causing swelling. She rushed to the hospital, where the physician palpated the small lymphoid masses found behind her knee. These masses are called the _____

3. These masses were normal, but the lymphoid tissue masses at the top of the swollen leg were swollen due to an infected cut in her upper thigh. These lymphoid masses are called the _____

➤ **Group B**

1. Mr R stepped on a rusty nail, resulting in a deep puncture wound. When he arrived home 2 hours later, he noticed swelling, heat, and redness in the area surrounding the painful wound. These classic symptoms indicate that a series of defensive processes are ocurring called the _____

2. Many of his symptoms are due to the release of a chemical that dilates blood vessels. This chemical is called _____

3. Mr R went to a medical clinic to have his wound treated. The nurse on duty inquired as to the status of Mr R's immunizations. Another term for immunization is _____

4. Mr R had never been immunized against tetanus, so he was injected with a substance to neutralize harmful secretions produced by the tetanus bacteria. These harmful secretions are called _____.

5. The injection will produce a short-term form of immunity called _____

III. Short Essays

1. Trace a lymph droplet from the interstitial fluid of the lower leg to the right atrium, based on the structures shown in Figure 15-4.

_____

_____

_____

2. Discuss the role of macrophages in specific and non-specific body defenses.

_____

_____

_____

Conceptual Thinking

1. Ms. Y, a healthy 24-year-old woman, is studying for her nursing final examinations. She has been sitting at her desk for 10 hours straight when she notices that her legs are swollen. Use your knowledge of the lymphatic system to explain the swelling, and suggest how she can prevent it in the future.

_____

_____

_____

2. Baby G was born without a thymus, but was otherwise normal. Speculate as to which aspects of her immune system will be affected by this deficiency, and which aspects will be unaffected.

_____

_____

_____

_____

_____

3. Mr. A stepped on a fish while beachcombing in the South Pacific. A spine was embedded in his foot, and he rapidly became dizzy and the foot swelled alarmingly. Mr. A was told by a local

doctor that the fish spine contains an incredibly potent poison, and that he will be dead in 8 hours unless the poison is neutralized.

    A. What would be the best treatment for Mr. A—vaccination with fish toxoid or an injection of an antitoxin? Defend your answer.

_____

_____

_____

_____

_____

_____

    B. What form of immunity will be induced by this treatment?

_____

    C. Will Mr. A be protected from future encounters with this particular fish poison? Explain why or why not.

_____

_____

_____

Expanding Your Horizons

A vaccine for AIDS? Although the treatments for AIDS have improved by leaps and bounds, the disease still results in enormous suffering. The "holy grail" of AIDS research is the development of a vaccine to protect individuals from the infection. However, the quest for a vaccine is not an easy one, as discussed in the following two articles.

Resource List

Baltimore D, Heilman C. HIV vaccines: prospects and challenges. Sci Am 1998;279:98–103.
Ezzell C. Hope in a vial. Will there be an AIDS vaccine anytime soon? Sci Am 2002;286:38–45.

chapter 16

Respiration

Overview

Oxygen is taken into the body and carbon dioxide is released by means of the organs and passageways that constitute the **respiratory system**. This system contains the **nasal cavities**, the **pharynx**, the **larynx**, the **trachea**, the **bronchi**, and the **lungs**.

Oxygen is obtained from the atmosphere and delivered to the cells by the process of **respiration**. The first phase of respiration is **pulmonary ventilation**, which normally is accomplished by breathing. During normal, quiet breathing, air enters the lungs (**inhalation**) because the diaphragm and intercostal muscles contract to expand the thoracic cavity. Air leaves the lungs (**exhalation**) when the muscles relax. Deeper breathing requires additional muscles during inhalation and exhalation. The other two phases of respiration are **external exchange of gases** between the alveoli of the lungs and the bloodstream and **internal exchange of gases** between the blood and the tissues. Oxygen is delivered to the cells, and carbon dioxide is transported to the lungs for elimination.

Oxygen is transported to the tissues almost entirely by the **hemoglobin** in red blood cells. Some carbon dioxide is transported in the red blood cells as well, but most is converted into **bicarbonate ions** and **hydrogen ions**. Bicarbonate ions are carried in plasma, and the hydrogen ions (along with hydrogen ions from other sources) increase the acidity of the blood.

Breathing is primarily controlled by the **respiratory control centers** in the medulla and the pons of the brain stem. These centers are influenced by **chemoreceptors** located outside the medulla that respond to changes in the acidity of the cerebrospinal fluid. The acidity reflects the concentration of carbon dioxide.

Learning the Language: Word Anatomy

Word Part	Meaning	Example
1. spir/o-	_____	_____
2. _____	nose	_____
3. -pnea	_____	_____
4. _____	carbon dioxide	_____
5. _____	lung	_____
6. _____	air, gas	_____
7. orth/o-	_____	_____
8. or/o	_____	_____

Addressing the Learning Outcomes

I. Writing Exercise

The learning outcomes for Chapter 16 are listed below. These learning outcomes provide an overview of the major topics covered in this chapter. On a separate piece of paper, try to write out an answer to each learning outcome. All of the answers can be found in the pages of the textbook. Learning Outcomes 2 and 6 are also addressed in the Coloring Atlas.

1. Define *respiration* and describe the three phases of respiration.
2. Name and describe all the structures of the respiratory system.
3. Explain the mechanism for pulmonary ventilation.
4. List the ways in which oxygen and carbon dioxide are transported in the blood.
5. Describe nervous and chemical controls of respiration.
6. Give several examples of altered breathing patterns.
7. Show how word parts are used to build words related to respiration.

II. Labeling and Coloring Atlas

EXERCISE 16-1: Respiratory System (text Fig. 16-2)

INSTRUCTIONS

1. Label the indicated parts.
2. Color all of the structures that encounter air green.
   Color structures containing oxygenated blood red.
   Color structures containing deoxygenated blood blue.

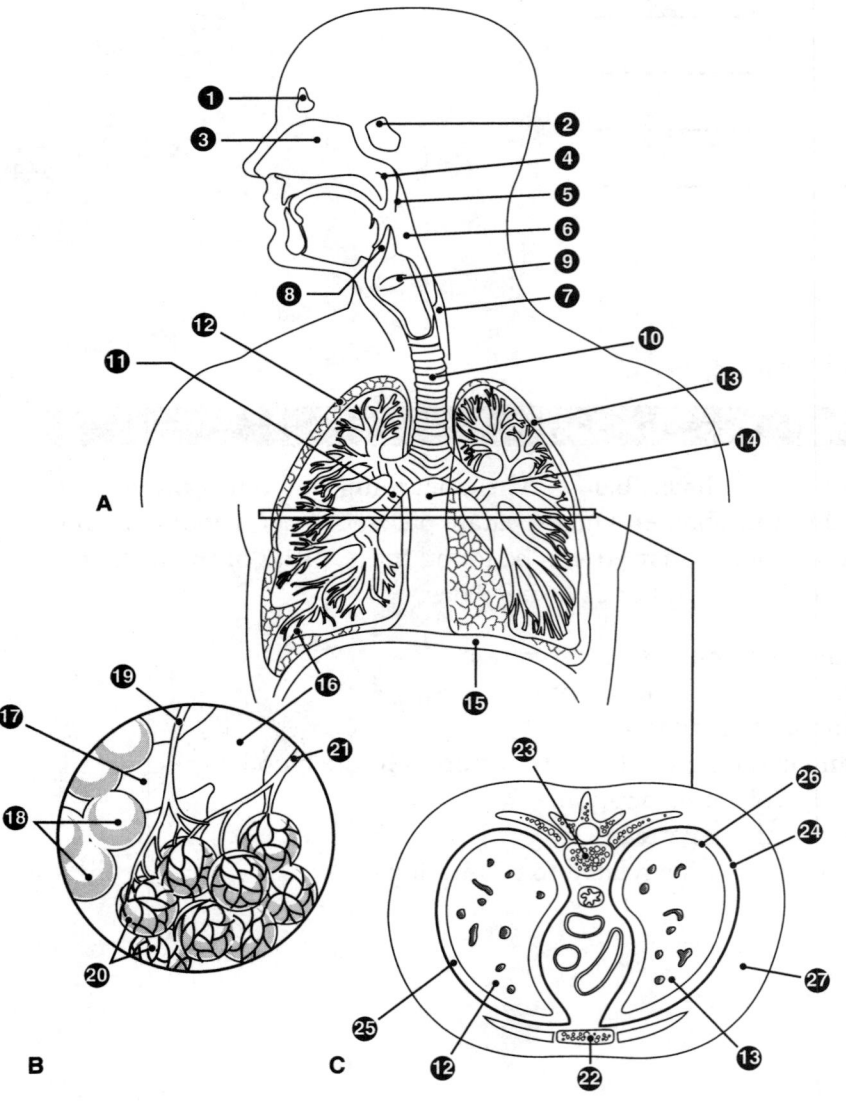

1. _____

2. _____

3. _____

4. _____

5. _____

6. _____

7. _____

8. _____

9. _____

10. _____

11. _____

12. _____

13. _____

14. _____

15. _____

16. _____

17. _____

18. _____

19. _____

20. _____

21. _____

22. _____

23. _____

24. _____

25. _____

26. _____

27. _____

EXERCISE 16-2: The Larynx (text Fig. 16-3)

INSTRUCTIONS

1. Write the name of each labeled part on the numbered lines in different colors.
2. Color the different parts on the diagram with the corresponding color.

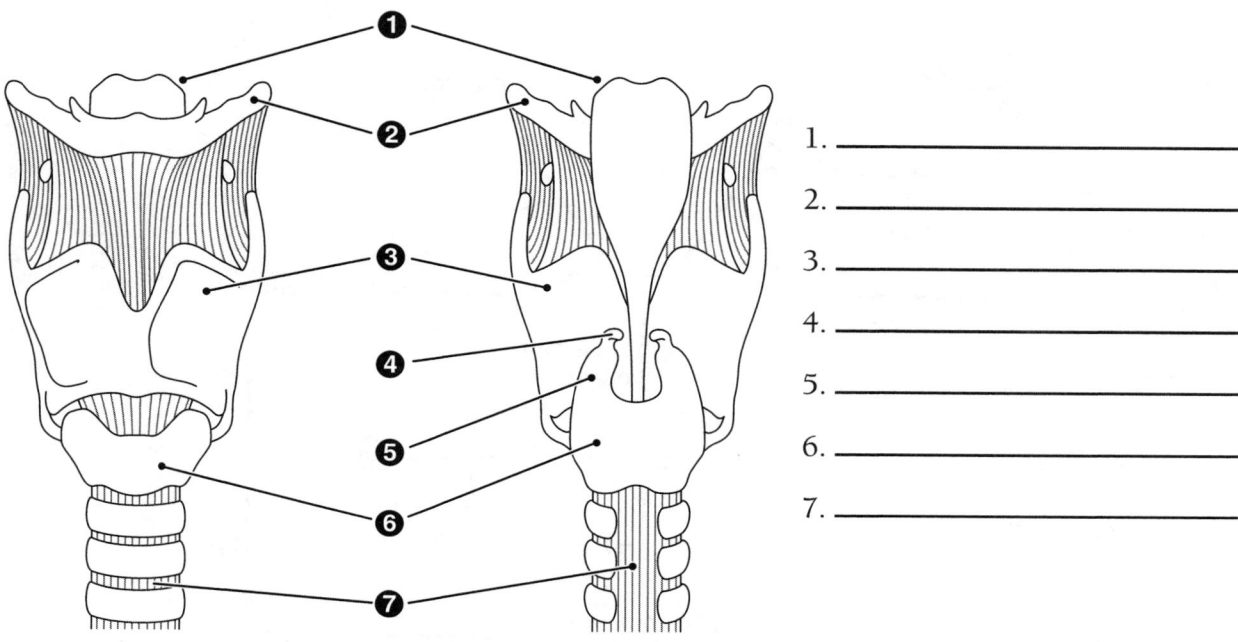

1. _____

2. _____

3. _____

4. _____

5. _____

6. _____

7. _____

EXERCISE 16-3: A Spirogram (text Fig. 16-9)

Write the names of the different lung volumes and capacities in the boxes on the diagram.

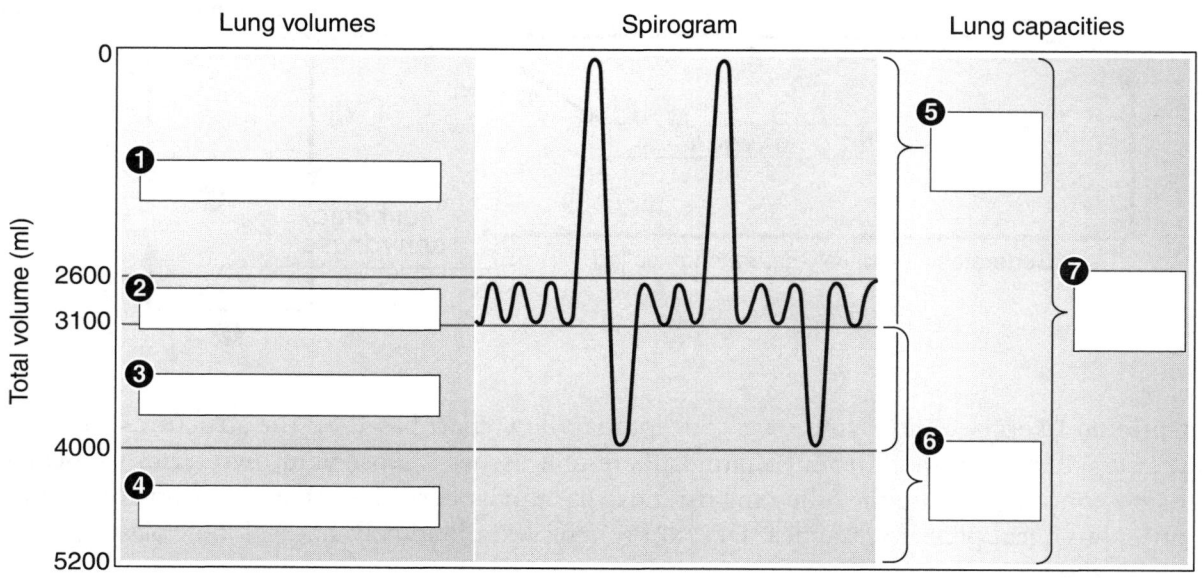

Making the Connections

The following concept map deals with the organization of the respiratory system. Each pair of terms is linked together by a connecting phrase into a sentence. The sentence should be read in the direction of the arrow. Complete the concept map by filling in the appropriate term or phrase. There is one right answer for each term. However, there are many correct answers for the connecting phrases (3, 5, 7, 9, 10–12, 15–19).

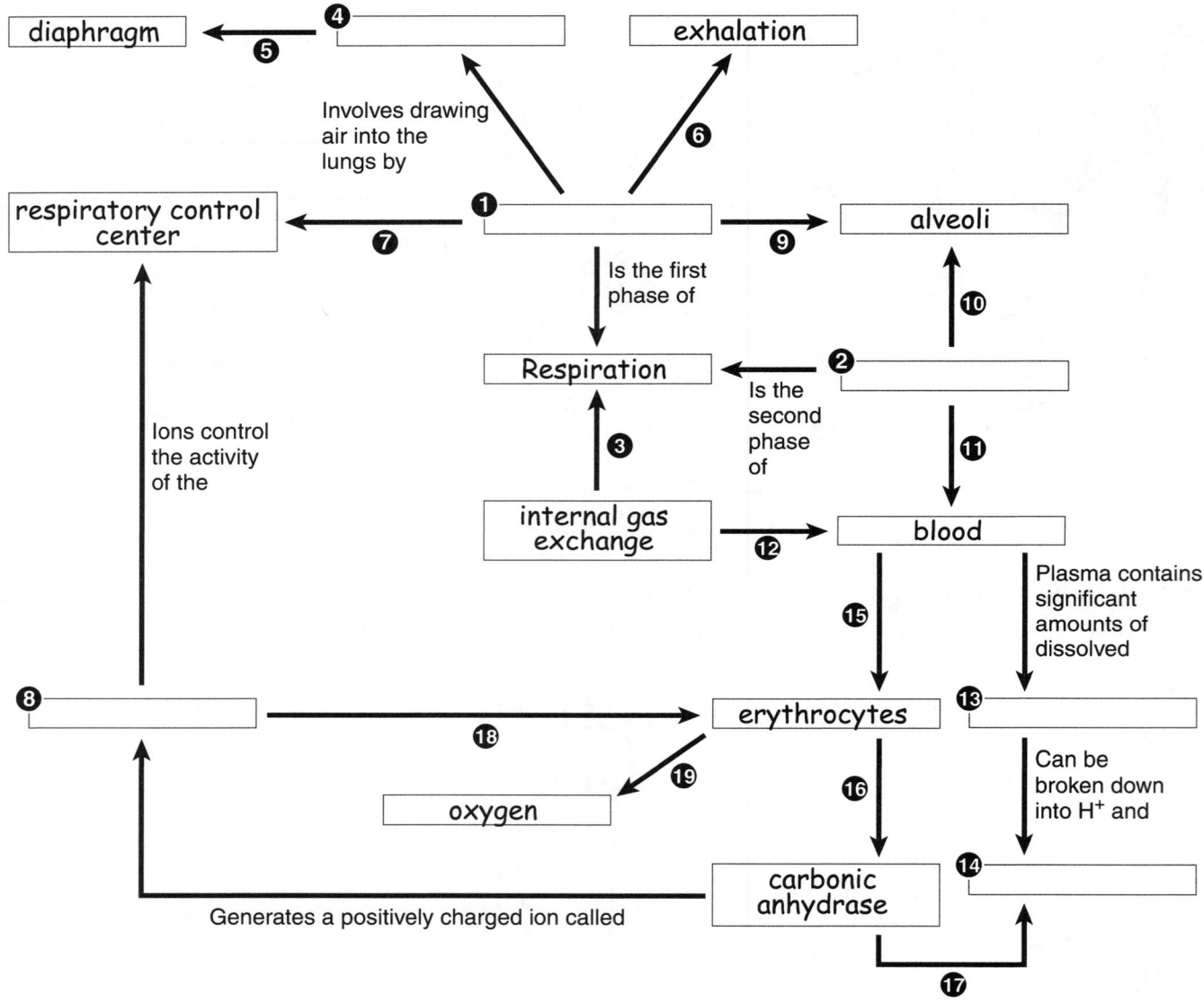

Optional Exercise: Make your own concept map/flow chart based on the structures an oxygen molecule will pass through from the atmosphere to a tissue. Choose your own terms to incorporate into your map, or use the following list: nostrils, atmosphere, nasopharynx, oropharynx, nasal cavities, laryngeal pharynx, trachea, larynx, bronchioles, blood cell, hemoglobin, plasma, tissue, bronchi, alveoli.

Testing Your Knowledge
Building Understanding

I. Matching Exercises

Matching only within each group, write the answers in the spaces provided.

➤ **Group A**

nares   conchae   pharynx   glottis   epiglottis
larynx   hilum   bronchus   bronchiole   sinus

1. The openings of the nose _____
2. The three projections arising from the lateral walls of each nasal cavity _____
3. The scientific name for the voice box _____
4. The leaf-shaped structure that helps to prevent the entrance of food into the trachea _____
5. One of the two branches formed by division of the trachea _____
6. The notch or depression where the bronchus, blood vessels, and nerves enter the lung _____
7. The area below the nasal cavities that is common to both the digestive and respiratory systems _____
8. A small air-conducting tube containing a smooth muscle layer but little or no cartilage _____

➤ **Group B**

alveoli   surfactant   pleura   inhalation   tidal volume
exhalation   intercostals   compliance   spirometer   vital capacity

1. The substance in the fluid lining the alveoli that prevents their collapse _____
2. The phase of pulmonary ventilation in which air is expelled from the alveoli _____
3. The phase of pulmonary ventilation in which the diaphragm contracts _____
4. The serous membrane around each lung _____

5. The only respiratory structures involved in external gas
   exchange   _____

6. The amount of air inhaled during a normal breath   _____

7. The ease with which the lungs and thorax can be expanded   _____

8. The maximum volume of air that can be inhaled after
   maximum expiration   _____

➤ **Group C**

bicarbonate ion	hemoglobin	carbonic anhydrase	carbon dioxide
diffusion	osmosis	hydrogen ion	oxygen

1. The process by which oxygen moves from the blood into
   tissues   _____

2. The substrate for carbonic anhydrase   _____

3. An important blood buffer produced from carbon dioxide   _____

4. The substance that carries most of the oxygen in the blood _____

5. The gas that is more concentrated in the blood than in
   metabolically active tissues   _____

6. An ion that renders blood more acidic   _____

➤ **Group D**

hydrogen ion	oxygen	brain stem	aortic arch	hypoxemia
hypercapnia	hypocapnia	carbon dioxide	hypoxia	dyspnea

1. A lower than normal concentration of oxygen in the tissues _____

2. The symptom of difficult or labored breathing   _____

3. The substance that acts directly on the central
   chemoreceptors to stimulate breathing   _____

4. The change in carbon dioxide concentration resulting from
   hyperventilation   _____

5. A lower than normal blood concentration of oxygen   _____

6. The location of the central chemoreceptors   _____

7. An increase in the blood carbon dioxide concentration   _____

8. The location of a peripheral chemoreceptor   _____

II. Multiple Choice

Select the best answer and write the letter of your choice in the blank.

1. Carbon dioxide will diffuse out of blood during the phase of
   respiration called: 1. _____
      a. internal exchange of gases
      b. external exchange of gases
      c. pulmonary ventilation
      d. none of the above
2. Gas exchange occurs in the: 2. _____
      a. alveoli
      b. bronchioles
      c. bronchi
      d. all of the above
3. Which of the following terms does NOT apply to the cells that line the
   conducting passages of the respiratory tract?   3. _____
      a. pseudostratified
      b. connective
      c. columnar
      d. ciliated
4. An increase in blood carbon dioxide levels would result in: 4. _____
      a. less bicarbonate ions in the blood
      b. more hydrogen ions in the blood
      c. more alkaline blood
      d. hypocapnia
5. The substance that reduces surface tension in the alveoli is: 5. _____
      a. surfactant
      b. bicarbonate
      c. exudate
      d. effusion
6. The residual volume is: 6. _____
      a. the amount of air that is always in the lungs, even after a
         maximal expiration
      b. the total amount of air in the lungs after a maximal inspiration
      c. the amount of air remaining in the lungs after a normal
         exhalation
      d. the amount of air that can be forced out of the lungs after a
         normal exhalation

III. Completion Exercise

Write the word or phrase that correctly completes each sentence.

1. The space between the vocal cords is called the   _____
2. An abnormal decrease in the depth and rate of respiration
   is termed   _____
3. A lower than normal level of oxygen in tissues is called   _____

4. Heart disease and other disorders may cause the bluish color of the skin and visible mucous membranes characteristic of a condition called _____

5. The space between the lungs is called the _____

6. The term that is used for the pressure of each gas in a mixture of gases is _____

7. Each heme region of a hemoglobin molecule contains an inorganic element called _____

8. The nerve that innervates the diaphragm is the _____

Understanding Concepts

I. True or False

For each question, write "T" for true or "F" for false in the blank to the left of each number. If a statement is false, correct it by replacing the underlined term and write the correct statement in the blank below the question.

_____ 1. Hypercapnia results in greater blood acidity.

_____

_____ 2. Most carbon dioxide in the blood is carried bound to hemoglobin.

_____

_____ 3. The wall of an alveolus is made of stratified squamous epithelium.

_____

_____ 4. During internal exchange of gases, oxygen moves down its concentration gradient out of blood.

_____

_____ 5. The receptors that detect changes in blood gas concentrations are called mechanoreceptors.

_____

_____ 6. Inhalation ALWAYS involves muscle contraction.

_____

_____ 7. Hyperventilation results in an increase of carbon dioxide in the blood.

_____

II. Practical Applications

Study each discussion. Then write the appropriate word or phrase in the space provided.

➤ **Group A**

1. Ms. L's symptoms included shortness of breath, a chronic cough productive of thick mucus, and a "chest cold" of 2 months' duration.

She was advised to quit smoking, a major cause of lung irritation. These symptoms were caused in part by the obstruction of groups of alveoli by mucous plugs. Ms. L was told that the mucus is not moving normally out of her airways because the toxins in cigarette smoke paralyze small cell extensions that beat to create an upward current. These extensions are called

_____

2. Ms. L's respiratory function was evaluated by quantifying different lung volumes and capacities using a machine called a(n)

_____

3. Evaluation of Ms. L's respiratory function showed a reduction in the amount of air that could be moved into and out of her lungs. The amount of air that can be expelled by maximum exhalation after maximum inhalation is termed the

_____

4. The other abnormality in Ms. L's evaluation was also characteristic of her disease. There was an increase in the amount of air remaining in her lungs after a normal expiration. This amount is the

_____

➤ **Group B**

1. Baby L was born at 32 weeks' gestation gestation. She is obviously struggling for breath, and her skin is bluish in color. This skin coloration is called

_____

2. This coloration reflects a lower than normal oxygen level in the blood, technically known as

_____

3. The obstetrician fears that one or both of her lungs are not able to inflate, so baby L is placed on pressurized oxygen to inflate the lung. The physician tells the worried parents that her lungs have not yet matured sufficiently to produce the lung substance that reduces the surface tension in alveoli. This substance is called

_____

III. Short Essays

1. Are lungs passive or active players in pulmonary ventilation? Explain.

_____

_____

2. Name some parts of the respiratory tract where gas exchange does NOT occur.

_____

_____

_____

Conceptual Thinking

1. A. Name the phase of respiration regulated by the respiratory control center.

_____

   B. Explain how the respiratory control center can alter this phase of respiration.

_____

_____

_____

   C. Name the chemical factor(s) that regulate(s) the activity of the control center.

_____

_____

_____

Expanding Your Horizons

Everyone would agree that oxygen is a very useful molecule. Commercial enterprises, working on the premise that more is better, market water supplemented with extra oxygen. They claim that consumption of hyperoxygenated water increases alertness and exercise performance. Do these claims make sense? Do we obtain oxygen from the lungs or from the digestive tract? A logical extension of this premise is that soda, supplemented with carbon dioxide, would increase carbon dioxide in the blood and increase the breathing rate! Is this true? You can read about another oxygen gimmick, oxygen bars, on the web site of the Food and Drug Administration (Bren L. Oxygen bars: is a breath of fresh air worth it? 2002. Available at: http://www.fda.gov/fdac/features/ 2002/ 602_air.html).

chapter 17

Digestion

Overview

The food we eat is made available to cells throughout the body by the complex processes of **digestion** and **absorption**. These are the functions of the **digestive system**, composed of the **digestive tract** and the **accessory organs**.

The digestive tract, consisting of the **mouth**, the **pharynx**, the **esophagus**, the **stomach**, and the small and large **intestine**, forms a continuous passageway in which ingested food is prepared for use by the body and waste products are collected to be expelled from the body. The accessory organs, the **salivary glands**, **liver**, **gallbladder**, and **pancreas**, manufacture and store various enzymes and other substances needed in digestion.

Digestion begins in the mouth with the digestion of starch. It continues in the stomach, where proteins are digested, and is completed in the small intestine. Most absorption of digested food also occurs in the small intestine through small projections of the lining called **villi**. The products of carbohydrate (monosaccharides) and protein (amino acids) digestion are absorbed into capillaries, but the products of fat digestion (glycerol and fatty acids) are absorbed into **lacteals**.

The process of digestion is controlled by both nervous and hormonal mechanisms, which regulate the activity of the digestive organs and the rate at which food moves through the digestive tract.

Learning the Language: Word Anatomy

Word Part	Meaning	Example
1. _____	starch	_____
2. mes/o-	_____	_____
3. _____	intestine	_____
4. chole	_____	_____
5. bil/i	_____	_____
6. _____	bladder, sac	_____
7. _____	stomach	_____
8. _____	away from	_____
9. hepat/o	_____	_____
10. lingu/o	_____	_____

Addressing the Learning Outcomes

I. Writing Exercise

The learning outcomes for Chapter 17 are listed below. These learning outcomes provide an overview of the major topics covered in this chapter. On a separate piece of paper, try to write out an answer to each learning outcome. All of the answers can be found in the pages of the textbook. Learning Outcomes 2–6 are also addressed in the Coloring Atlas.

1. Name the three main functions of the digestive system.
2. Describe the four layers of the digestive tract wall.
3. Differentiate between the two layers of the peritoneum.
4. Name and locate the different types of teeth.
5. Name and describe the functions of the organs of the digestive tract.
6. Name and describe the functions of the accessory organs of digestion.
7. Describe how bile functions in digestion.
8. Name and locate the ducts that carry bile from the liver into the digestive tract.
9. Explain the role of enzymes in digestion and give examples of enzymes.
10. Name the digestion products of fats, proteins, and carbohydrates.
11. Define *absorption*.
12. Define *villi* and state how villi function in absorption.
13. Explain the use of feedback in regulating digestion and give several examples.
14. List several hormones involved in regulating digestion.
15. Show how word parts are used to build words related to digestion.

II. Labeling and Coloring Atlas

EXERCISE 17-1: The Wall of the Small Intestine (text Fig. 17-1)

INSTRUCTIONS

1. Write the names of the intestinal layers and associated structures on the appropriate numbered lines in different colors. Use the same color for parts 6 and 7.
2. Color the layers and structures on the diagram with the appropriate color.

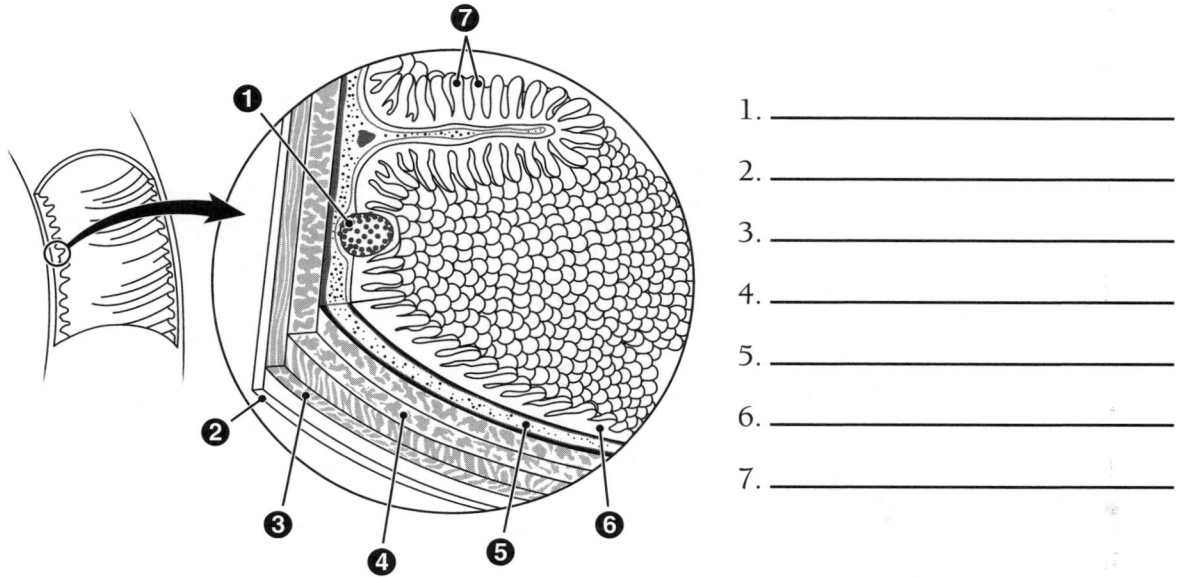

1. _____

2. _____

3. _____

4. _____

5. _____

6. _____

7. _____

Exercise 17-2: Abdominal Cavity Showing Peritoneum (text Fig. 17-3)

Instructions

1. Write the names of the abdominal organs on the appropriate numbered lines 1–9 in different colors. Use the same color for parts 3 and 4.
2. Color the organs on the diagram with the appropriate color.
3. Label the parts of the peritoneum (lines 10–14). Color the greater and lesser peritoneal cavities in contrasting colors.

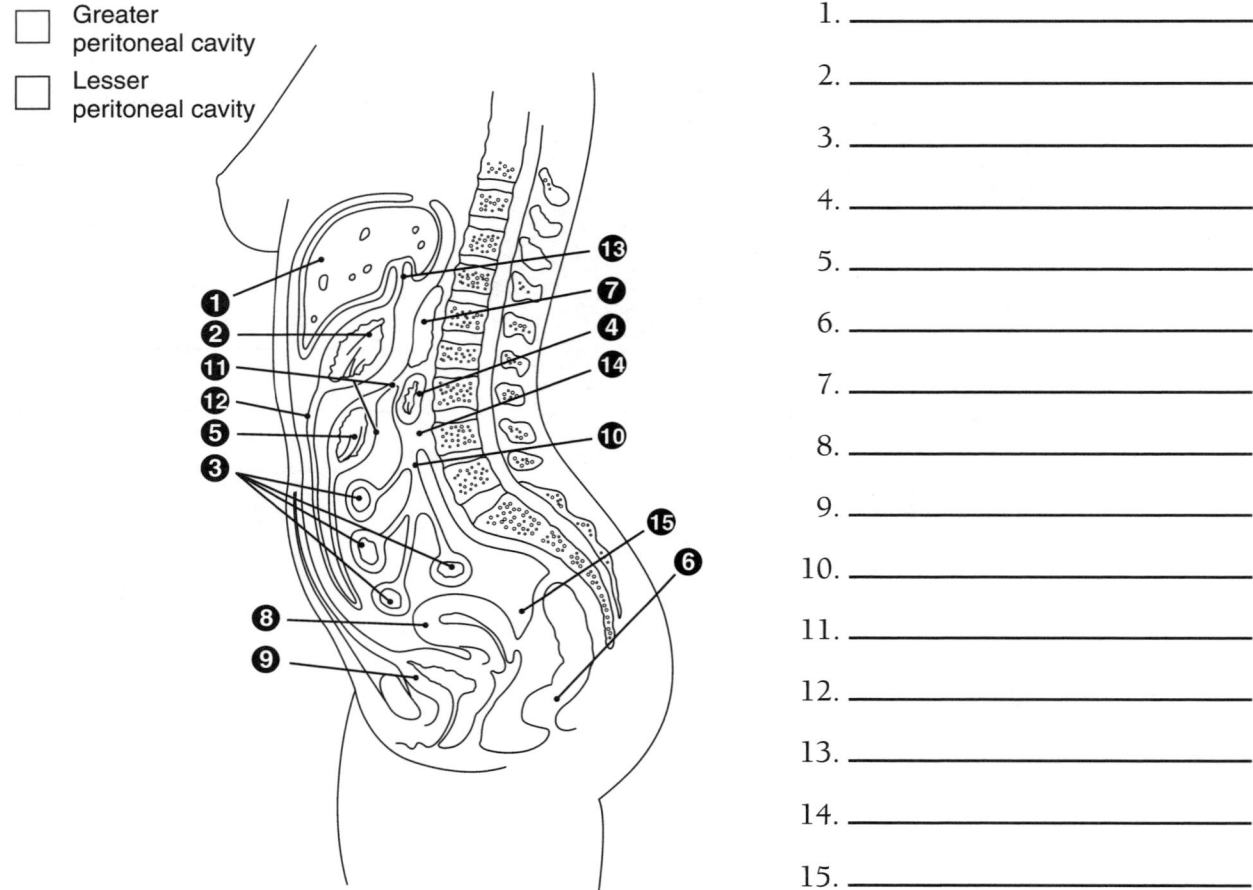

☐ Greater peritoneal cavity

☐ Lesser peritoneal cavity

1. _____

2. _____

3. _____

4. _____

5. _____

6. _____

7. _____

8. _____

9. _____

10. _____

11. _____

12. _____

13. _____

14. _____

15. _____

EXERCISE 17-3: Digestive System (text Fig. 17-4)

INSTRUCTIONS

1. Trace the path of food through the digestive tract by labeling parts 1–12. You can color all of these structures orange.
2. Write the names of the accessory organs and ducts on the appropriate lines in different colors. Use black for structure 20, because it will not be colored.
3. Color the accessory organs on the diagram with the appropriate colors.

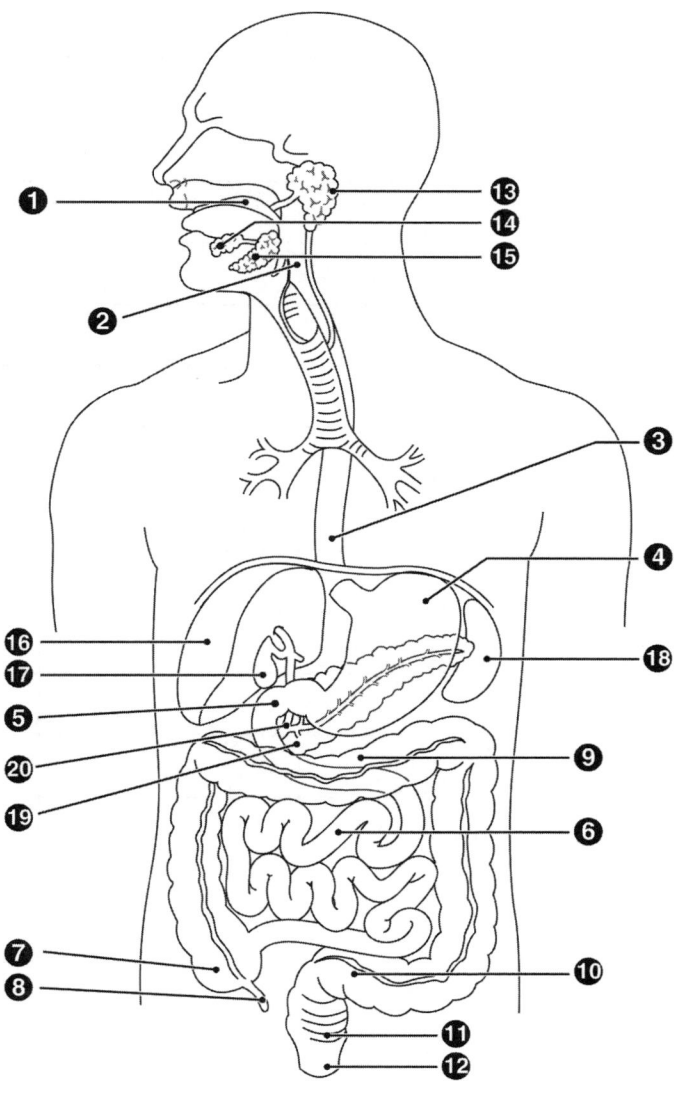

1. _____

2. _____

3. _____

4. _____

5. _____

6. _____

7. _____

8. _____

9. _____

10. _____

11. _____

12. _____

13. _____

14. _____

15. _____

16. _____

17. _____

18. _____

19. _____

20. _____

EXERCISE 17-4: The Mouth (text Fig. 17-5)

INSTRUCTIONS

1. Write the names of the teeth on the appropriate lines 1–6 in different colors. Use the same color to label parts 5 and 6.
2. Color all of the teeth with the appropriate colors.
3. Label the other parts of the mouth.

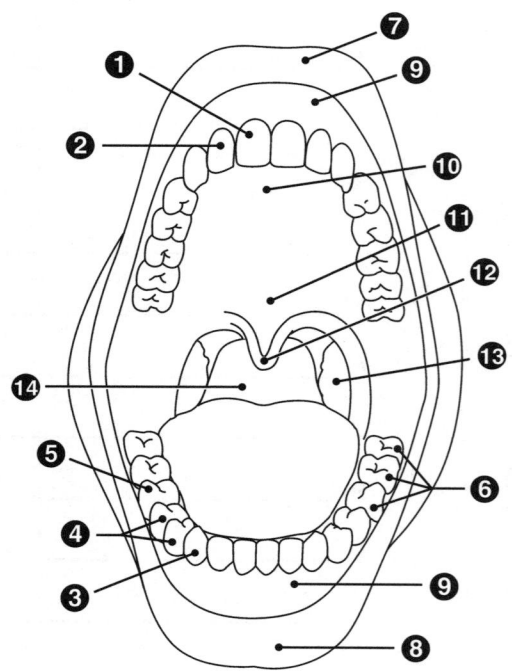

1. _____
2. _____
3. _____
4. _____
5. _____
6. _____
7. _____
8. _____
9. _____
10. _____
11. _____
12. _____
13. _____
14. _____

EXERCISE 17-5: Molar (text Fig. 17-6)

INSTRUCTIONS

1. Write the names of the two divisions of a tooth in the numbered boxes.
2. Write the names of the parts of the tooth and gums on the appropriate numbered lines in different colors. Use the same color for parts 3 and 4 and for 6 and 7. Use a dark color for structure 8, because it will be outlined.
3. Label the other parts of the mouth.

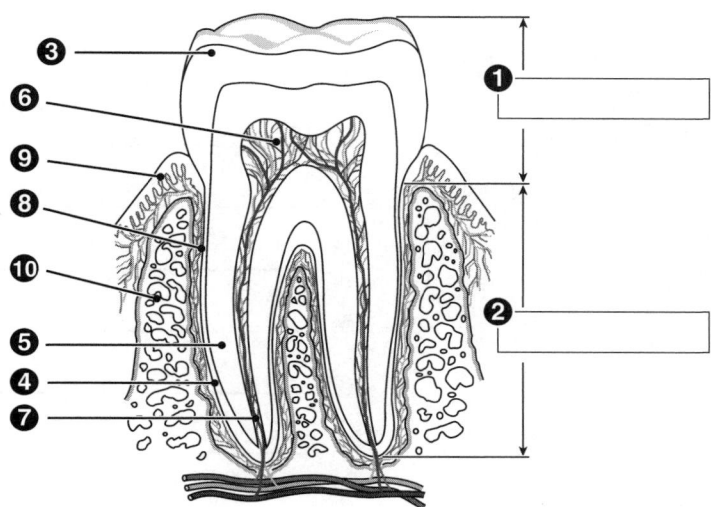

3. _____

4. _____

5. _____

6. _____

7. _____

8. _____

9. _____

10. _____

EXERCISE 17-6: Longitudinal Section of the Stomach (text Fig. 17-7)

INSTRUCTIONS

1. Label the parts of the stomach, esophagus, and duodenum (parts 1–7).
2. Label the layers of the stomach wall (parts 8–11). You can use colors to highlight the different muscular layers.
3. Label the two stomach curvatures (labels 12 and 13).

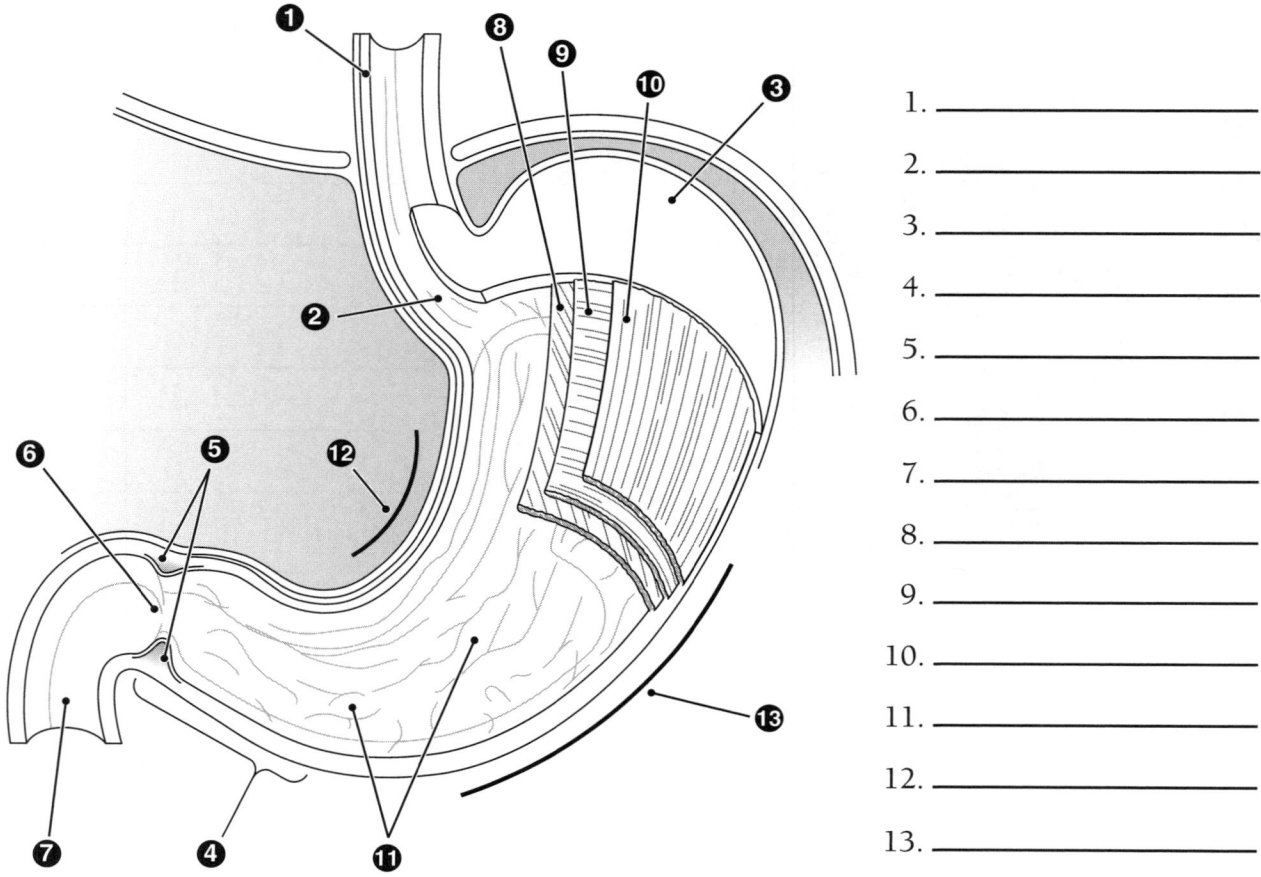

1. _____

2. _____

3. _____

4. _____

5. _____

6. _____

7. _____

8. _____

9. _____

10. _____

11. _____

12. _____

13. _____

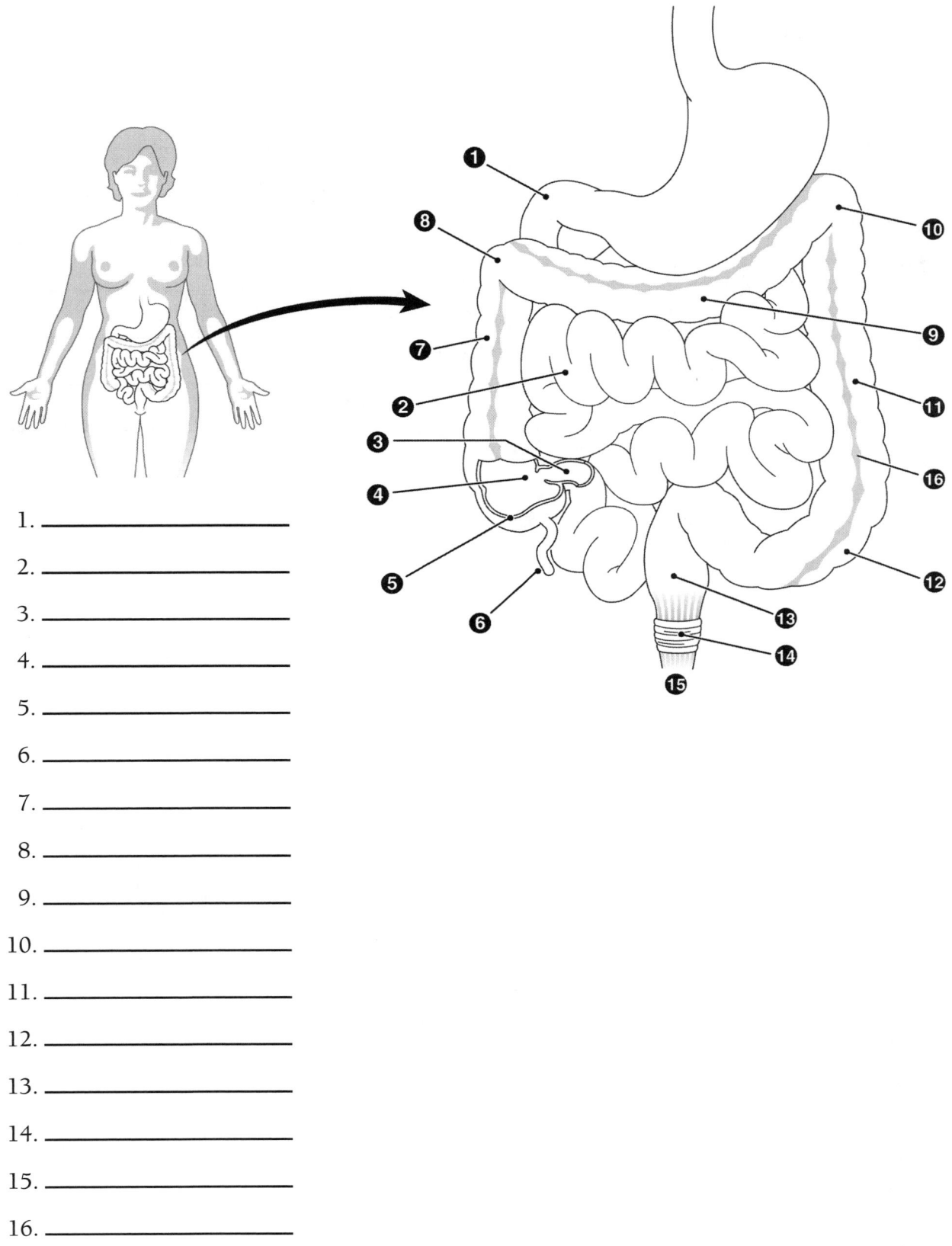

EXERCISE 17-7: The Small and Large Intestines (text Fig. 17-8)
Label the indicated parts.

1. _____

2. _____

3. _____

4. _____

5. _____

6. _____

7. _____

8. _____

9. _____

10. _____

11. _____

12. _____

13. _____

14. _____

15. _____

16. _____

EXERCISE 17-8: Accessory Organs (text Fig. 17-10)

INSTRUCTIONS

1. Write the names of the labeled parts on the appropriate lines in different colors.
2. Color the structures on the diagram.

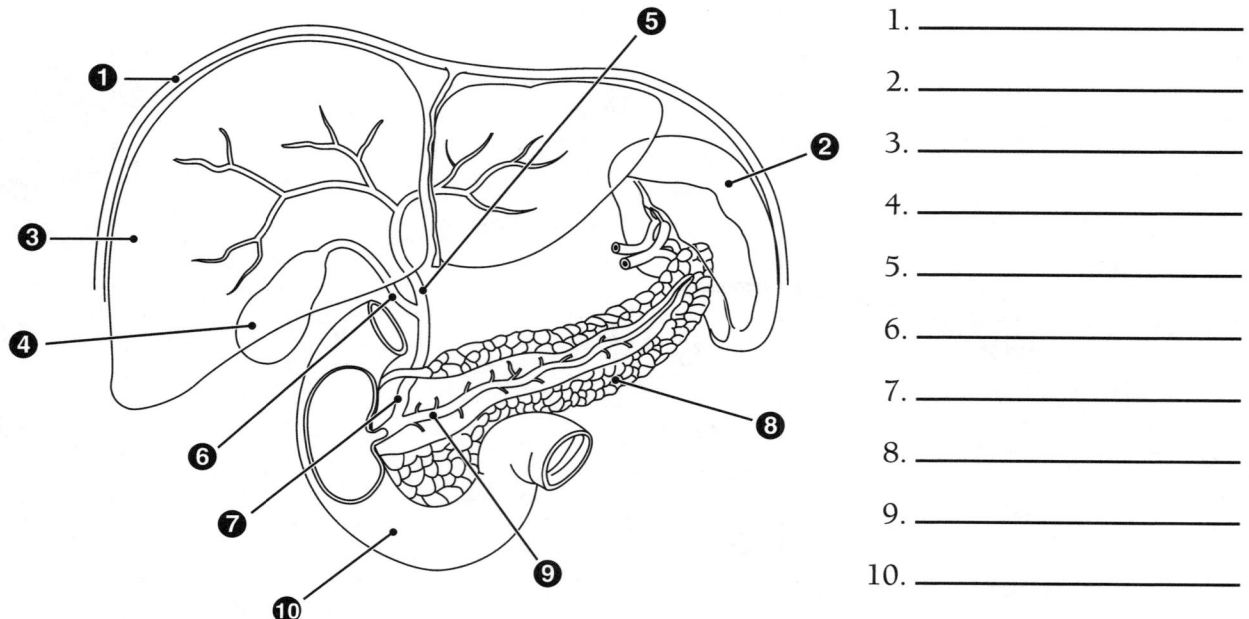

1. _____
2. _____
3. _____
4. _____
5. _____
6. _____
7. _____
8. _____
9. _____
10. _____

Making the Connections

The following concept map deals with the structure and regulation of the gastrointestinal system. Each pair of terms is linked together by a connecting phrase into a sentence. The sentence should be read in the direction of the arrow. Complete the concept map by filling in the appropriate term or phrase. There is one right answer for each term (1, 2, 4, 7, 15–17). However, there are many correct answers for the connecting phrases. Write the phrase beside the appropriate number (if space permits) or on a separate sheet of paper.

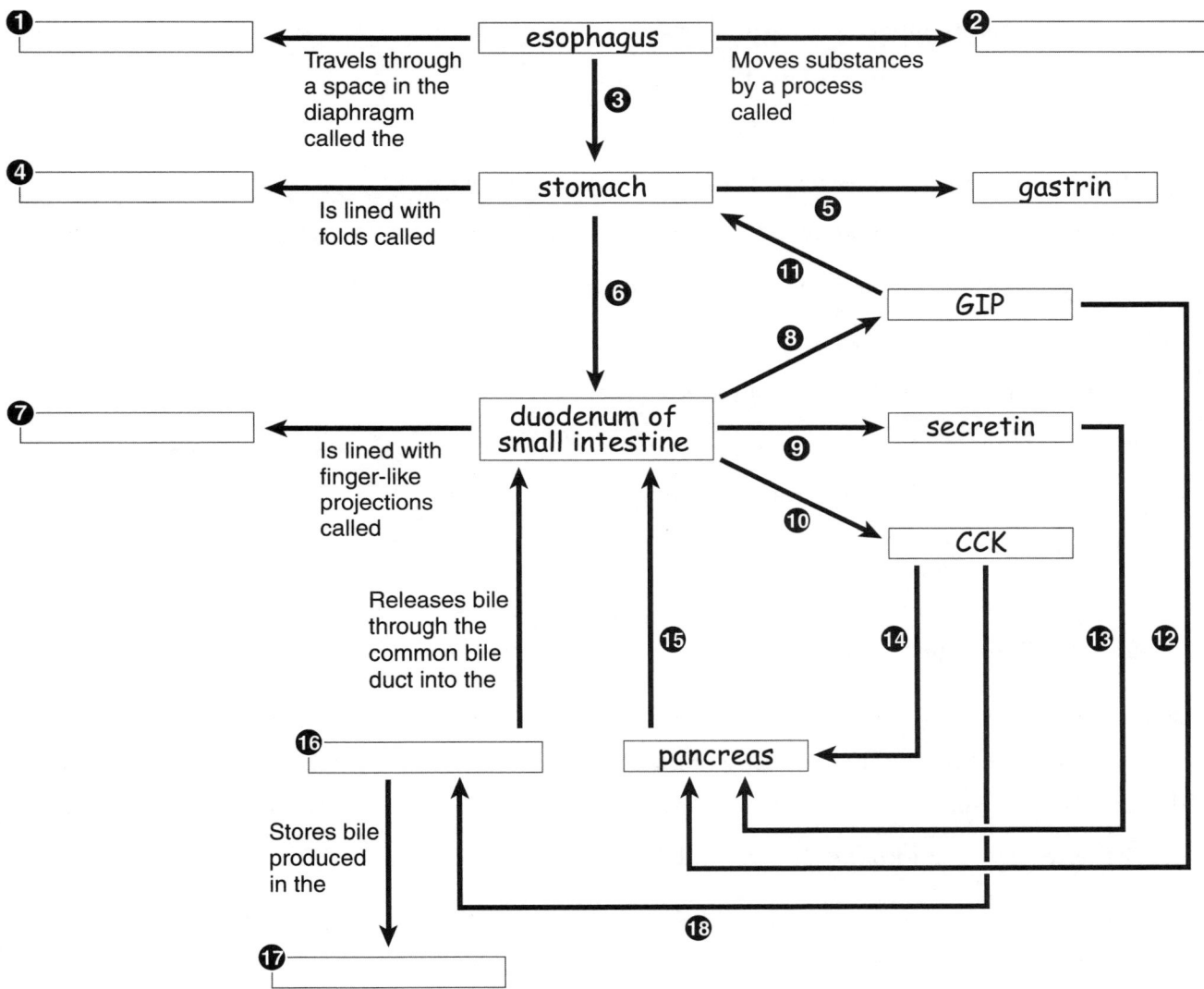

Optional Exercise: Make your own concept map based on the three processes of digestion and how they apply to proteins, sugars, and fats. Choose your own terms to incorporate into your map, or use the following list: digestion, absorption, elimination, stomach, small intestine, large intestine, fats, carbohydrates, proteins, amylase, lipase, bile, hydrochloric acid, pepsin, trypsin, peptidase, maltase.

Testing Your Knowledge
Building Understanding

I. Matching Exercises

Matching only within each group, write the answers in the spaces provided.

➤ **Group A**

digestion	absorption	elimination	mucous membrane	submucosa
serosa	smooth muscle	parietal peritoneum	visceral peritoneum	

1. The transfer of nutrients into the bloodstream _____

2. The serous membrane layer attached to the abdominal wall _____

3. The layer of connective tissue beneath the mucous membrane
   in the wall of the digestive tract _____

4. The layer of the digestive tract wall that is responsible
   for peristalsis _____

5. The breakdown of food into small particles that can
   pass through intestinal cells _____

6. The innermost layer of the serous membrane lining
   the abdominopelvic cavity _____

7. The layer of the digestive tract wall that contains villi
   in the small intestine _____

➤ **Group B**

mesocolon	greater omentum	lesser omentum	deglutition	mastication
deciduous	cuspids	incisors	dentin	gingiva

1. The term that describes the baby teeth, based on the fact
   that they are lost _____

2. The process of chewing _____

3. The act of swallowing _____

4. The layer of the peritoneum extending between the stomach
   and liver _____

5. The medical term for the gum _____

6. The eight cutting teeth located in the anterior of
   the oral cavity _____

7. A calcified substance making up most of the tooth

   structure   _____

8. A large double serous membrane that contains fat and hangs

   over the front of the intestine   _____

➤ Group C

| ileum | hard palate | soft palate | epiglottis | pyloric sphincter |
| LES | rugae | chyme | duodenum | jejunum |

1. The valve between the distal end of the stomach and

   the small intestine   _____

2. The structure that guards the entrance into the stomach   _____

3. A structure that covers the opening of the larynx

   during swallowing   _____

4. The part of the oral cavity roof that extends to form the uvula   _____

5. The final, and longest, section of the small intestine   _____

6. The section of the small intestine that receives gastric juices

   and food from the stomach   _____

7. The mixture of gastric juices and food that enters the

   small intestine   _____

8. Folds in the stomach that are absent if the stomach is full _____

➤ Group D

| villi | lacteal | microvilli | teniae coli | cecum | transverse colon |
| vermiform appendix | sigmoid colon | rectum | ileocecal valve | | |

1. The part of the large intestine just before the anus   _____

2. The small blind tube attached to the first part of the

   large intestine   _____

3. The sphincter that prevents food moving from the large

   intestine into the small intestine   _____

4. Fingerlike extensions of the mucosa in the small intestine   _____

5. A blind-ended lymphatic vessel that absorbs fat   _____

6. Bands of longitudinal muscle in the large intestine   _____

7. The portion of the large intestine that extends across the

   abdomen   _____

8. The most proximal part of the large intestine   _____

➤ Group E

parotid glands	submandibular glands	sublingual glands	gallbladder
liver	pancreas	sodium bicarbonate	lipase
maltose	trypsin	maltase	

1. A pancreatic enzyme that splits proteins into amino acids   _____

2. An enzyme that breaks fats into simpler compounds   _____

3. An organ that stores nutrients and releases them as needed

   into the bloodstream   _____

4. The accessory organ that stores bile   _____

5. An enzyme that acts on a particular type of disaccharide   _____

6. The salivary glands that are inferior and anterior to the ear   _____

7. A substance released into the small intestine that neutralizes

   the acidity in chyme   _____

8. Glands found under the tongue that secrete into the oral cavity   _____

➤ Group F

| bilirubin | glycogen | urea | protein | common bile duct |
| common hepatic duct | cystic duct | hydrolysis | fat | |

1. The splitting of food molecules by the addition of water   _____

2. The form in which glucose is stored in the liver   _____

3. A waste product produced from the destruction of red

   blood cells   _____

4. A waste product synthesized by the liver as a result of

   protein metabolism   _____

5. The duct connecting the hepatic duct to the gallbladder   _____

6. Bile participates in the digestion of this nutrient   _____

7. The nutrient type that is partially digested by gastric juice   _____

➤ **Group G**

| gastrin | cholecystokinin | secretin | gastric-inhibitory peptide |
| nuclease | pepsin | trypsin | |

1. A hormone that stimulates the secretion of gastric juice and

   increases stomach motility   _____

2. A hormone released from the duodenum that stimulates the

   pancreas to release bicarbonate solution   _____

3. An intestinal hormone that causes the gallbladder to contract,

   releasing bile   _____

4. A substance that digests DNA   _____

5. An enzyme that digests proteins in the stomach   _____

II. Multiple Choice

Select the best answer and write the letter of your choice in the blank.

1. Which teeth would NOT be found in a 20-year-old male?   1. _____
   a. bicuspid
   b. cuspid
   c. deciduous
   d. incisor
2. Which of the following is the correct order of tissue from the innermost
   to the outermost layer in the wall of the digestive tract?   2. _____
   a. submucosa, serous membrane, smooth muscle, mucous membrane
   b. smooth muscle, serous membrane, mucous membrane, submucosa
   c. serous membrane, smooth muscle, submucosa, mucosa
   d. mucous membrane, submucosa, smooth muscle, serous membrane
3. The parotid salivary gland is located: 3. _____
   a. inferior and anterior to the ear
   b. under the tongue
   c. in the cheek
   d. in the oropharynx
4. Which of the following is NOT a portion of the peritoneum?   4. _____
   a. mesocolon
   b. mesentery
   c. hiatus
   d. greater omentum
5. The active ingredients in gastric juice are: 5. _____
   a. amylase and pepsin
   b. pepsin and hydrochloric acid
   c. maltase and secretin
   d. bile and trypsin

6. Gastric-inhibitory peptide stimulates the release of: 6. _____
   a. gastric juice
   b. insulin
   c. bicarbonate
   d. none of the above
7. In the adult, fats are digested in the: 7. _____
   a. mouth
   b. stomach
   c. small intestine
   d. all of the above
8. Which of the following does NOT occur in the mouth?   8. _____
   a. mastication
   b. digestion of starch
   c. absorption of nutrients
   d. ingestion
9. Which of the following is an enzyme?   9. _____
   a. bile
   b. gastrin
   c. trypsin
   d. secretin
10. Which of the following is associated with the intestine?   10. _____
   a. rugae
   b. lacteals
   c. LES
   d. greater curvature

III. Completion Exercise

Write the word or phrase that correctly completes each sentence.

1. The process by which ingested nutrients are broken down
   into smaller components is called   _____

2. The lower part of the colon bends into an S shape, so this
   part is called the   _____

3. A temporary storage section for indigestible and unabsorbable
   waste products of digestion is a tube called the   _____

4. The wavelike movement created by alternating muscle
   contractions in the esophagus is called   _____

5. Most of the digestive juices contain substances that cause the
   chemical breakdown of foods without entering into the
   reaction themselves. These catalytic agents are   _____

6. The portion of the peritoneum extending between the
   stomach and liver is called the   _____

7. The process of swallowing is called   _____

8. Teeth are largely composed of a calcified substance called   _____

9. The esophagus passes through the diaphragm at a point
   called the   _____

10. The hormone that stimulates gallbladder contraction is called   _____

11. Small projecting folds in the plasma membrane of intestinal epithelial cells are called _____

12. The stomach enzyme involved in protein digestion is called _____

Understanding Concepts

I. True or False

For each question, write "T" for true or "F" for false in the blank to the left of each number. If a statement is false, correct it by replacing the underlined term and write the correct statement in the blank below the question.

_____ 1. There are 32 deciduous teeth.

_____ 2. The layer of the peritoneum attached to the liver is the visceral peritoneum.

_____ 3. Ms. Q is deficient in lactase. She will be unable to digest some carbohydrates.

_____ 4. Trypsin is secreted by the gastric glands.

_____ 5. Increased acidity in the chyme could be neutralized by the actions of the hormone gastrin.

_____ 6. Fats are absorbed into capillaries in the intestinal villi.

_____ 7. The middle section of the small intestine is called the jejunum.

_____ 8. Folds in the stomach wall are called villi.

_____ 9. The common bile duct delivers bile from the gall bladder into the duodenum.

_____ 10. Amylase is involved in the digestion of carbohydrates.

_____ 11. The pancreas is responsible for the synthesis of urea.

II. Practical Applications

Study each discussion. Then write the appropriate word or phrase in the space provided.

1. Mr. P, age 42, came to the clinic reporting pain in the "pit of the stomach." He was a tense man who divided his long working hours with coffee and cigarette breaks. When asked about his alcohol consumption, Mr. C mentioned that he drank 3 or 4 beers and 1 glass of wine each night, and significantly more on the weekends. Endoscopy showed inflammation of the innermost layer of the stomach. This layer is called the _____

2. A damaged area was also found in the most proximal part of the small intestine. This section of the small intestine is called the _____

3. Mr. P had an ulcer diagnosed and was given a prescription for antibiotics. The antibiotics will eliminate the *H. pylori* bacterium involved in ulcer formation. Mr. P was also given a medication to inhibit the release of the hormone that stimulates gastric juice secretion. This hormone is called _____

4. The physician had almost completed her physical examination of Mr. P when she felt the edge of his liver only 5 cm (2 in) below the ribs. She also noticed that the whites of his eyes were tinged with yellow. The yellow coloration results from the release of a hepatic secretion into the bloodstream. This secretion, which is needed for the digestion of fat, is called _____

5. Based on her clinical findings and Mr. P's self-reported alcohol abuse, the physician suspected that Mr. P has cirrhosis, a chronic liver disease. However, further testing revealed that Mr. P's liver function was normal. His jaundice was due to a blockage in the duct that empties bile into the duodenum, the _____

III. Short Essays

1. Describe some features of the small intestine that increase the surface area for absorption of nutrients.

_____

_____

_____

2. List four differences between the digestion and/or absorption of fats and proteins.

_____

_____

_____

Conceptual Thinking

1. Ms. M is taking a drug that blocks the action of cholecystokinin. Discuss the impact of this drug on digestion.

_____

_____

_____

2. Is bile an enzyme? Explain your answer.

_____

_____

_____

Expanding Your Horizons

A growing number of young women (and even some young men) are "dying to be thin." Because of eating disorders, they starve themselves and/or binge-and-purge, sometimes to death. You can learn more about eating disorders by viewing the PBS Nova program "Dying to Be Thin," which is available through the PBS web site (http://shop.wgbh.org). The following two journal articles discuss eating disorders from a nurse's perspective.

Resource List

Clark-Stone S, Joyce H. Understanding eating disorders. Nurs Times 2003;99:20–23.
Murphy B, Manning Y. An introduction to anorexia nervosa and bulimia nervosa. Nurs Stand 2003;18:45–52.

chapter 18

Metabolism, Nutrition, and Body Temperature

Overview

The nutrients that reach the cells after digestion and absorption are used to maintain life. All the physical and chemical reactions that occur within the cells make up **metabolism**, which has two phases: a breakdown phase, or **catabolism**, and a building phase, or **anabolism**. Nutrients are oxidized to yield energy for the cells in the form of ATP using catabolic reactions. This process, termed **cellular respiration**, occurs in two steps: the first is **anaerobic** (does not require oxygen) and produces a small amount of energy; the second is **aerobic** (requires oxygen). This second step occurs within the mitochondria of the cells. It yields a large amount of the energy contained in the nutrient plus carbon dioxide and water.

By the various pathways of metabolism, the breakdown products of food can be built into substances needed by the body. The **essential** amino acids and fatty acids cannot be manufactured internally and must be ingested in food. **Minerals** and **vitamins** are also needed in the diet for health. A balanced diet includes carbohydrates, proteins, and fats consumed in amounts relative to individual activity levels.

The rate at which energy is released from nutrients is termed the **metabolic rate**. It is affected by many factors including age, size, sex, activity, and hormones. Some of the energy in nutrients is released in the form of heat. Heat production is greatly increased during periods of increased muscular or glandular activity. Most heat is lost through through the skin, but heat is also dissipated through exhaled air and eliminated waste products (urine and feces). The **hypothalamus** maintains body temperature at approximately 37°C (98.6°F) by altering blood flow through the surface blood vessels and the activity of sweat glands and muscles.

Learning the Language: Word Anatomy

Word Part	Meaning	Example
1. -lysis	_____	_____
2. _____	sugar, sweet	_____

Addressing the Learning Outcomes

I. Writing Exercise

The learning outcomes for Chapter 18 are listed below. These learning outcomes provide an overview of the major topics covered in this chapter. On a separate piece of paper, try to write out an answer to each Learning Outcome. All of the answers can be found in the pages of the textbook.

1. Differentiate between catabolism and anabolism.
2. Differentiate between the anaerobic and aerobic phases of cellular respiration and give the end products and the relative amount of energy released by each.
3. Define metabolic rate and name several factors that affect the metabolic rate.
4. Explain the roles of glucose and glycogen in metabolism.
5. Compare the energy contents of fats, proteins, and carbohydrates.
6. Define essential amino acid.
7. Explain the roles of minerals and vitamins in nutrition and give examples of each.
8. List the recommended percentages of carbohydrate, fat, and protein in the diet.
9. Distinguish between simple and complex carbohydrates, giving examples of each.
10. Compare saturated and unsaturated fats.
11. List some adverse effects of alcohol consumption.
12. Explain how heat is produced and lost in the body.
13. Describe the role of the hypothalamus in regulating body temperature.
14. Show how word parts are used to build words related to metabolism, nutrition, and body temperature.

Making the Connections

The following concept map deals with nutrition and metabolism. Each pair of terms is linked together by a connecting phrase into a sentence. The sentence should be read in the direction of the arrow. Complete the concept map by filling in the appropriate term or phrase. There is one right answer for each term (1–3, and 8). However, there are many correct answers for the connecting phrases. Write your phrases beside the appropriate number (if space permits) or on a separate piece of paper.

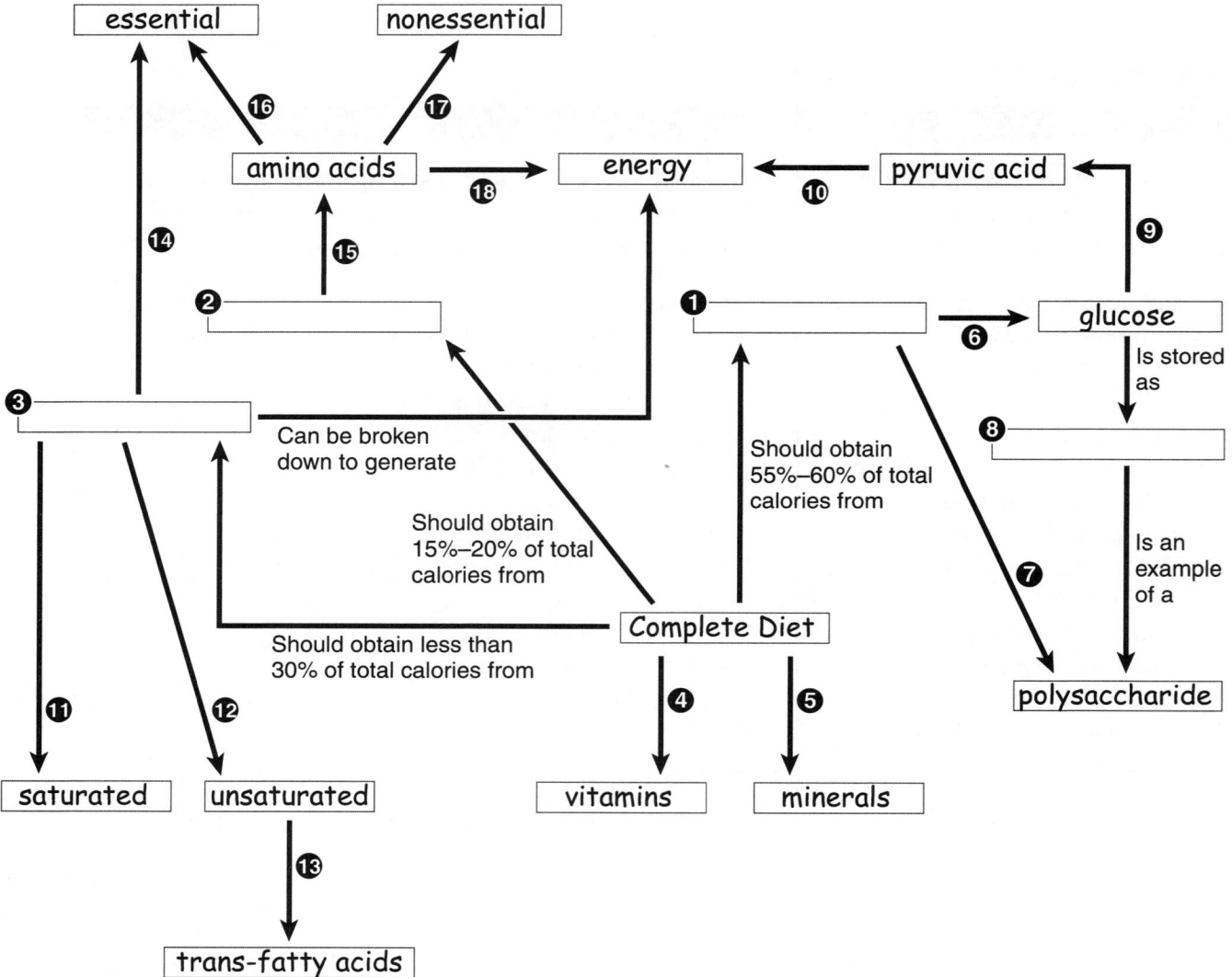

Optional Exercise: Make your own concept map based on the regulation of body temperature. Choose your own terms to incorporate into your map, or use the following list: body temperature, hypothalamus, sweating, shivering, dilation, constriction, skin, respiratory system, radiation, convection, conduction, evaporation.

Testing Your Knowledge
Building Understanding

I. Matching Exercises

Matching only within each group, write the answers in the spaces provided.

➤ Group A

anabolism	catabolism	glycolysis	lactic acid	pyruvic acid
anaerobic	aerobic	glycogen	deamination	

1. A term that describes any reaction that does not require oxygen _____

2. The metabolic breakdown of complex compounds _____

3. The storage form of glucose _____

4. The metabolic building of simple compounds into substances needed by cells _____

5. A modification of amino acids that occurs before they can be oxidized for energy _____

6. An organic product of glucose catabolism that can be completely oxidized within the mitochondria _____

7. An organic substance produced when a muscle is generating energy in the absence of oxygen _____

8. The first anaerobic phase of cellular respiration _____

➤ Group B

trans-fatty acids	unsaturated fats	essential amino acids	nonessential amino acids
monosaccharides	vitamins	minerals	antioxidants
saturated fats	polysaccharides		

1. Fats that are usually of animal origin and are solid at room temperature _____

2. Fats that are artificially saturated to prevent rancidity _____

3. Complex organic molecules that are essential for metabolism _____

4. Protein components that must be taken in as part of the diet _____

5. Inorganic elements needed for proper nutrition _____

6. Protein building blocks that can be manufactured by the body _____

7. A class of substances that stabilizes free radicals _____

8. Carbohydrates with a low glycemic effect _____

➤ Group C

zinc	iodine	iron	potassium	calcium
folate	calciferol	riboflavin	vitamin A	vitamin K

1. The vitamin that prevents dry, scaly skin and night blindness _____

2. The vitamin needed to prevent anemia, digestive disorders,

    and neural tube defects in the embryo _____

3. Another name for vitamin D_3, the vitamin required for

    normal bone formation _____

4. The mineral component of thyroid hormones _____

5. A mineral important in blood clotting and muscle contraction _____

6. The characteristic element in hemoglobin, the oxygen-

    carrying compound in the blood _____

7. A mineral that promotes carbon dioxide transport and

    energy metabolism _____

8. A vitamin involved in the synthesis of blood clotting factors

    that can be synthesized by colonic bacteria _____

➤ Group D

evaporation	conduction	epinephrine	dilation	constriction
98	37	radiation		

1. A response in the superficial blood vessels that increases

    heat loss _____

2. A normal body temperature measured by the Celsius scale _____

3. The transfer of heat to the surrounding air _____

4. The change that occurs in blood vessels of the skin if too much

    heat is being lost from the body _____

5. Heat loss resulting from the conversion of a liquid, such as

    perspiration, to a vapor _____

II. Multiple Choice

Select the best answer and write the letter of your choice in the blank.

1. The brain region involved in temperature regulation is the: 1. _____
    a. thalamus
    b. cerebral cortex
    c. hippocampus
    d. hypothalamus

2. A complete protein contains: 2. _____
    a. all the amino acids
    b. all the essential fatty acids
    c. a variety of minerals
    d. all the essential amino acids

3. Deamination is: 3. _____
    a. an anabolic reaction
    b. the conversion of proteins into amino acids
    c. the conversion of glucose into glycogen
    d. the removal of a nitrogen group from an amino acid

4. Conventional nutritional guidelines suggest that daily caloric intake
  should be divided between the three nutrient types as follows: 4. _____
    a. 55% protein, 30% fat, 15% carbohydrate
    b. 33% protein, 33% fat, 33% carbohydrate
    c. 60% carbohydrate, 25% fat, 15% protein
    d. 55% carbohydrate, 30% protein, 15% fat

5. The end product of the anaerobic phase of glucose metabolism is: 5. _____
    a. glycogen
    b. pyruvic acid
    c. folic acid
    d. tocopherol

6. Trace elements in the diet are: 6. _____
    a. sugars with a high glycemic effect
    b. vitamins needed in very small amounts
    c. minerals needed in large quantity
    d. minerals needed in very small amounts

7. Profuse sweating increases heat lost by the process of: 7. _____
    a. radiation
    b. evaporation
    c. convection
    d. none of the above

8. Unsaturated fats: 8. _____
    a. are generally healthier than saturated fats
    b. can be converted into trans fats
    c. contain double bonds between the carbon atoms
    d. all of the above

9. Which of the following is an example of an anabolic reaction?   9. _____
    a. glycerol and fatty acids are used to form a fat
    b. starches and glycogen are converted into glucose
    c. a short peptide is converted into arginine and cysteine
    d. glucose is completely oxidized to carbon dioxide and water

III. Completion Exercise

Write the word or phrase that correctly completes each sentence.

1. The unit used to measure energy is the   _____
2. The amount of energy needed to accomplish necessary cell
  functions at rest is termed the   _____

3. Shivering generates additional body heat by increasing the
   activity of the _____

4. Organic substances needed in small amounts in the diet
   are the _____

5. The most important heat-regulating center is a section of the
   brain called the _____

6. The series of reactions that results in the release of energy
   from nutrients is called _____

7. Heat that is moved away from the skin by the wind is lost by
   the process of _____

8. Glycolysis occurs in the part of the cell called the _____

9. Fatty acids that must be consumed in the diet are called _____

Understanding Concepts

I. True or False

For each question, write "T" for true or "F" for false in the blank to the left of each number. If a statement is false, correct it by replacing the underlined term and write the correct statement in the blank below the question.

_____ 1. A body temperature of 35°C is abnormally low.

_____

_____ 2. Grapeseed oil is liquid at room temperature. This oil is most likely a saturated fat.

_____

_____ 3. The conversion of glycogen into glucose is an example of a catabolic reaction.

_____

_____ 4. Most heat loss in the body occurs through the skin.

_____

_____ 5. The element nitrogen is found in all sugars.

_____

_____ 6. Mr. B is training for an upcoming road race by doing sprints. His leg muscles are working anaerobically. The pyruvic acid accumulating in his muscles may be responsible for
   the fatigue he is experiencing.

_____

_____ 7. The rate at which energy is released from nutrients in Mr. B's cells during his sprints is
   called his basal metabolism.

_____

_____ 8. Pernicious anemia is caused by a deficiency in vitamin B12.

_____

_____ 9. Linoleic acid is an example of an <u>essential amino acid</u>.

_____

_____ 10. Copper and calcium are examples of <u>vitamins</u>.

_____

_____ 11. Body temperature is regulated by the <u>medulla oblongata</u> in the brain.

_____

II. Practical Applications

Ms. S is researching penguin behavior at a remote location in Antarctica. She will be camping on the ice for 2 months. Study each discussion. Then write the appropriate word or phrase in the space provided.

1. Ms. S is spending her first night on the ice. She is careful to wear many layers of clothing to avoid a dangerous drop in body temperature. The extra clothing will reduce the direct transfer of heat from Ms S's body to the surrounding air by the process of _____

2. She is out for a moonlight walk to greet the penguins when she surprises an elephant seal stalking a penguin. Frightened, she sprints back to her tent. Her muscles are generating ATP by an oxygen-independent pathway. Each glucose molecule is generating a small number of ATP molecules or, to be exact, _____

3. The next morning, Ms. S has soreness in her leg muscles. She attributes the soreness to the accumulation of a byproduct of anaerobic metabolism called _____

4. This byproduct must be converted into another substance before it can be completely oxidized. This substance is called _____

5. After 2 weeks on the ice, Ms. S is out of fresh fruits and vegetables, and the penguins have stolen her multivitamin supplements. She has been reading accounts of early explorers with scurvy and fears she will experience the same fate. Scurvy is caused by a deficiency of _____

6. Ms. S's diet is now reduced to luncheon meat and crackers. The crackers are still tasty because they contain significant amounts of artificially hydrogenated fats, known as _____

7. She looks forward to eating her normal diet when she returns home, which is rich in fruits, vegetables, and complex carbohydrates, also known as _____

8. Ms. S hikes to a distant penguin colony on her final day on the ice. She is dressed very warmly, and the sun is very bright. After several hours of hiking, Ms. S is sweating profusely, so she removes some clothing to cool off. Some excess heat will be lost through the evaporation of sweat. The wind will also increase heat loss by the process called _____

III. Short Essays

1. Is alcohol a nutrient? Defend your answer.

_____

_____

_____

2. A glucose molecule has been transported into a muscle cell. This cell has ample supplies of oxygen. Discuss the steps involved in using this glucose to produce energy. For each step, describe its location and oxygen requirements and name the substances produced.

_____

_____

_____

Conceptual Thinking

1. Your friend wants to lose some weight. She is following a diet that contains 20% carbohydrates, 40% fat, and 40% protein. Why is this diet designed to limit fat deposition? You may have to review the actions of pancreatic hormones (see Chapter 12) to answer this question.

_____

_____

_____

Expanding Your Horizons

The classic food pyramid emphasizes the consumption of high levels of carbohydrates and low levels of fat. However, most modern diet plans (_e.g._, the Atkins diet, the Zone, the South Beach diet) are low-carbohydrate and often high-fat, reflecting recent research into fat metabolism and the glycemic effect. Which approach is best? The following article discusses a new food pyramid that incorporates the new research but does not ignore the sound physiological ideas behind the original food pyramid.

Resource List

Willett WC, Stampfer MJ. Rebuilding the food pyramid. Sci Am 2003;288:64–71.

chapter 19

The Urinary System and Body Fluids

Overview

The urinary system comprises two **kidneys**, two **ureters**, one **urinary bladder**, and one **urethra.** This system is thought of as the body's main excretory mechanism; it is, in fact, often called the **excretory system.** The kidney, however, performs other essential functions; it aids in maintaining water and electrolyte balance and in regulating the acid–base balance (pH) of body fluids. The kidneys also secrete a hormone that stimulates red blood cell production and an enzyme that acts to increase blood pressure.

The functional unit of the kidney is the **nephron.** It is the nephron that produces **urine** from substances filtered out of the blood through a cluster of capillaries, the **glomerulus.** The processes involved in urine formation in addition to filtration are tubular reabsorption, tubular secretion, and concentration of urine. Oxygenated blood is brought to the kidney by the **renal artery.** The arterial system branches through the kidney until the smallest subdivision, the **afferent arteriole**, carries blood into the glomerulus. Blood leaves the glomerulus by means of the **efferent arteriole** and eventually leaves the kidney by means of the **renal vein.** Before blood enters the venous network of the kidney, exchanges occur between the filtrate and the blood through the **peritubular capillaries** that surround each nephron.

The majority (50% to 70%) of a person's body weight is **water**. This water serves as a solvent, a transport medium, and a participant in metabolic reactions. A variety of substances are dissolved in this water, including electrolytes, nutrients, gases, enzymes, hormones, and waste products. Body fluids are distributed in two main compartments: (1) the **intracellular fluid** compartment located within the cells, and (2) the **extracellular fluid** compartment located outside the cells. The latter category includes blood plasma, interstitial fluid, lymph, and fluids in special compartments, such as the humors of the eye, cerebrospinal fluid, serous fluids, and synovial fluids.

Water balance is maintained by matching fluid intake with fluid output. Fluid intake is stimulated by the thirst center in the **hypothalamus,** although humans often consume inadequate or insufficient fluids. Normally, the amount of fluid taken in with food and beverages equals the amount of fluid lost through the skin and the respiratory, digestive, and urinary tracts.

The composition of intracellular and extracellular fluids is an important factor in homeostasis. These fluids must have the proper levels of electrolytes and must be kept at a constant pH. The kidneys are the main regulators of body fluids. Other factors that aid in regulation include hormones, buffers, and respiration. The normal pH of body fluids is a slightly alkaline 7.4.

Learning the Language: Word Anatomy

Word Part	Meaning	Example
1. _____	night	_____
2. intra-	_____	_____
3. _____	partial, half	_____
4. osmo-	_____	_____
5. nephr/o-	_____	_____
6. _____	many	_____
7. _____	backward, behind	_____
8. _____	next to	_____
9. ren/o	_____	_____
10. extra-	_____	_____

Addressing the Learning Outcomes

I. Writing Exercise

The learning outcomes for Chapter 19 are listed below. These learning outcomes provide an overview of the major topics covered in this chapter. On a separate piece of paper, try to write out an answer to each learning outcome. All of the answers can be found in the pages of the textbook. Learning Outcomes 2–6 and 10–12 are also addressed in the Coloring Atlas.

1. List the systems that eliminate waste and name the substances eliminated by each.
2. Describe the parts of the urinary system and give the functions of each.
3. Trace the path of a drop of blood as it flows through the kidney.
4. Describe a nephron.
5. Describe the components and functions of the juxtaglomerular (JG) apparatus.
6. Name the four processes involved in urine formation and describe the action of each.
7. Identify the role of ADH in urine formation.
8. Describe the process of micturition.
9. Name three normal constituents of urine.
10. Compare intracellular and extracellular fluids.
11. List four types of extracellular fluids.
12. Name the systems that are involved in water balance.
13. Explain how thirst is regulated.
14. Define *electrolytes* and describe some of their functions.
15. Describe the role of hormones in electrolyte balance.
16. Describe three methods for regulating the pH of body fluids.
17. Show how word parts are used to build words related to the urinary system and body fluids.

II. Labeling and Coloring Atlas

EXERCISE 19-1: Male Urinary System (text Fig. 19-1)

INSTRUCTIONS

1. Write the names of the arteries on the appropriate numbered lines in red, and color the arteries (except for the small box) on the diagram.
2. Write the names of the veins on the appropriate numbered lines in blue, and color the veins (except for the small box) on the diagram.
3. Write the names of the remaining structures on the appropriate numbered lines in different colors, and color the structures on the diagram.
4. Put arrows in the small boxes to indicate the direction of blood/urine movement.

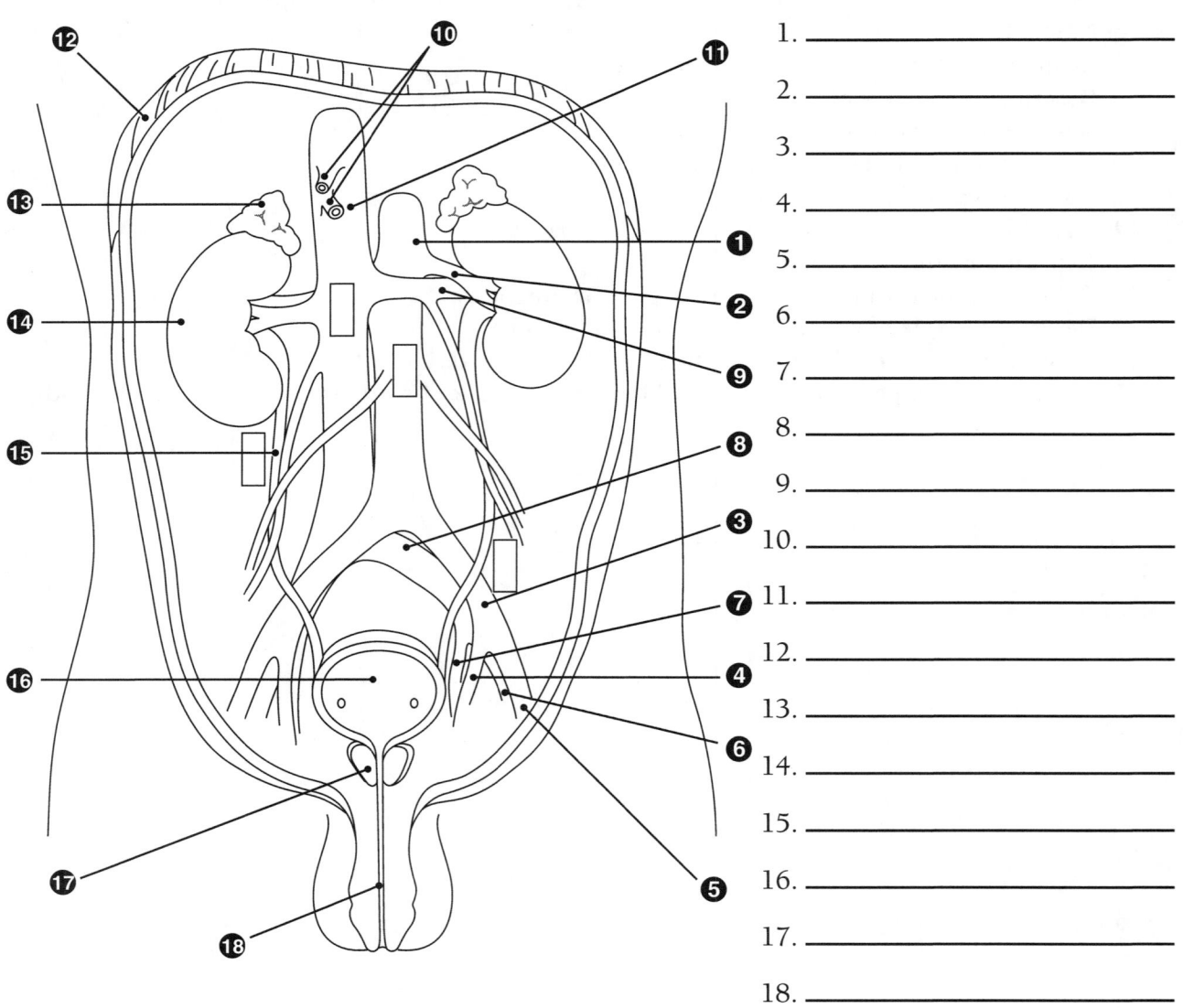

1. _____
2. _____
3. _____
4. _____
5. _____
6. _____
7. _____
8. _____
9. _____
10. _____
11. _____
12. _____
13. _____
14. _____
15. _____
16. _____
17. _____
18. _____

EXERCISE 19-2: Longitudinal Section Through the Kidney (text Figs. 19-2 & 19-3)

INSTRUCTIONS

1. Write the names of the blood vessels on lines 1 and 2 (vessel 1 drains from the abdominal aorta and vessel 2 drains into the inferior vena cava). Use red for the artery and blue for the vein.
2. Color the artery and arterioles on the diagram red and the veins and venules blue.
3. Write the names of the remaining structures on the appropriate numbered lines in different colors, and color the structures on the diagram. Use the same, dark color for structures 3 and
4. Use the same color for structures 6 and 7. Use yellow for structures 8 to 10.

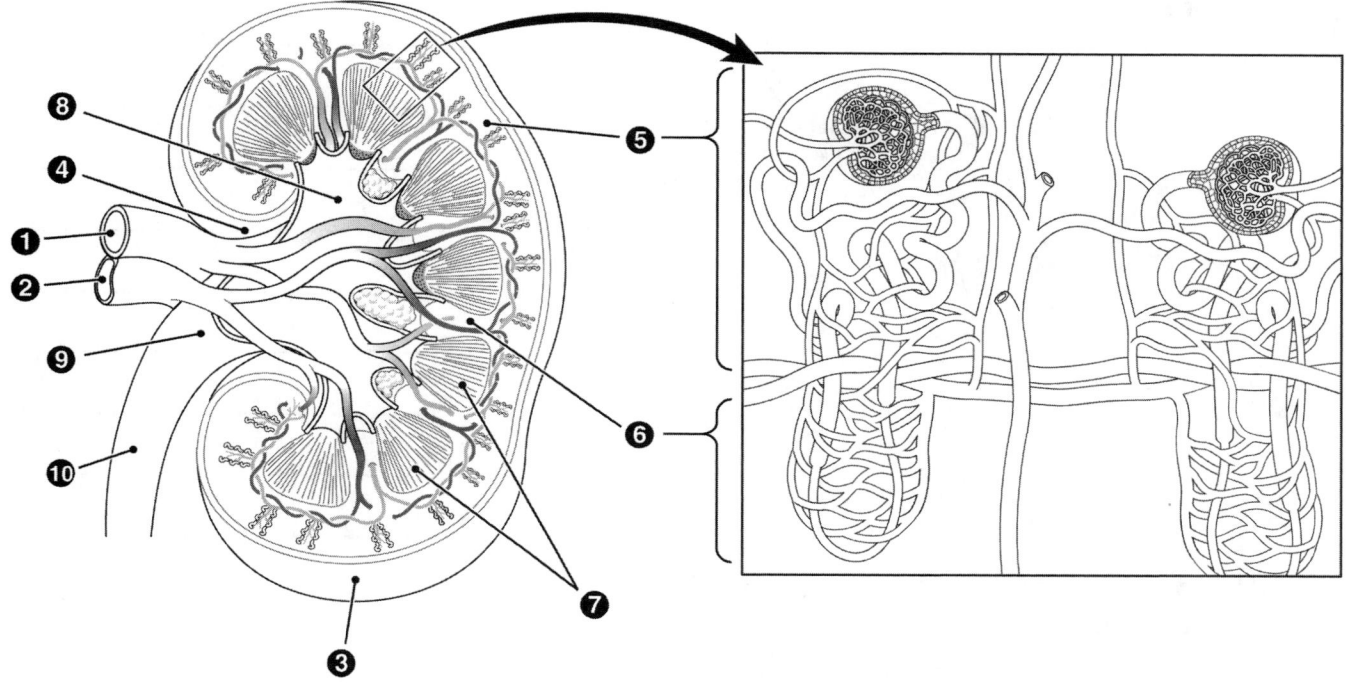

1. _____

2. _____

3. _____

4. _____

5. _____

6. _____

7. _____

8. _____

9. _____

10. _____

EXERCISE 19-3: A Nephron and its Blood Supply (text Fig. 19-4)

INSTRUCTIONS

1. Follow the passage of blood by labeling structures 1 to 6. Use different shades of red for the arteries/arterioles, purple for the capillaries, and blue for the venules/veins. Lines indicate the boundaries between different vessels.
2. Follow the passage of filtrate through the nephron by labeling structures 7 to 13. Use different colors (perhaps shades of yellow and orange) for the different structures. Lines indicate the boundaries between the different nephron parts.

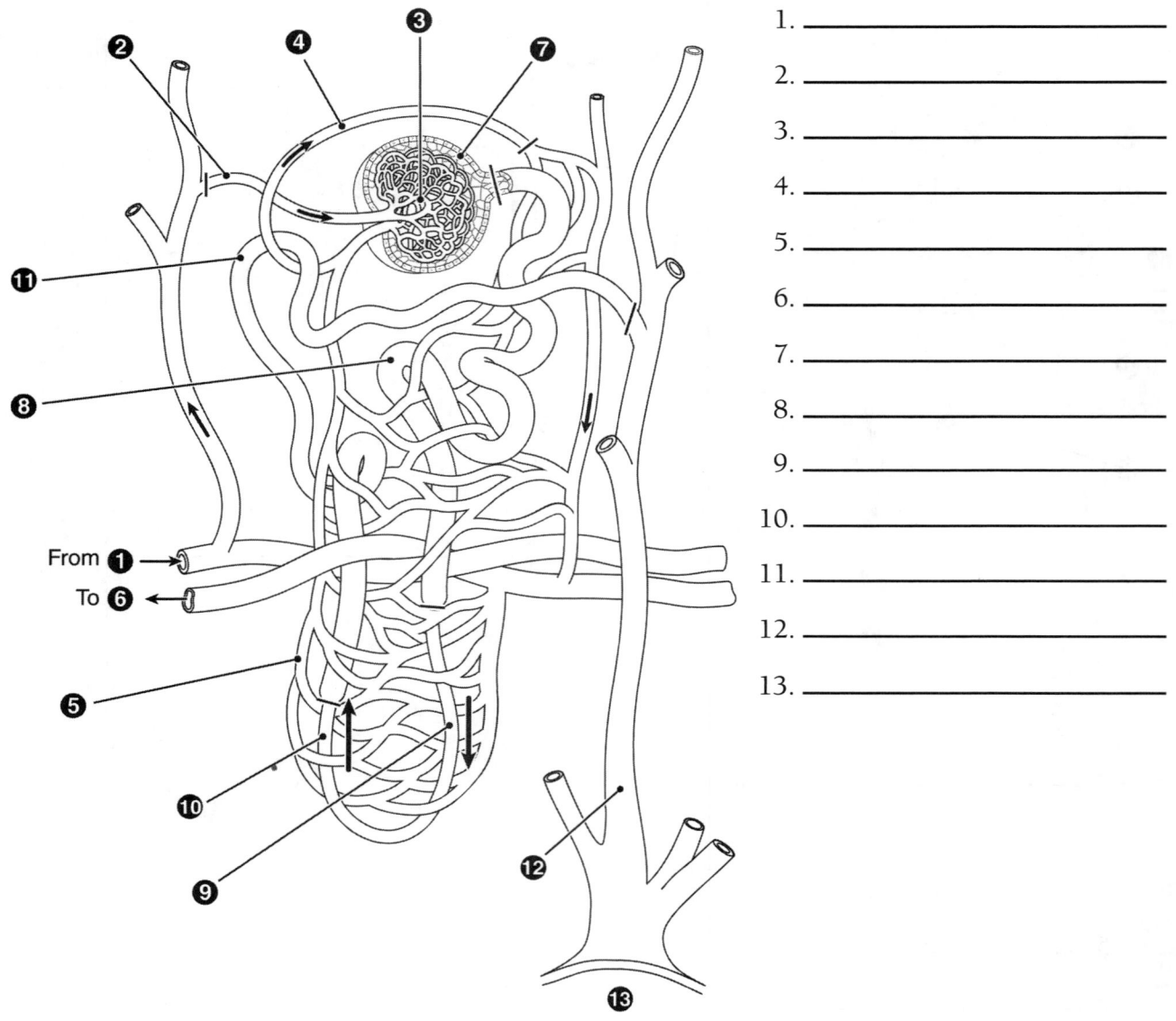

1. _____
2. _____
3. _____
4. _____
5. _____
6. _____
7. _____
8. _____
9. _____
10. _____
11. _____
12. _____
13. _____

EXERCISE 19-4: Structure of the Juxtaglomerular (JG) Apparatus (text Fig. 19-6)
INSTRUCTIONS

1. Write the names of the different structures on the appropriate numbered lines in different colors, and color the structures on the diagram.
2. Use different shades of red for structures 1 to 3. Use a dark color for structure 8. Some structures have appeared on earlier diagrams. You may want to use the same color scheme.

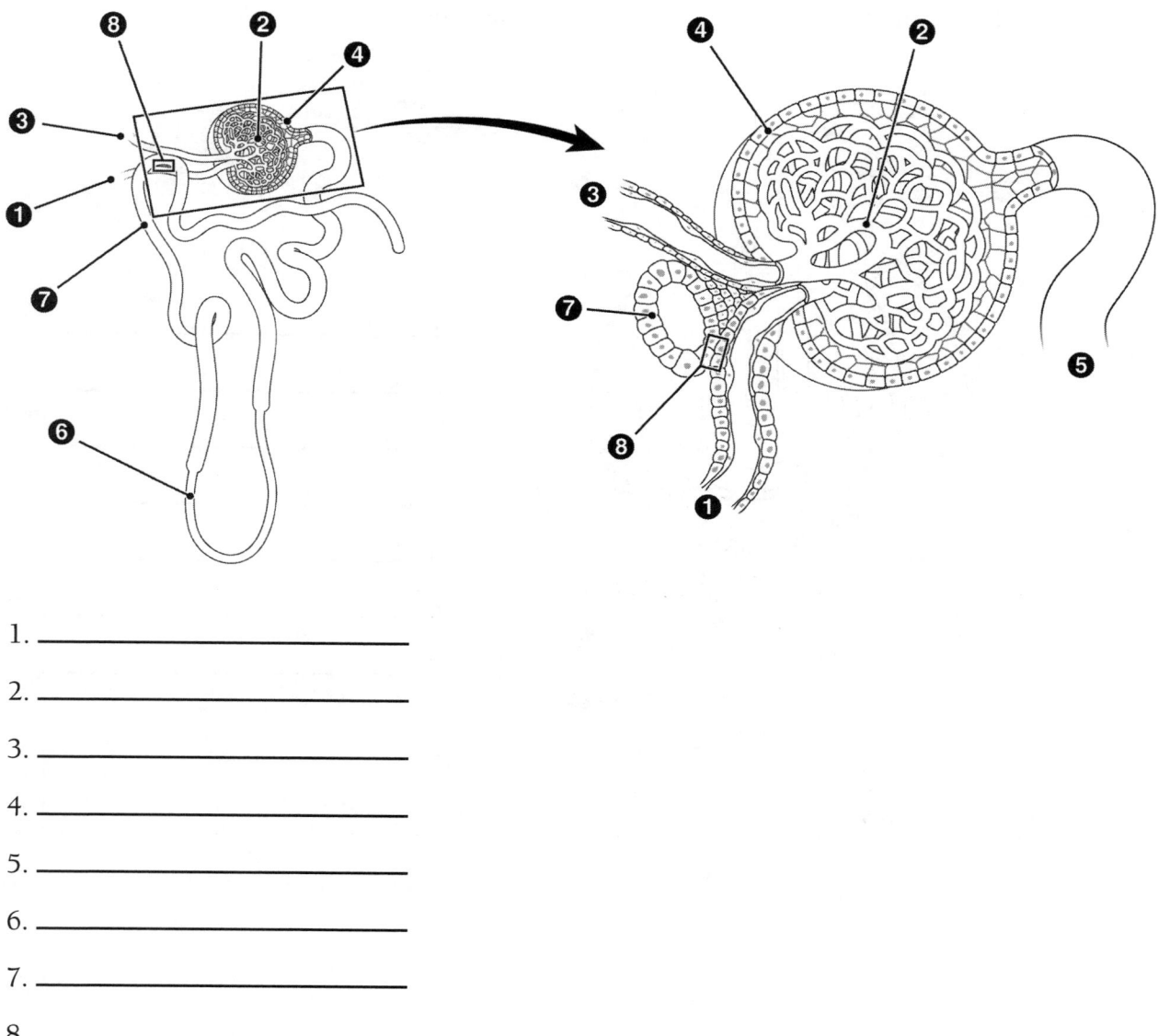

1. _____

2. _____

3. _____

4. _____

5. _____

6. _____

7. _____

8. _____

EXERCISE 19-5: Filtration Process (text Fig. 19-7)

INSTRUCTIONS

1. Write the names of the different parts on the appropriate numbered lines in different colors, and color them on the diagram. Use different shades of red for structures 1 to 3, and yellow for part 7. Do not color over the symbols. Some structures have appeared on earlier diagrams. You may want to use the same color scheme.
2. Color the symbols beside "soluble molecules," "proteins," and "blood cells" in different dark colors and color the corresponding symbols on the diagram.

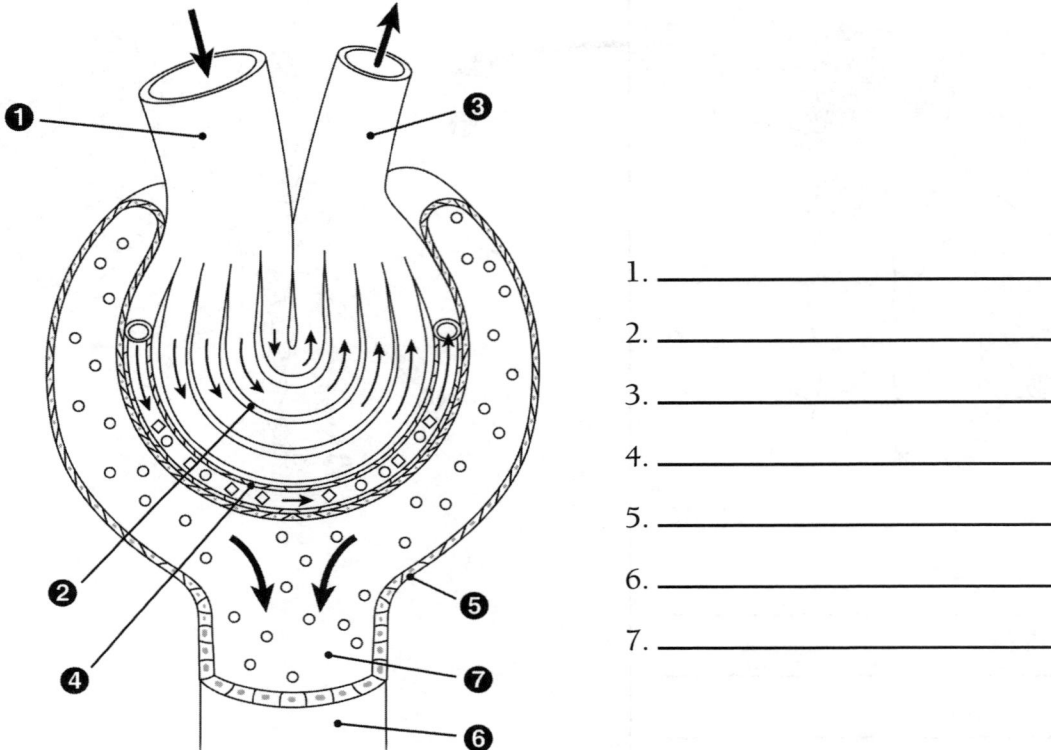

1. _____

2. _____

3. _____

4. _____

5. _____

6. _____

7. _____

○ Soluble molecules
◇ Proteins
○ Blood cells

EXERCISE 19-6: Summary of Urine Formation (text Fig. 19-9)

INSTRUCTIONS

1. Label the structures and fluids by writing the appropriate terms on lines 5 to 11.
2. Write the name of the hormone that controls water reabsorption in the distal tubule and collecting duct on line 12.
3. In boxes 1 to 4, name the process that is occurring.

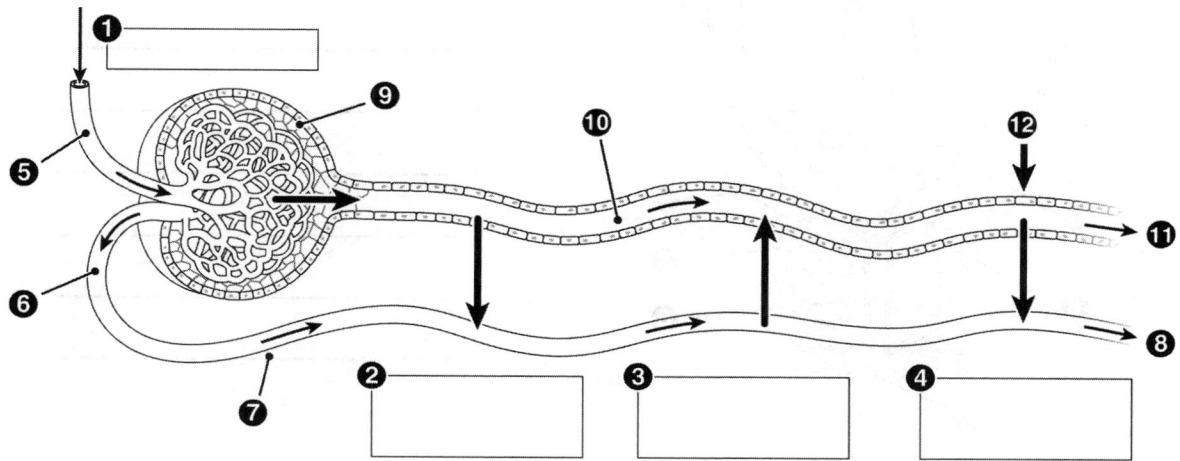

5. _____

6. _____

7. _____

8. _____

9. _____

10. _____

11. _____

12. _____

EXERCISE 19-7: Interior of the Male Urinary Bladder (text Fig. 19-10)
Label the indicated parts.

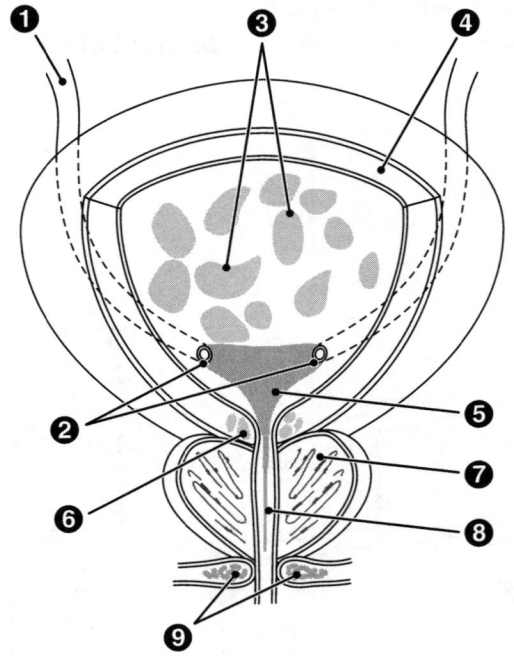

1. _____

2. _____

3. _____

4. _____

5. _____

6. _____

7. _____

8. _____

9. _____

EXERCISE 19-8: Main Fluid Compartments (text Fig. 19-11)

Label the different fluid compartments.

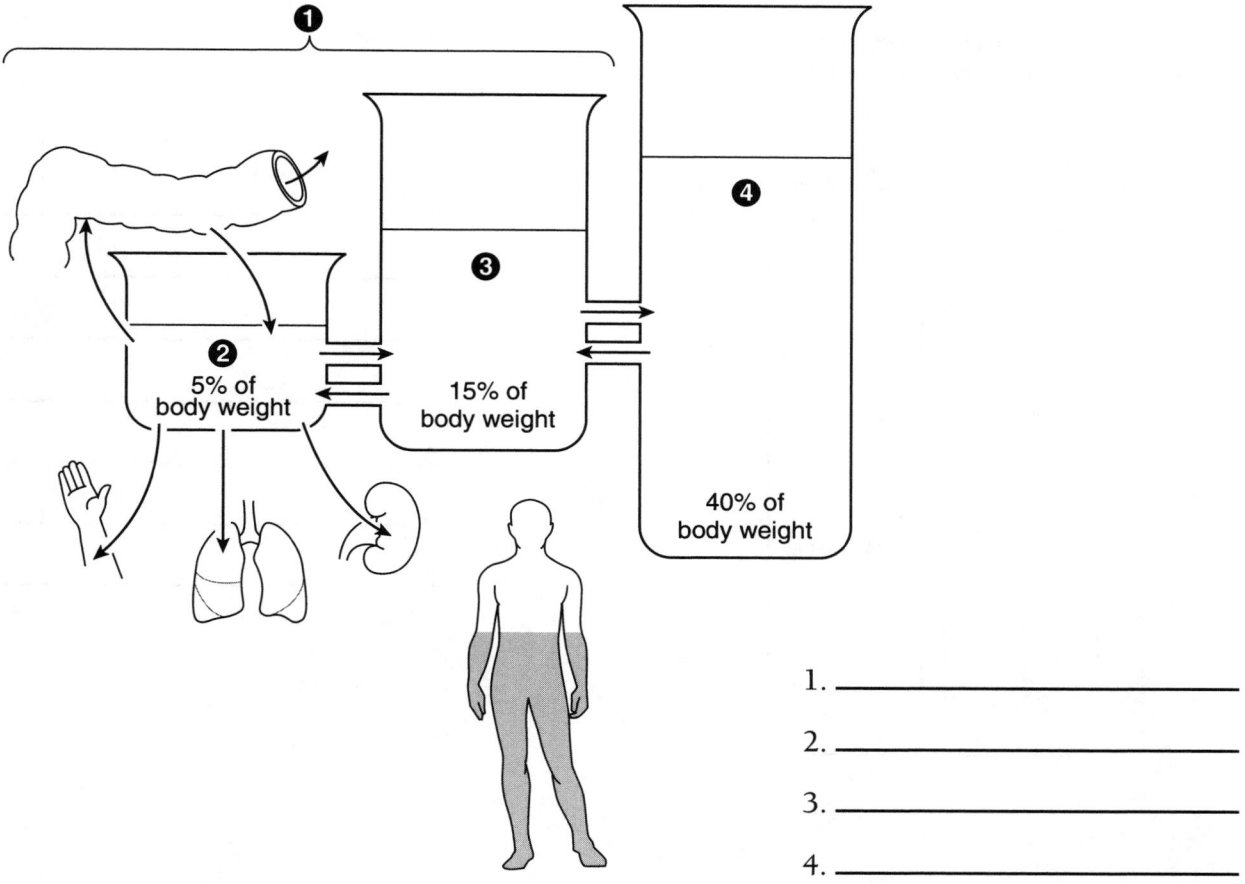

1. _____

2. _____

3. _____

4. _____

EXERCISE 19-9: Daily Gain and Loss of Water (text Fig. 19-12)

Write the names of the different sources of water gain and loss on the appropriate numbered lines in different colors. Color the diagram with the appropriate colors.

Water gain
2500 mL/day

Water loss
2500 mL/day

❶ 200 mL

❷ 700 mL

❸ 1600 mL

❹ 200 mL

❺ 300 mL

❻ 500 mL

❼ 1500 mL

1. _____

2. _____

3. _____

4. _____

5. _____

6. _____

7. _____

Making the Connections

The following concept maps deal with the organization of the kidney (Map A) and the distribution of body fluids (Map B). Each pair of terms is linked together by a connecting phrase into a sentence. The sentence should be read in the direction of the arrow. Complete the concept map by filling in the appropriate term or phrase. There is one right answer for each term. However, there are many correct answers for the connecting phrases. Three phrases in Map A (13, 15, and 16) involve three terms. For each of these phrases, build a single sentence linking the three terms together. For instance, use terms 4 and 8 and filtration to build phrase 13, term 12, peritubular capillaries, and secretion to build phrase 15, and term 9, reabsorption, and peritubular capillaries to build phrase 16. Write the phrase beside the appropriate number (if space permits) or on a separate piece of paper.

MAP A

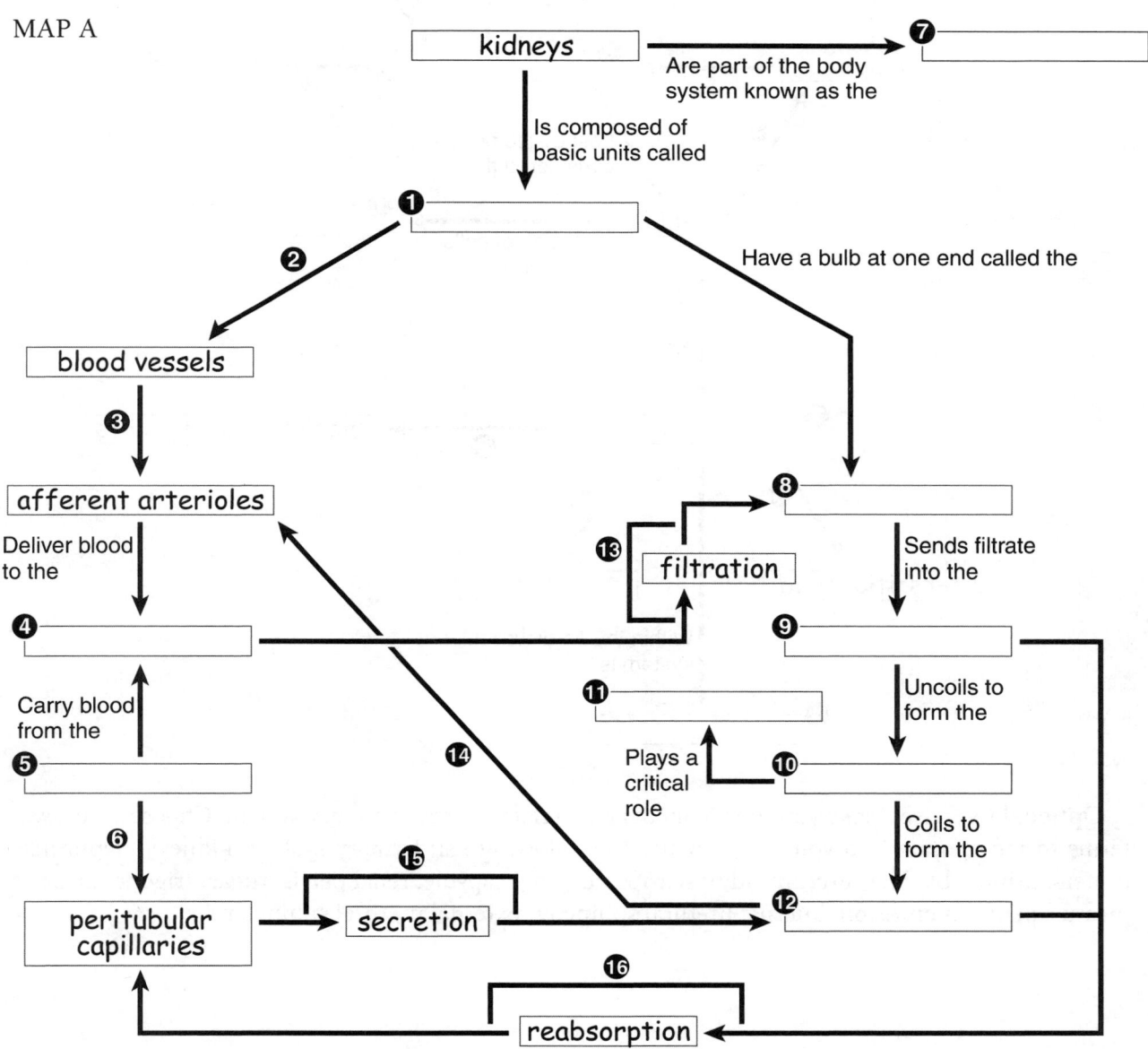

MAP B

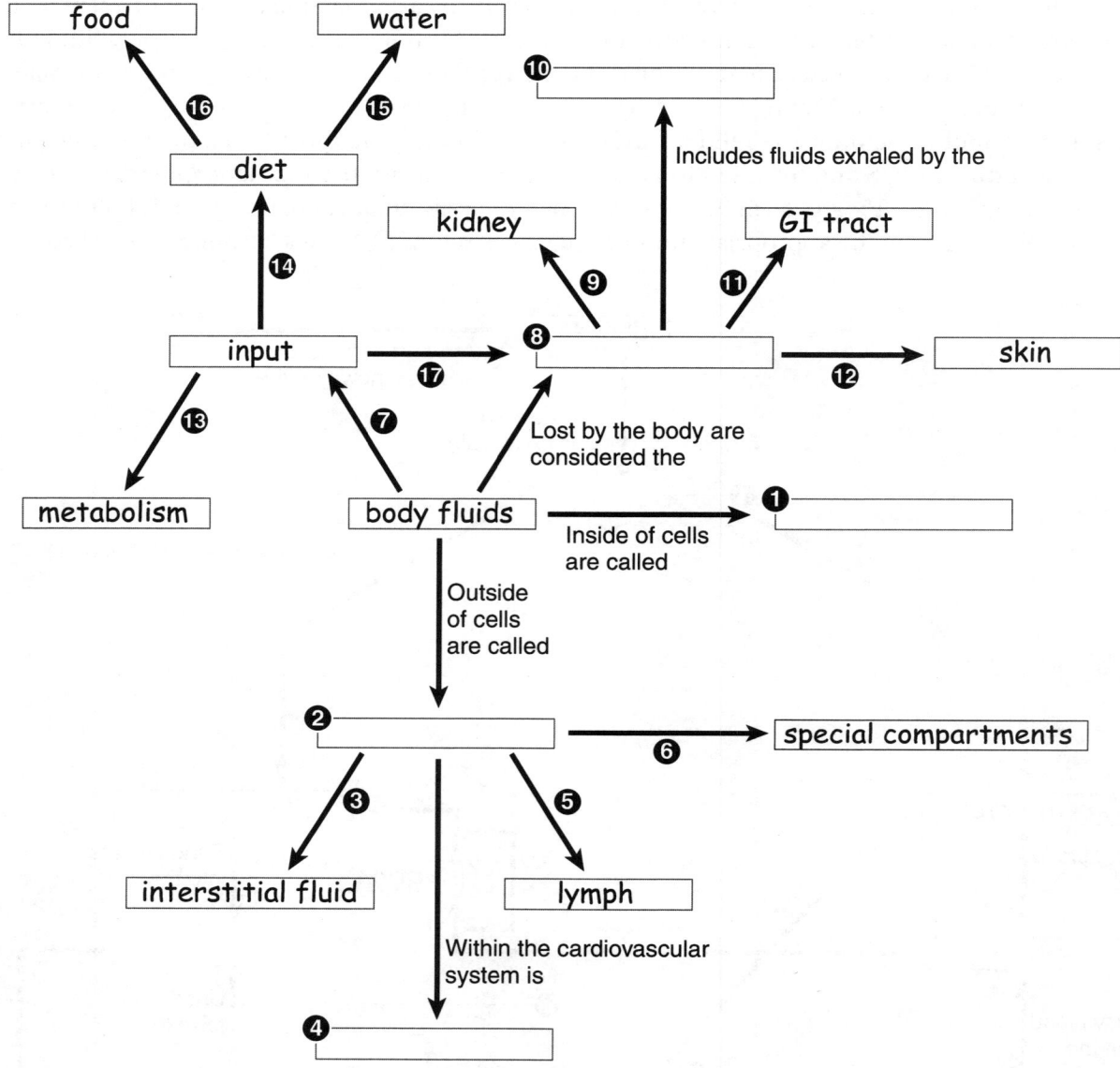

Optional Exercise: Make your own concept map related to the excretory system. Choose your own terms to incorporate into your map, or use the following list: Urinary system, kidneys, nephrons, ureters, urinary bladder, urethra, adipose capsule, renal capsule, renal pelvis, rugae, trigone, urinary meatus, penis, micturition, internal urethral sphincter, external urethral sphincter.

Testing Your Knowledge
Building Understanding

I. Matching Exercises

Matching only within each group, write the answers in the spaces provided.

➤ **Group A**

ureter	urinary bladder	urethra	renal capsule	renal cortex
retroperitoneal space	nephron	renal pelvis	adipose capsule	renal medulla

1. A funnel-shaped basin that collects urine from collecting ducts _____

2. The tube that carries urine from the bladder to the outside _____

3. The area behind the peritoneum that contains the ureters

    and the kidneys _____

4. A microscopic functional unit of the kidney _____

5. A tube connecting a kidney with the bladder _____

6. The crescent of fat that helps to support the kidney _____

7. The inner region of the kidney _____

8. The outer region of the kidney _____

➤ **Group B**

afferent arteriole	proximal convoluted tubule	peritubular capillaries	loop of Henle
glomerulus	glomerular capsule	efferent arteriole	renal artery
renal vein	collecting duct		

1. A hollow bulb at the proximal end of the nephron _____

2. The blood vessels connecting the afferent and efferent

    arterioles _____

3. The portion of the nephron receiving filtrate from the

    Bowman capsule _____

4. The vessel that branches to form the glomerulus _____

5. The vessel that drains the kidney _____

6. The blood vessels that exchange substances with the nephron _____

7. A tube that receives urine from the distal convoluted tubule _____

8. The portion of the nephron that dips into the medulla _____

➤ **Group C**

renin   juxtaglomerular apparatus   urea   EPO   angiotensin
filtration   tubular reabsorption   tubular secretion   antidiuretic hormone   aldosterone

1. An enzyme produced by the kidney   _____

2. The hormone that increases sodium reabsorption in the DCT   _____

3. The process that returns useful substances in the filtrate to
   the bloodstream   _____

4. The process by which substances leave the glomerulus and
   enter the glomerular capsule   _____

5. The structure in the kidney that produces renin   _____

6. The hormone produced in the kidney that stimulates
   erythrocyte synthesis by the bone marrow   _____

7. The process by which the renal tubule actively moves
   substances from the blood into the nephron to be excreted   _____

8. The hormone that increases the permeability of the DCT
   and collecting duct to water   _____

➤ **Group D**

interstitial   intracellular   extracellular   water   potassium
electrolyte   sodium   calcium   hypothalamus   brain stem

1. The most abundant ion inside cells   _____

2. The substance that makes up 50% to 70% of a person's
   body weight   _____

3. The part of the brain that controls the sense of thirst   _____

4. The term that specifically describes fluids in the microscopic
   spaces between cells   _____

5. A compound that forms ions in solution   _____

6. A term that describes the fluid within the body cells   _____

7. An ion involved in bone formation   _____

8. The most abundant ion in the fluid surrounding cells   _____

➤ **Group E**

cation   anion   buffer   hydrogen ion   dextrose

parathyroid hormone   aldosterone   antidiuretic hormone   calcitonin   normal saline

1. A hormone secreted from the pituitary that causes the

   kidney to reabsorb water   _____

2. A substance that aids in maintaining a constant pH   _____

3. The substance that directly determines the acidity or alkalinity

   of a fluid   _____

4. The adrenal hormone that promotes the reabsorption of sodium   _____

5. A hormone that causes the kidney to reabsorb calcium   _____

6. An ion with a negative electrical charge   _____

7. A sugar that is often administered intravenously   _____

8. An isotonic solution that is the first administered in

   emergencies   _____

II. Multiple Choice

Select the best answer and write the letter of your choice in the blank.

1. Select the correct order of urine flow from its source to the
   outside of the body.   1. _____
      a. urethra, bladder, kidney, ureter
      b. bladder, kidney, urethra, ureter
      c. kidney, ureter, bladder, urethra
      d. kidney, urethra, bladder, ureter
2. Select the correct order of filtrate flow through the nephron.   2. _____
      a. loop of Henle, distal convoluted tubule, proximal
         convoluted tubule, collecting duct
      b. glomerular capsule, proximal convoluted tubule,
         loop of Henle, distal convoluted tubule
      c. proximal convoluted tubule, distal convoluted
         tubule, loop of Henle, glomerular capsule
      d. glomerular capsule, distal convoluted tubule,
         proximal convoluted tubule, collecting duct
3. The enzyme renin raises blood pressure by activating: 3. _____
      a. urea
      b. glomerular filtration
      c. angiotensin
      d. erythropoietins

4. The juxtaglomerular apparatus consists of cells in the: 4. _____
    a. proximal convoluted tubule and efferent arteriole
    b. renal artery and afferent arteriole
    c. collecting tubules and renal vein
    d. distal convoluted tubule and afferent arteriole

5. Which of the following is NOT a function of the kidneys?   5. _____
    a. red blood cell destruction
    b. blood pressure regulation
    c. elimination of nitrogenous wastes
    d. modification of body fluid composition

6. The movement of a substance from the distal convoluted
   tubule to the peritubular capillaries occurs by the
   process of: 6. _____
    a. secretion
    b. filtration
    c. reabsorption
    d. excretion

7. Urine does NOT usually contain: 7. _____
    a. sodium
    b. hydrogen
    c. casts
    d. urea

8. The process of expelling urine is called: 8. _____
    a. reabsorption
    b. micturition
    c. dehydration
    d. defecation

9. Aldosterone is produced by the: 9. _____
    a. hypothalamus
    b. pituitary
    c. kidney
    d. adrenal gland

10. Antidiuretic hormone: 10. _____
    a. increases salt excretion by the kidney
    b. inhibits thirst
    c. decreases urine production
    d. increases calcium reabsorption by the kidney

11. Normal bone formation requires: 11. _____
    a. calcium
    b. phosphate
    c. neither calcium nor phosphate
    d. both calcium and phosphate

12. Which of the following is NOT a buffer?   12. _____
    a. hemoglobin
    b. bicarbonate
    c. oxygen
    d. phosphate

13. Which of the following fluids is NOT in the extracellular compartment?   13. _____
    a. cytoplasm
    b. cerebrospinal fluid
    c. lymph
    d. interstitial fluid

III. Completion Exercise

Write the word or phrase that correctly completes each sentence.

1. A negatively charged ion is called a(n)   _____
2. The receptors that detect an increase in the concentration of body fluids are called   _____
3. The ion that plays the largest role in maintaining body fluid volume is   _____
4. Water balance is partly regulated by a thirst center located in a region of the brain called the   _____
5. When the bladder is empty, its lining is thrown into the folds known as   _____
6. The vessel that brings blood to the glomerulus is the   _____
7. The most distal portion of the nephron is the   _____
8. The inner portion of the kidney is called the   _____
9. The hormone that increases water absorption in the collecting duct is   _____

Understanding Concepts

I. True or False

For each question, write "T" for true or "F" for false in the blank to the left of each number. If a statement is false, correct it by replacing the underlined term and write the correct statement in the blank below the question.

_____ 1. The movement of hydrogen ions from the peritubular capillaries into the distal convoluted tubule is an example of <u>tubular secretion</u>.

_____

_____ 2. Urine with a specific gravity of 0.05 is <u>more</u> concentrated than urine with a specific gravity of 0.04.

_____

_____ 3. Aldosterone tends to <u>decrease</u> the amount of urine produced.

_____

_____ 4. Adults can control the <u>internal</u> urethral sphincter.

_____

_____ 5. The triangular region in the floor of the bladder is called the <u>renal pelvis</u>.

_____

_____ 6. Most water loss occurs through the actions of the <u>digestive</u> system.

_____

_____ 7. The exhalation of carbon dioxide makes the blood more <u>acidic</u>.

_____

_____ 8. The fluids found in joint capsules and in the eyeball are examples of <u>extracellular</u> fluids.

_____

_____ 9. A solution with a pH of 9 is said to be <u>alkaline</u>.

_____

_____10. Urine exits the body through the <u>ureter</u>.

_____

II. Practical Applications

Study each discussion. Then write the appropriate word or phrase in the space provided.

➤ Group A

1. Ms. S, age 26, was teaching English in rural India. She developed severe diarrhea, probably as a result of a questionable pakora from a road-side stand. On admission to a hospital, she was found to be severely dehydrated. Ms S's blood will contain high levels of a hormone synthesized by the hypothalamus called _____

2. The physician's first concern was to increase Ms. S's plasma volume. Her fluid deficit was addressed by administering a 0.9% sodium chloride solution. This solution contains the same concentration of solutes as Ms. S's cells and is thus termed _____

3. Next, the physician addressed Ms. S's acid–base balance. The pH of a blood sample was tested. The laboratory technician was looking for a pH value outside the normal range. The normal pH of blood is _____

4. Ms. S's blood pH was found to be abnormal, and sodium bicarbonate was added to her IV. Bicarbonate is an example of a substance that helps maintain a constant pH. These substances are known as _____

➤ Group B

1. Young S, age 1, was brought to the hospital with an enlarged abdomen. His blood pressure was abnormally high, suggesting that S may suffer from hypertension. This disorder can result from abnormally high levels of renin. Renin is produced by a specialized region of the kidney called the _____

2. S was administered a medication that blocks the activation of the renin substrate. Renin activates a substance called _____

3. Further testing showed that S was suffering from the irreversible loss of the small units of the kidney that produce urine. These units are the _____

4. S's enlarged abdomen is due to the accumulation of fluid outside cells. Body fluids that are not intracellular are termed _____

5. S was also quite lethargic, due to a deficiency in red blood cells. This deficiency probably reflects the fact that the kidney synthesizes a hormone called _____

III. Short Essays

1. Compare and contrast the processes of filtration and secretion. Name at least one similarity and two differences.

_____

_____

_____

2. Explain why breath holding will increase blood acidity, and how the kidney would respond to repeated episodes of breath holding.

_____

_____

_____

Conceptual Thinking

1. Ms. W has just eaten a large bag of salty popcorn. Her blood is now too salty and must be diluted. Is it possible for the kidney to increase water reabsorption without increasing salt absorption? Explain.

_____

_____

_____

2. Mr. R is taking penicillin to cure a throat infection. He must take the drug frequently, because the kidney clears penicillin very efficiently. That is, all of the penicillin that enters the renal artery leaves the kidney in the urine. However, only some penicillin molecules will be filtered into the glomerular capsule. How can the kidney excrete all of the penicillin it receives?

_____

_____

_____

3. Ms. J is stranded on a desert island with limited water supplies. A. How will the volume and concentration of her body fluids change? B. How will her hypothalamus and pituitary gland respond to these changes? C. What will be the net effect of these responses?

_____

_____

_____

Expanding your Horizons

"Space. The final frontier." The classic statement from the show *Star Trek* remains valid in terms of human physiology. The effects of prolonged weightlessness and space travel on the human body remain an area of hot research. One effect of weightlessness is a dramatic redistribution of body fluids. You can read all about this and other effects of space travel in the following Scientific American article.

Resource List

White RJ. Weightlessness and the human body. Sci Am 1998;279:58–63.

chapter 20

The Male and Female Reproductive Systems

Overview

Reproduction is the process by which life continues. Human reproduction is **sexual**, that is, it requires the union of two different **germ cells** or **gametes**. (Some simple forms of life can reproduce without a partner in the process of **asexual** reproduction.) These germ cells, the **spermatozoon** in males and the **ovum** in females, are formed by **meiosis**, a type of cell division in which the chromosome number is reduced by half. When fertilization occurs and the gametes combine, the original chromosome number is restored.

The reproductive glands or **gonads** manufacture the gametes and also produce hormones. These activities are continuous in the male but cyclic in the female. The male gonad is the **testis**. The remainder of the male reproductive tract consists of passageways for storage and transport of spermatozoa; the male organ of copulation, the **penis**; and several glands that contribute to the production of **semen**.

The female gonad is the **ovary**. The ovum released each month at the time of **ovulation** travels through the **oviducts** to the **uterus**, where the egg, if fertilized, develops. If no fertilization occurs, the ovum, along with the built-up lining of the uterus, is eliminated through the **vagina** as the **menstrual flow**.

Reproduction is under the control of hormones from the **anterior pituitary**, which, in turn, is controlled by the **hypothalamus** of the brain. These organs respond to **feedback** mechanisms, which maintain proper hormone levels.

Aging causes changes in both the male and female reproductive systems. A gradual decrease in male hormone production begins as early as age 20 and continues throughout life. In the female, a more sudden decrease in activity occurs between ages 45 and 55 and ends in **menopause**, the cessation of menstruation and of the childbearing years.

Learning the Language: Word Anatomy

Word Part	Meaning	Example
1. _____	extreme end	_____
2. semin/o-	_____	_____
3. _____	egg	_____
4. metr/o	_____	_____
5. fer	_____	_____
6. test/o	_____	_____
7. _____	around	_____
8. ovar, ovari/o	_____	_____
9. test/o	_____	_____

Addressing the Learning Outcomes

I. Writing Exercise

The learning outcomes for Chapter 20 are listed below. These learning outcomes provide an overview of the major topics covered in this chapter. On a separate piece of paper, try to write out an answer to each learning outcome. All of the answers can be found in the pages of the textbook. Learning Outcomes 1, 3, 5, and 6 are also addressed in the Coloring Atlas.

1. Name the male and female gonads and describe the function of each.
2. State the purpose of meiosis.
3. List the accessory organs of the male and female reproductive tracts and cite the function of each.
4. Describe the composition and function of semen.
5. Draw and label a spermatozoon.
6. List in the correct order the hormones produced during the menstrual cycle and cite the source of each.
7. Describe the functions of the main male and female sex hormones.
8. Explain how negative feedback regulates reproductive function in both males and females.
9. Describe the changes that occur during and after menopause.
10. Cite the main methods of birth control in use.
11. Show how word parts are used to build words related to the male and female reproductive systems.

II. Labeling and Coloring Atlas

EXERCISE 20-1: Male Reproductive System (text Fig. 20-1)

INSTRUCTIONS

1. Write the names of the structures that are not part of the reproductive system on the appropriate lines 1 to 6 in different colors. Use the same color for structures 1 and 2 and for structures 4 and 5. Color the structures on the diagram.
2. Write the names of the parts of the male reproductive system on the appropriate lines 7 to 20 in different colors. Use the same color for structures 10 and 11. Color the structures on the diagram.

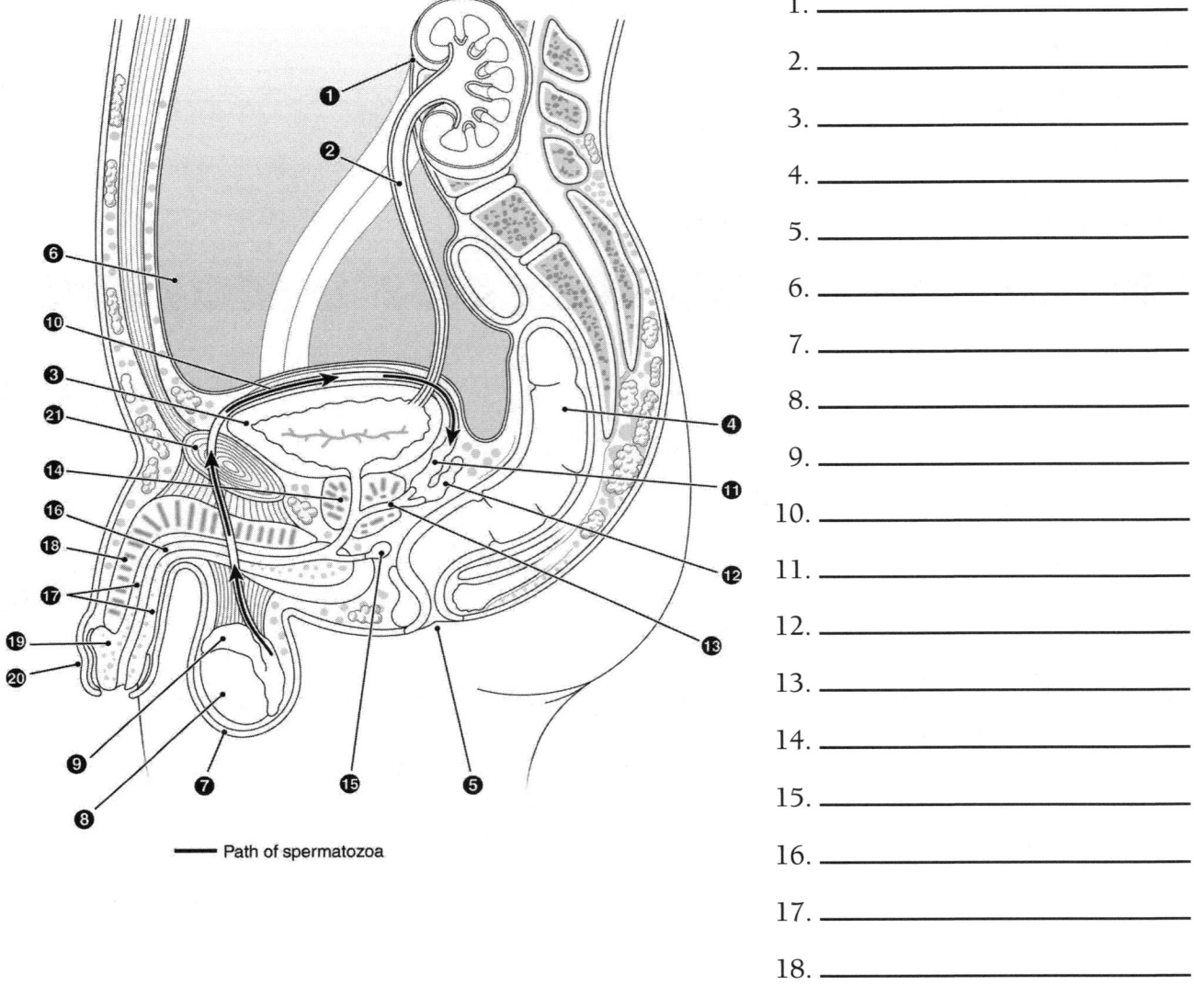

Path of spermatozoa

1. _____

2. _____

3. _____

4. _____

5. _____

6. _____

7. _____

8. _____

9. _____

10. _____

11. _____

12. _____

13. _____

14. _____

15. _____

16. _____

17. _____

18. _____

19. _____

20. _____

EXERCISE 20-2: Structure of the Testis (text Fig. 20-2)

Label the indicated parts. (Hint: the vein is more branched than the artery).

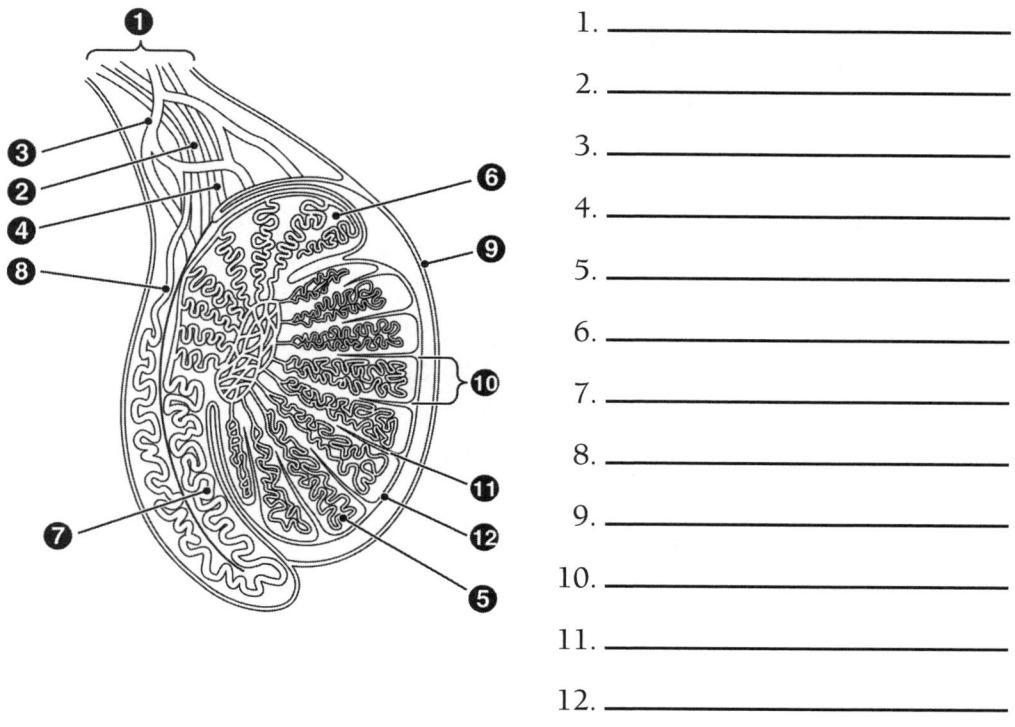

1. _____
2. _____
3. _____
4. _____
5. _____
6. _____
7. _____
8. _____
9. _____
10. _____
11. _____
12. _____

EXERCISE 20-3: Diagram of a Human Spermatozoon (text Fig. 20-4)

INSTRUCTIONS

1. Write the names of the parts on the appropriate lines in different colors. Use black for structures 1 to 3, because they will not be colored.
2. Color the structures on the diagram.

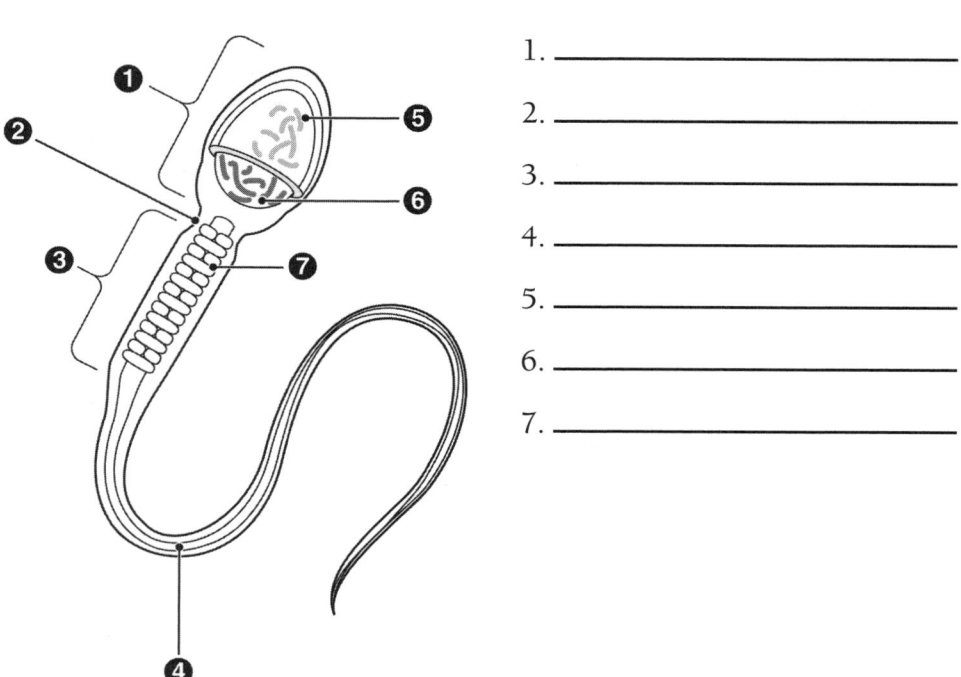

1. _____
2. _____
3. _____
4. _____
5. _____
6. _____
7. _____

EXERCISE 20-4: Cross-section of the Penis (text Fig. 20-5)

INSTRUCTIONS

1. Write the names of the parts on the appropriate lines in different colors. (Hint: the nerve is solid and the veins have larger lumens.)
2. Color the structures on the diagram.

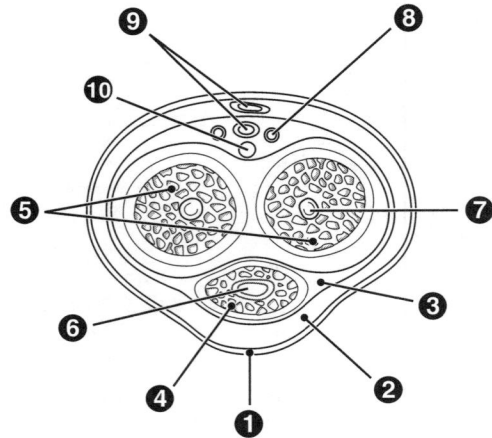

1. _____   6. _____

2. _____   7. _____

3. _____   8. _____

4. _____   9. _____

5. _____   10. _____

EXERCISE 20-5: Female Reproductive System (text Fig. 20-6)

INSTRUCTIONS

1. Write the names of the parts on the appropriate lines in different colors. Use the same color for parts 8 and 9, for parts 10, 11, and 13, and for parts 14 and 15.
2. Color the structures on the diagram.

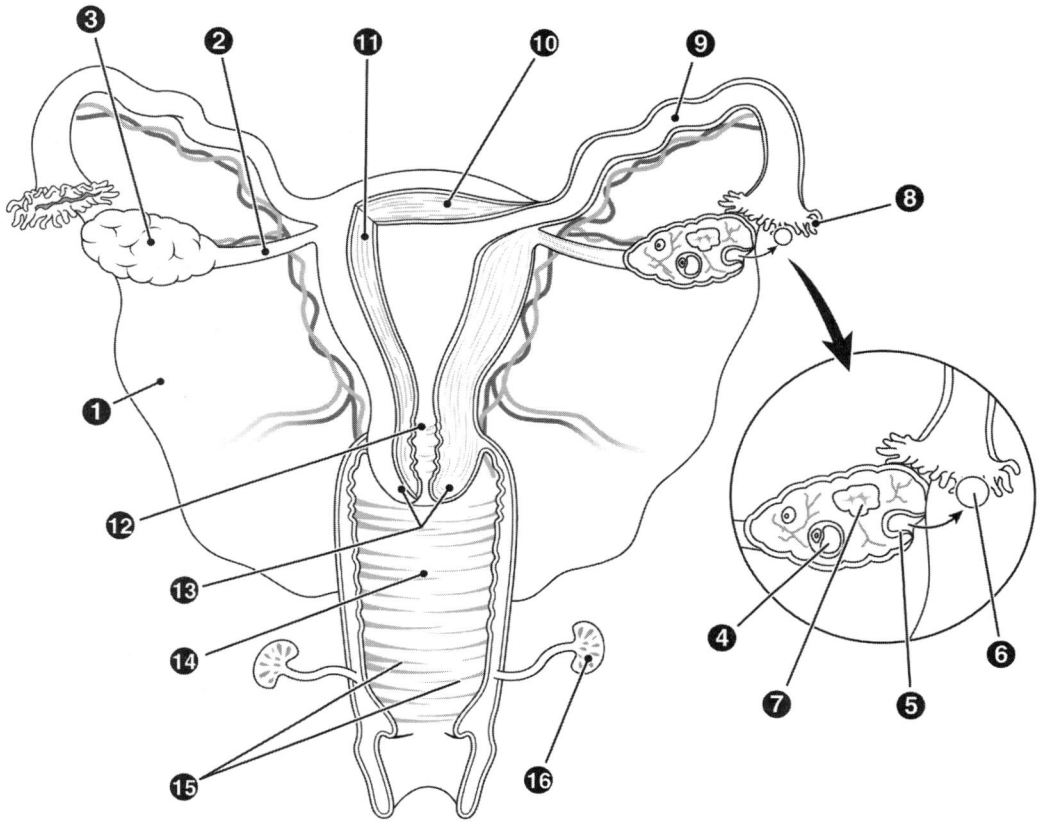

1. _____   9. _____

2. _____   10. _____

3. _____   11. _____

4. _____   12. _____

5. _____   13. _____

6. _____   14. _____

7. _____   15. _____

8. _____   16. _____

EXERCISE 20-6: Female Reproductive System (Sagittal Section) (text Fig. 20-9)

INSTRUCTIONS

1. Write the names of the structures that are not part of the reproductive system on the appropriate lines 1 to 8 in different colors. Use the same color for structures 1 and 2, for structures 3 and 4, and for structures 5 and 6. Color the structures on the diagram.
2. Write the names of the parts of the female reproductive system and supporting ligaments on the appropriate lines 9 to 19 in different colors. Use the same color for structures 15 and 16. Color the structures on the diagram.

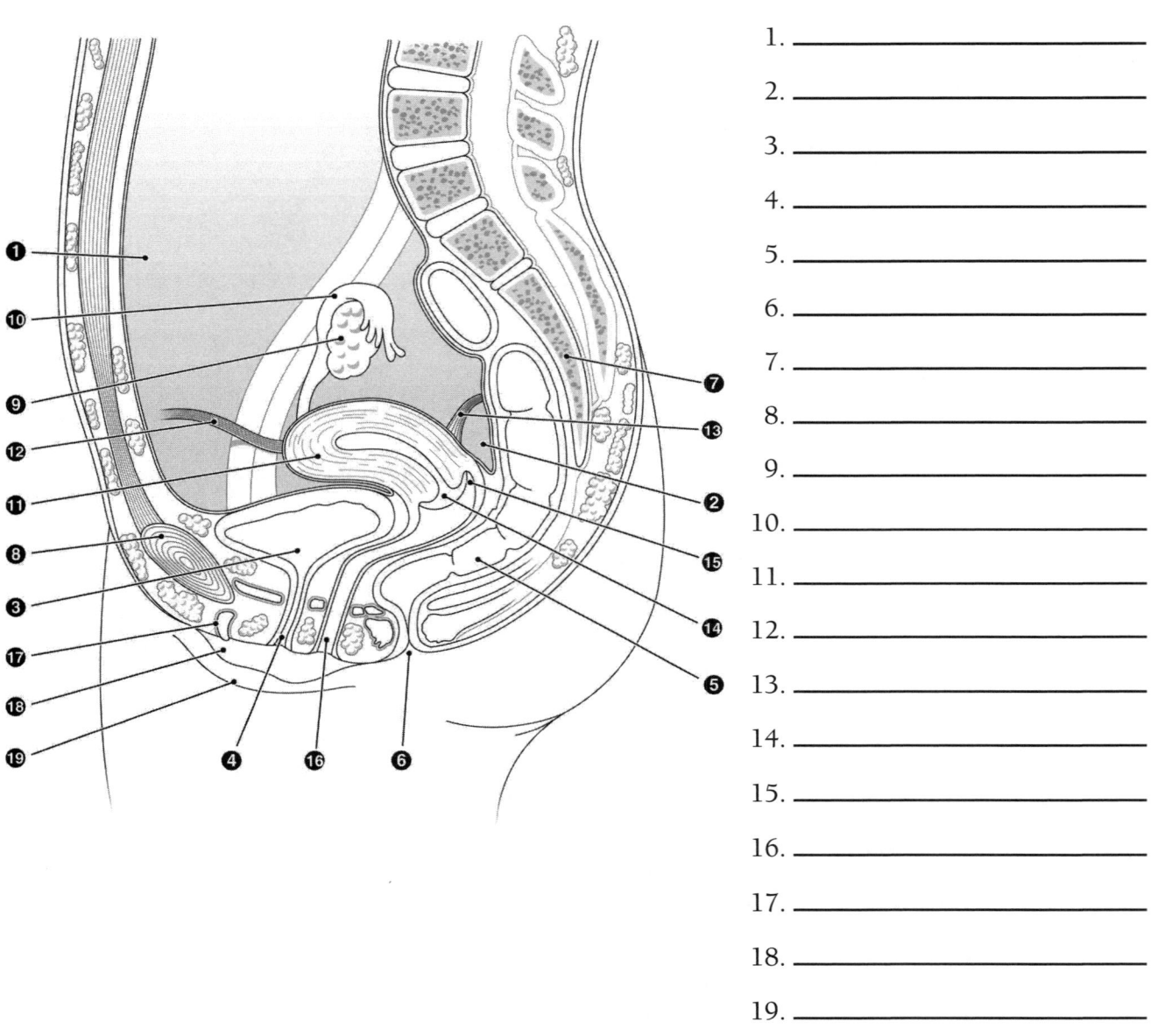

1. _____
2. _____
3. _____
4. _____
5. _____
6. _____
7. _____
8. _____
9. _____
10. _____
11. _____
12. _____
13. _____
14. _____
15. _____
16. _____
17. _____
18. _____
19. _____

EXERCISE 20-7: External Parts of the Female Reproductive System (text Fig. 20-10)
Label the indicated parts.

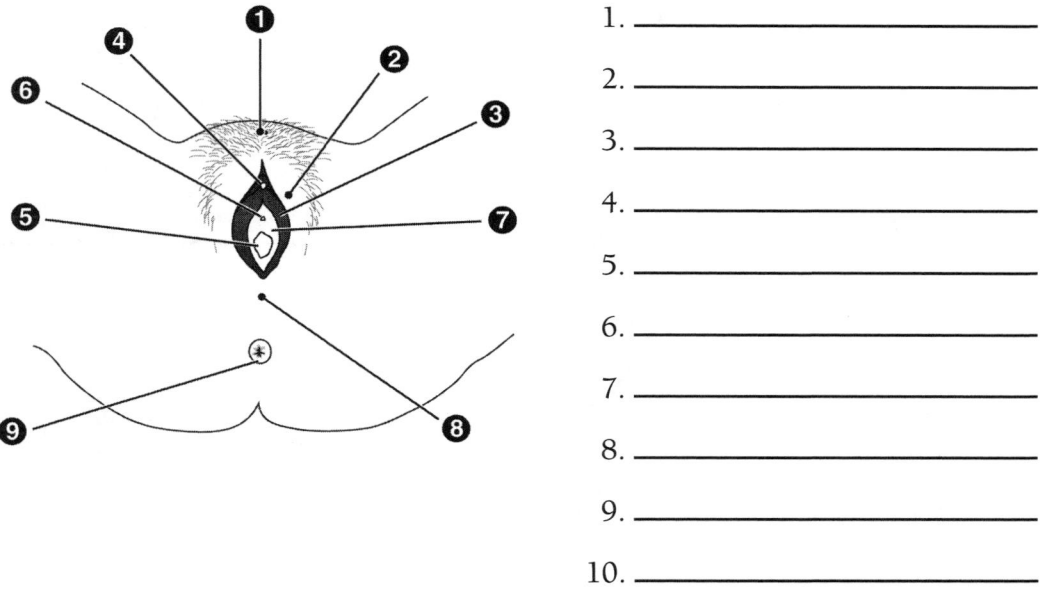

1. _____

2. _____

3. _____

4. _____

5. _____

6. _____

7. _____

8. _____

9. _____

10. _____

EXERCISE 20-8: The Menstrual Cycle (text Fig. 20-11)

INSTRUCTIONS

1. Identify the hormone responsible for each of the numbered lines in graph A, and write the
   hormone names on the appropriate lines in different colors. Trace over the lines in the graph
   with the appropriate color.
2. Write the names of the phases of the ovarian cycle (part B) and the uterine cycle (part C) on
   the appropriate lines.

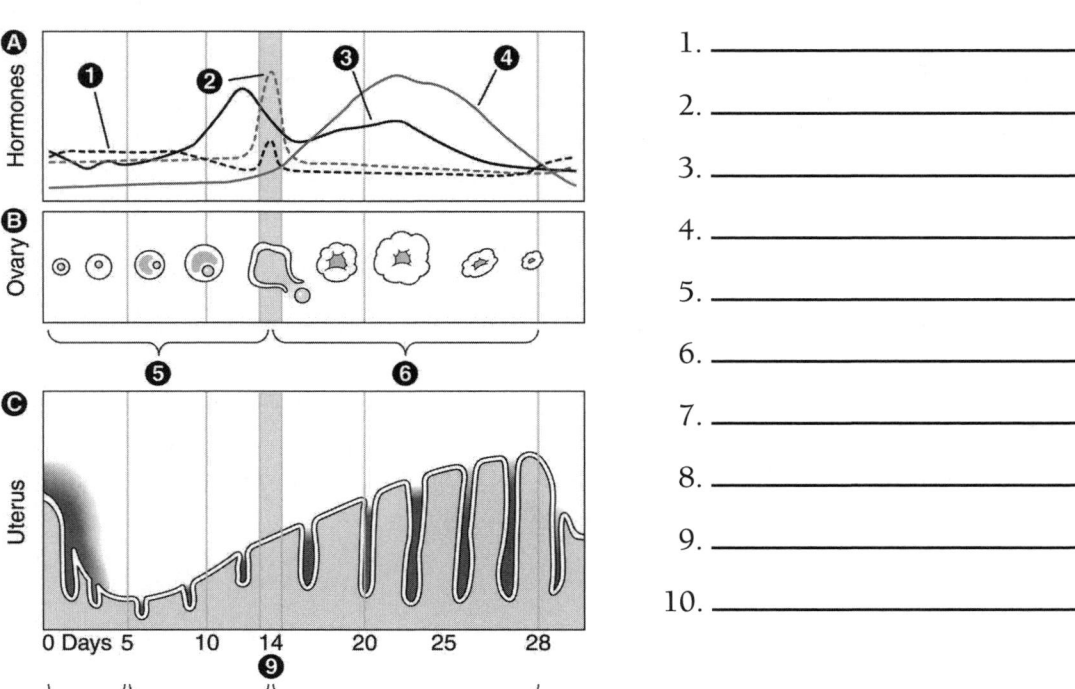

1. _____

2. _____

3. _____

4. _____

5. _____

6. _____

7. _____

8. _____

9. _____

10. _____

Making the Connections

The following concept map deals with the organization of the nervous system. Each pair of terms is linked together by a connecting phrase into a sentence. The sentence should be read in the direction of the arrow. Complete the concept map by filling in the appropriate term or phrase. There is one right answer for each term (1, 2, 4, 5, 14). However, there are many correct answers for the connecting phrases. Write each phrase beside the appropriate number (if space permits) or on a separate piece of paper.

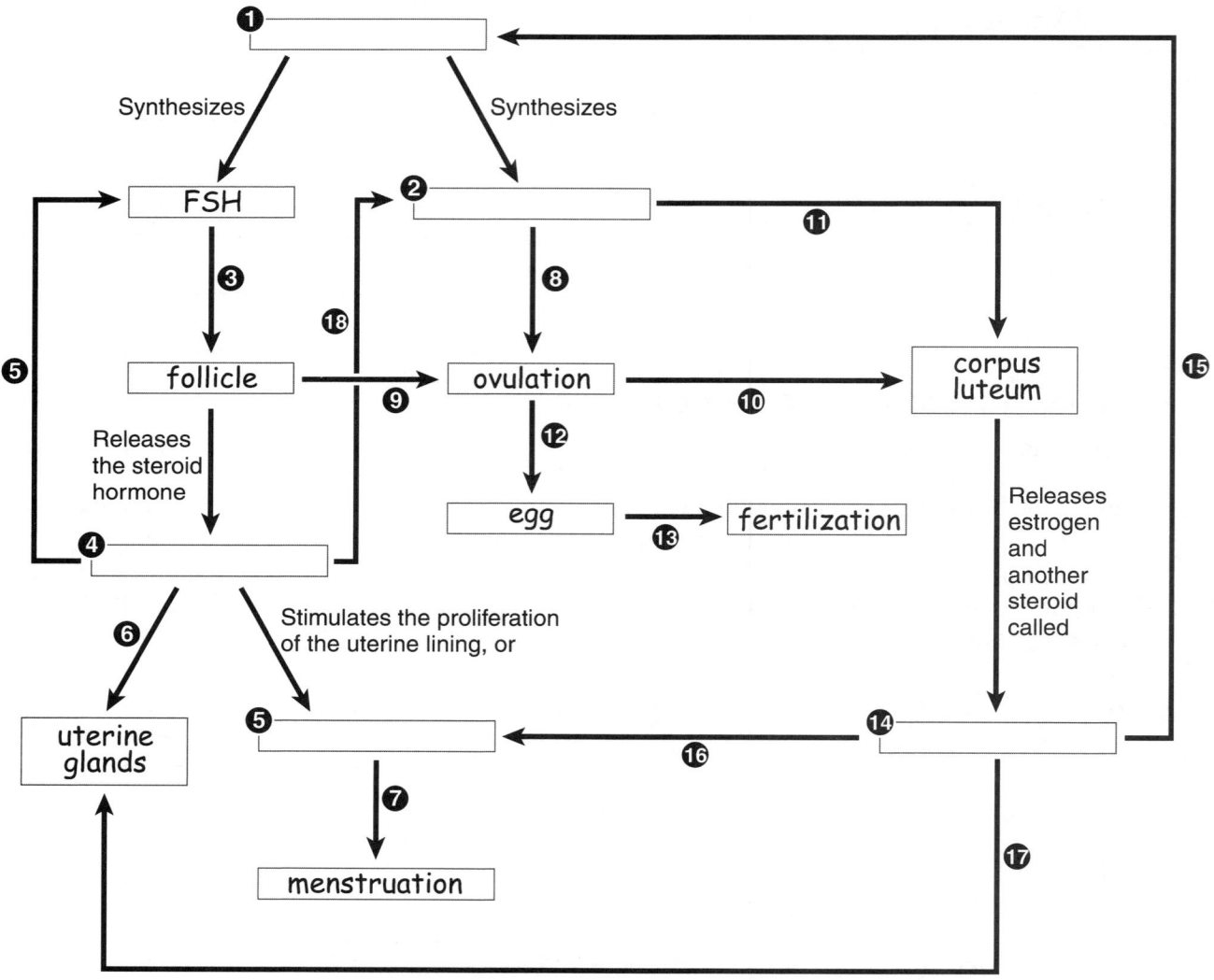

Optional Exercise: Make your own concept map, based on male reproductive anatomy and physiology. Choose your own terms to incorporate into your map, or use the following list: spermatozoon, testosterone, testis, FSH, LH, interstitial cell, epididymis, vas deferens, seminiferous tubule, Sertoli cell, prostate gland, bulbourethral gland, penis.

Testing Your Knowledge
Building Understanding

I. Matching Exercises

Matching only within each group, write the answers in the spaces provided.

➤ Group A

spermatozoon	ejaculatory duct	acrosome	interstitial cell	sustentacular cell
seminiferous tubule	epididymis	vas deferens	seminal vesicle	prostate gland

1. A cell that nourishes and protects developing spermatozoa   _____

2. A cell that secretes testosterone   _____

3. The germ cell of the male   _____

4. The coiled tube in which spermatozoa are stored as they mature and become motile   _____

5. A coiled duct in which germ cells develop in the testes   _____

6. One of the two glands that secrete a thick, yellow, alkaline secretion   _____

7. A caplike covering over the head of the spermatozoon that aids in penetration of the ovum   _____

8. The gland that secretes a thin alkaline secretion and that can contract to aid in ejaculation   _____

➤ Group B

fimbriae	oviduct	fundus	cervix	myometrium
endometrium	fornix	hymen	perineum	vestibule

1. The Bartholin glands secrete into this area   _____

2. Fringelike extensions that sweep the ovum into the uterine tube   _____

3. The specialized tissue that lines the uterus   _____

4. The small, rounded part of the uterus located above the openings of the oviducts   _____

5. A fold of membrane found at the opening of the vagina   _____

6. The necklike part of the uterus that dips into the upper vagina   _____

7. The muscular wall of the uterus   _____

8. The tube that transports the ova to the uterus   _____

➤ Group C

luteinizing hormone	follicle stimulating hormone	testosterone	estrogen
progesterone	ovarian follicle	corpus luteum	ovum
ovulation	menstruation		

1. A hormone that is only produced during the luteal phase of the menstrual cycle _____

2. A cell cluster within which the ovum matures _____

3. A hormone produced by the testicular interstitial cells _____

4. Discharge of an ovum from the surface of the ovary _____

5. The hormone that stimulates sustentacular cells _____

6. The female gamete _____

7. The structure formed by the ruptured follicle after ovulation _____

8. The portion of the menstrual cycle when the endometrium is degenerating _____

➤ Group D

IUD	broad ligament	vulva	clitoris
Emergency contraceptive pill	mefipristone	ovarian ligament	diaphragm

1. A large, flat ligament that supports the uterus and ovaries _____

2. A term describing all of the external parts of the female reproductive system _____

3. A synthetic progesterone taken after unprotected intercourse to reduce the risk of pregnancy _____

4. A cap that fits over the cervix preventing sperm entry _____

5. A device implanted into the uterus that prevents fertilization and implantation _____

6. A progesterone blocker that can be used to terminate an early pregnancy _____

II. Multiple Choice

Select the best answer and write the letter of your choice in the blank.

1. The corpus luteum secretes:
    a. testosterone
    b. estrogen
    c. FSH
    d. LH

1. _____

2. Which of the following is **NOT** part of the uterus?
    a. cervix
    b. fimbriae
    c. endometrium
    d. corpus

2. _____

3. Spermatozoa develop in the walls of the:
    a. prostate gland
    b. penis
    c. seminal vesicles
    d. seminiferous tubules

3. _____

4. The glans penis is formed from the:
    a. corpus spongiosum
    b. corpus cavernosum
    c. pubic symphysis
    d. vas deferens

4. _____

5. The ovum develops within the:
    a. corpus luteum
    b. ovarian follicle
    c. interstitial cells
    d. Sertoli cells

5. _____

6. Which of the following glands is found in the female?
    a. vestibular glands
    b. bulbourethral glands
    c. Cowper glands
    d. prostate gland

6. _____

7. Semen does NOT contain:
    a. seminal fluid
    b. a high concentration of hydrogen ions
    c. sugar
    d. sperm

7. _____

III. Completion Exercise

Write the word or phrase that correctly completes each sentence.

1. The enzyme-containing cap on the head of a spermatozoon is called the _____
2. The hormone that promotes development of spermatozoa in the male and development of ova in the female is _____
3. The process of cell division that reduces the chromosome number by half is _____
4. The testes are contained in an external sac called the _____
5. The main male sex hormone is _____
6. The pelvic floor in both males and females is called the _____
7. The hormone that stimulates ovulation is _____
8. In the male, the tube that carries urine away from the bladder also carries sperm cells. This tube is the _____
9. The surgical removal of the foreskin of the penis is called _____

Understanding Concepts

I. True or False

For each question, write "T" for true or "F" for false in the blank to the left of each number. If a statement is false, correct it by replacing the underlined term and write the correct statement in the blank below the question.

_____ 1. The urethra is contained in the corpus spongiosum of the penis.

_____

_____ 2. When estrogen and progesterone levels are high, luteinizing hormone secretion is inhibited.

_____

_____ 3. Gametes are produced by the process of mitosis.

_____

_____ 4. Estrogen and progesterone levels are lowest during the follicular phase of the menstrual cycle.

_____

_____ 5. Progesterone is the first ovarian hormone produced in the menstrual cycle.

_____

_____ 6. A deficiency in luteinizing hormone would result in testosterone deficiency.

_____

II. Practical Applications

Study each discussion. Then write the appropriate word or phrase in the space provided.

➤ **Group A**

1. Ms. J, age 22, reported painful menstrual cramps and excessive menstrual flow. Menstruation is the shedding of the uterine layer called the

2. The physician suggested anti-inflammatory medication, but Ms. J had previously tried medication to no avail. An alternate approach was tried, in which the passageway between the vagina and the uterus was artificially dilated. The part of the uterus containing this passageway is the

3. It was also suggested that Ms J take contraceptive pills. These pills contain two ovarian steroids, progesterone and

4. These hormones prevent ovulation by inhibiting the secretion of a pituitary hormone called.

➤ **Group B**

1. Mr. and Ms. S, both age 35, had been trying to conceive for 2 years with no success. Analysis of Mr. S's semen revealed a low concentration of the male gametes, known as

2. Blood tests were performed, revealing a deficiency in the pituitary hormone that acts on sustentacular cells. This hormone is called

3. Conversely, testosterone production was normal. The cells that produce testosterone are called

4. Mr. S's hormone deficiency was successfully treated, and Mr. and Ms. S became the proud parents of triplets. Mr. S went to the clinic soon after the birth, and the duct extending from the epididymis to the ejaculatory duct was cut to prevent further conceptions. This duct is called the

III. Short Essays

1. Discuss changes occurring in the ovary and in the uterus during the follicular phase of the menstrual cycle.

_____

_____

_____

2. Compare and contrast the male and female gametes. Discuss their structure and their production.

_____

_____

_____

Conceptual Thinking

1. Mr. S is taking synthetic testosterone to improve his wrestling performance. To his alarm, he notices that his testicles are shrinking. Explain why this is happening.

_____

_____

_____

2. Compare and contrast the role of FSH in the regulation of the male and female gonad.

_____

_____

_____

Expanding Your Horizons

Have you heard of kamikaze sperm? Based on studies in animals, some animal behavior researchers have hypothesized that semen contains a population of spermatozoa that is is capable of destroying spermatozoa from a competing male. These "kamikaze spermatozoa" seek out and destroy spermatozoa from other males. Other sperm are "blockers," which are misshapen spermatozoa with multiple tails and/or heads. A very small population of egg-getting spermatozoa attempt to fertilize the ovum. Although some aspects of this hypothesis have been challenged, the presence of sperm subpopulations is now well established. You can read more about the kamikaze sperm hypothesis in the following scientific articles.

Resource List

Baker RR, Bellis MA. Elaboration of the Kamikaze sperm hypothesis: a reply to Harcourt. Animal Behav 1989;37:865–867.
Moore HD, Martin M, Birkhead TR. No evidence for killer sperm or other selective interactions between human spermatozoa in ejaculates of different males in vitro. Proc R Soc Lond B Biol Sci 1999;266:2343–2350.

chapter 21

Development and Heredity

Overview

Pregnancy begins with fertilization of an ovum by a spermatozoon to form a **zygote**. Over the next 38 weeks of **gestation**, the offspring develops first as an **embryo** and then as a **fetus**. During this period, it is nourished and maintained by the **placenta**, formed from tissues of both the mother and the embryo. The placenta secretes a number of hormones, including progesterone, estrogen, human chorionic gonadotropin, human placental lactogen, and relaxin. These hormones induce changes in the uterus and breasts to support the pregnancy and prepare for parturition and lactation.

Childbirth or **parturition** occurs in four stages, beginning with contractions of the uterus and dilation of the cervix. Subsequent stages include delivery of the infant, delivery of the afterbirth, and control of bleeding. Milk production, or **lactation**, is stimulated by the hormones prolactin and oxytocin. Removal of milk from the breasts is the stimulus for continued production.

The scientific study of heredity has advanced with amazing speed in the past 50 years. Nevertheless, many mysteries remain. Gregor Mendel was the first person known to have performed formal experiments in genetics. He identified independent units of heredity, which he called factors and which we now call **genes**.

The chromosomes in the nucleus of each cell are composed of a complex molecule, **DNA**. This material makes up the many thousands of genes that determine a person's traits and are passed on to offspring at the time of fertilization. Genes direct the formation of **enzymes**, which, in turn, make possible all the chemical reactions of metabolism. Defective genes, produced by **mutation**, may disrupt normal enzyme activity and result in hereditary disorders. Some human traits are determined by a single pair of genes (one gene from each parent), but most are controlled by multiple pairs of genes acting together.

Genes may be classified as **dominant** or **recessive**. If one parent contributes a dominant gene, then any offspring who receives that gene will show the trait (e.g., Huntington disease). Traits carried by recessive genes may remain hidden for generations and be revealed only if they are contributed by both parents (e.g., albinism, cystic fibrosis, PKU, and sickle cell anemia).

Learning the Language: Word Anatomy

Word Part	Meaning	Example
1. _____	color	_____
2. zyg/o	_____	_____
3. _____	labor	_____
4. ox/y	_____	_____
5. chori/o	_____	_____
6. _____	body	_____
7. phen/o	_____	_____
8. _____	self	_____
9. _____	other, different	_____
10. homo-	_____	_____

Addressing the Learning Outcomes

I. Writing Exercise

The learning outcomes for Chapter 21 are listed below. These learning outcomes provide an overview of the major topics covered in this chapter. On a separate piece of paper, try to write out an answer to each learning outcome. All of the answers can be found in the pages of the textbook. Learning Outcomes 2 and 3 are also addressed in the Coloring Atlas.

1. Describe fertilization and the early development of the fertilized egg.
2. Describe the structure and function of the placenta.
3. Briefly describe changes that occur in the fetus and the mother during pregnancy.
4. Briefly describe the four stages of labor.
5. Compare fraternal and identical twins.
6. Cite the advantages of breast-feeding.
7. Briefly describe the mechanism of gene function.
8. Explain the difference between dominant and recessive genes.
9. Compare phenotype and genotype and give examples of each.
10. Describe what is meant by a carrier of a genetic trait.
11. Define meiosis and explain its function in reproduction.
12. Explain how sex is determined in humans.
13. Describe what is meant by the term *sex-linked* and list several sex-linked traits.
14. List several factors that may influence the expression of a gene.
15. Define mutation.
16. Show how word parts are used to build words related to development and heredity.

II. Labeling and Coloring Atlas

EXERCISE 21-1: Fetal Circulation (text Fig. 21-2)

INSTRUCTIONS

1. Label the parts of the fetal circulation and placenta. Hint: you can differentiate between the uterine arterioles and uterine venules by following the path of the vessels into the umbilical arteries and vein.
2. Color the boxes in the legend using the following color scheme. Color the oxygen-rich blood box red, the oxygen-poor blood box blue, and the mixed blood box purple.
3. As much as possible, color the blood vessels on the diagram with the appropriate color, based on the oxygen content of the blood.

1. _____

2. _____

3. _____

4. _____

5. _____

6. _____

7. _____

8. _____

9. _____

10. _____

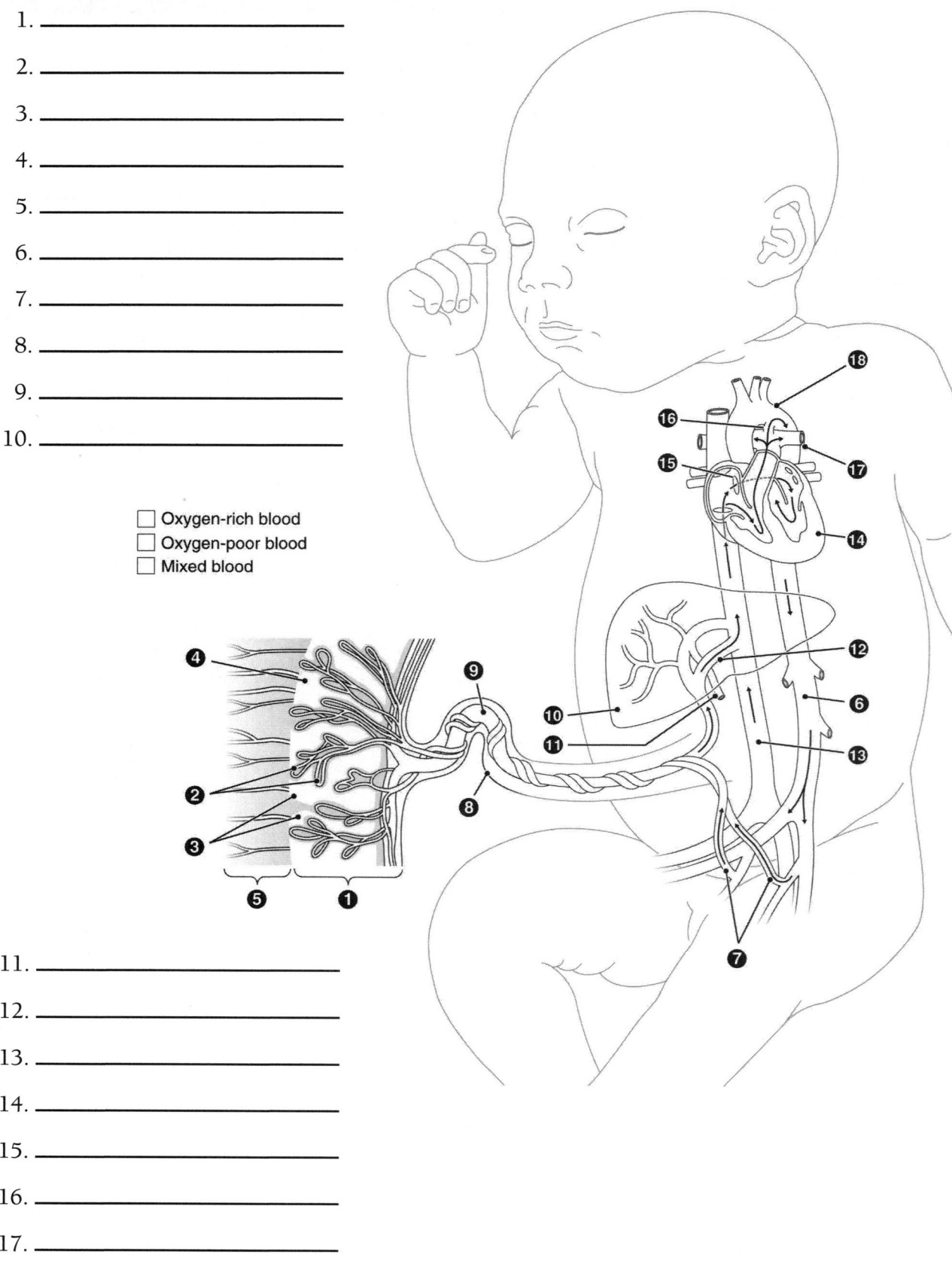

☐ Oxygen-rich blood
☐ Oxygen-poor blood
☐ Mixed blood

11. _____

12. _____

13. _____

14. _____

15. _____

16. _____

17. _____

18. _____

EXERCISE 21-2: Midsagittal Section of a Pregnant Uterus (text Fig. 21-5)
Write the name of each labeled part on the numbered lines.

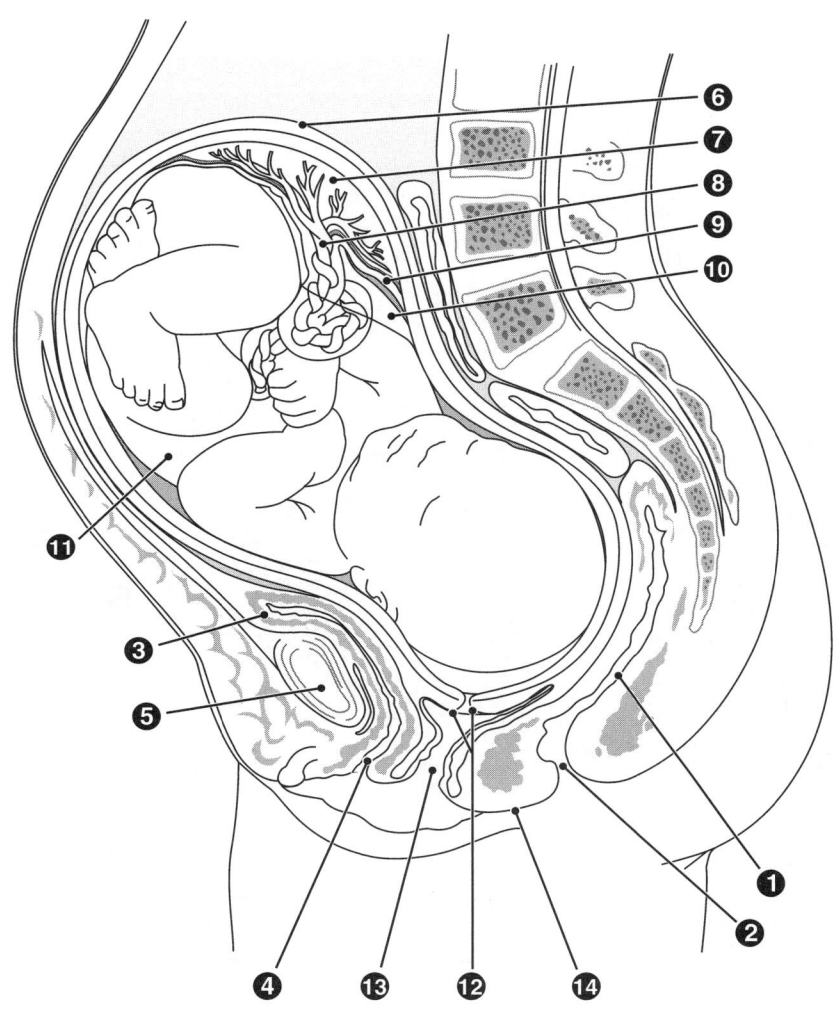

1. _____   8. _____

2. _____   9. _____

3. _____   10. _____

4. _____   11. _____

5. _____   12. _____

6. _____   13. _____

7. _____   14. _____

EXERCISE 21-3: Section of the Breast (text Fig. 21-7)

Write the name of each labeled part on the numbered lines.

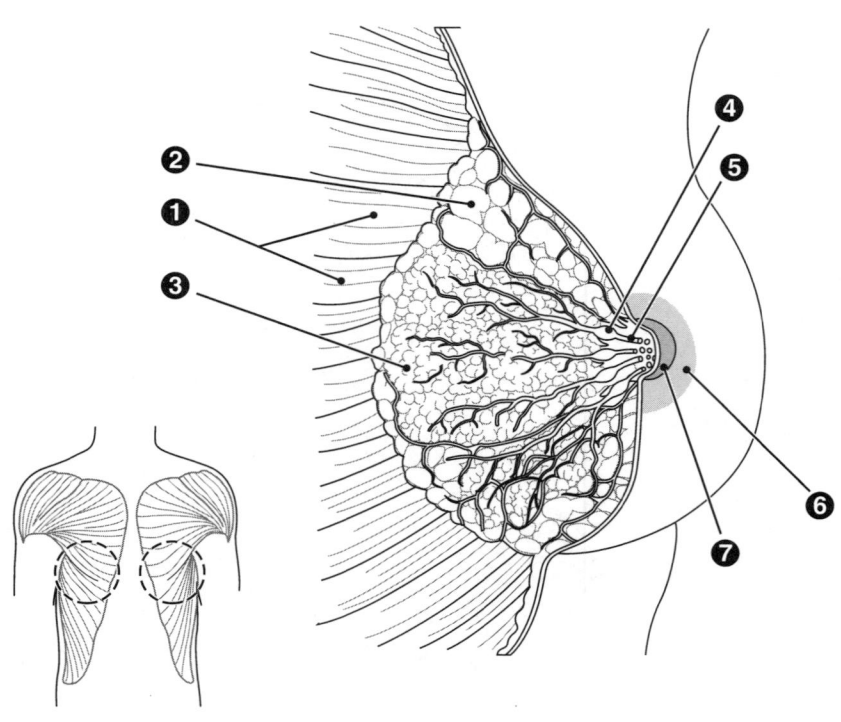

1. _____

2. _____

3. _____

4. _____

5. _____

6. _____

7. _____

Making the Connections

The following concept maps deal with different aspects of development (Map A) and heredity (Map B). Each pair of terms is linked together by a connecting phrase into a sentence. The sentence should be read in the direction of the arrow. Complete the concept map by filling in the appropriate term or phrase. There is one right answer for each term. However, there are many correct answers for the connecting phrases. Write each phrase beside the appropriate number (if space permits) or on a separate sheet of paper

MAP A

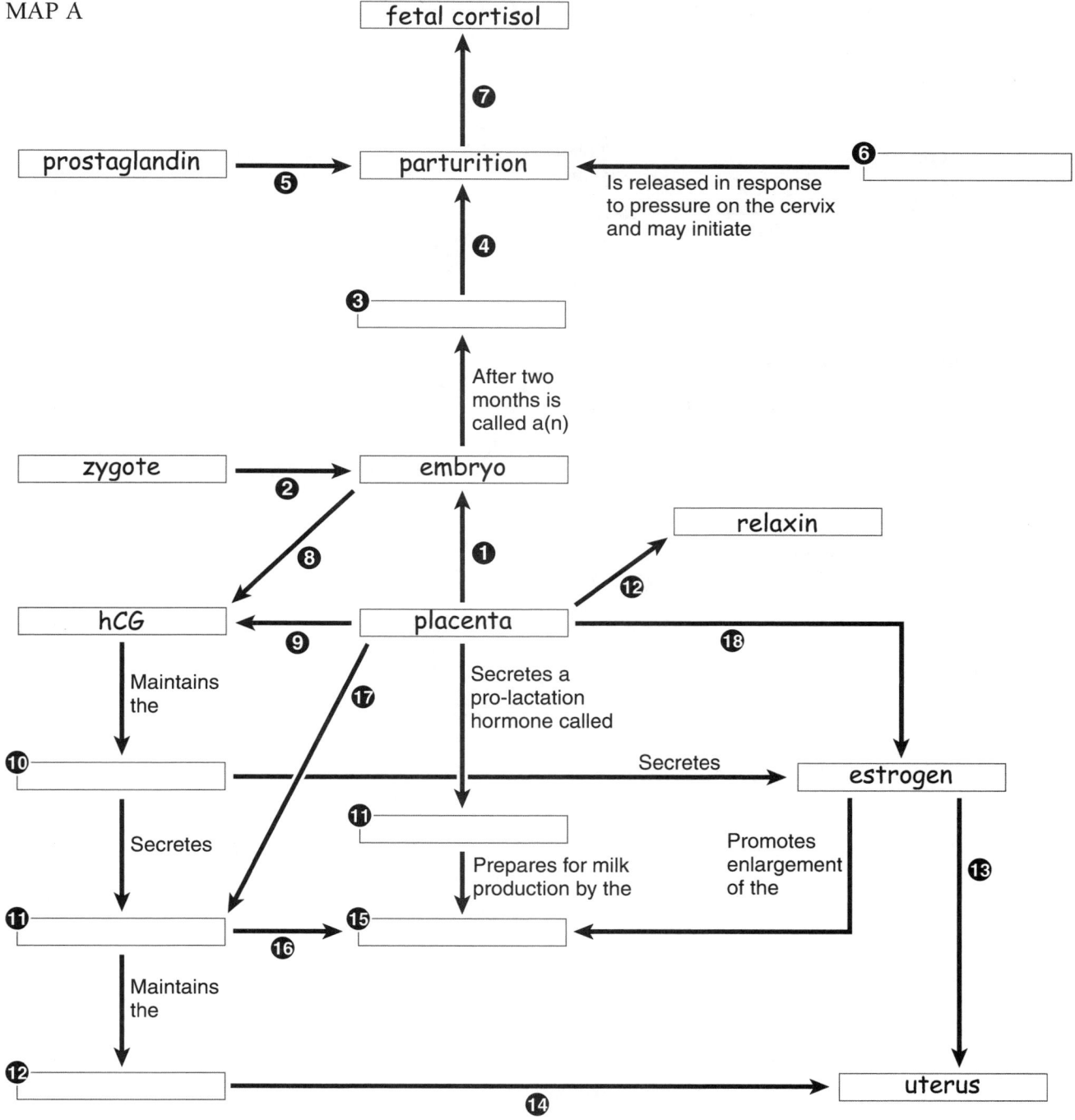

MAP B

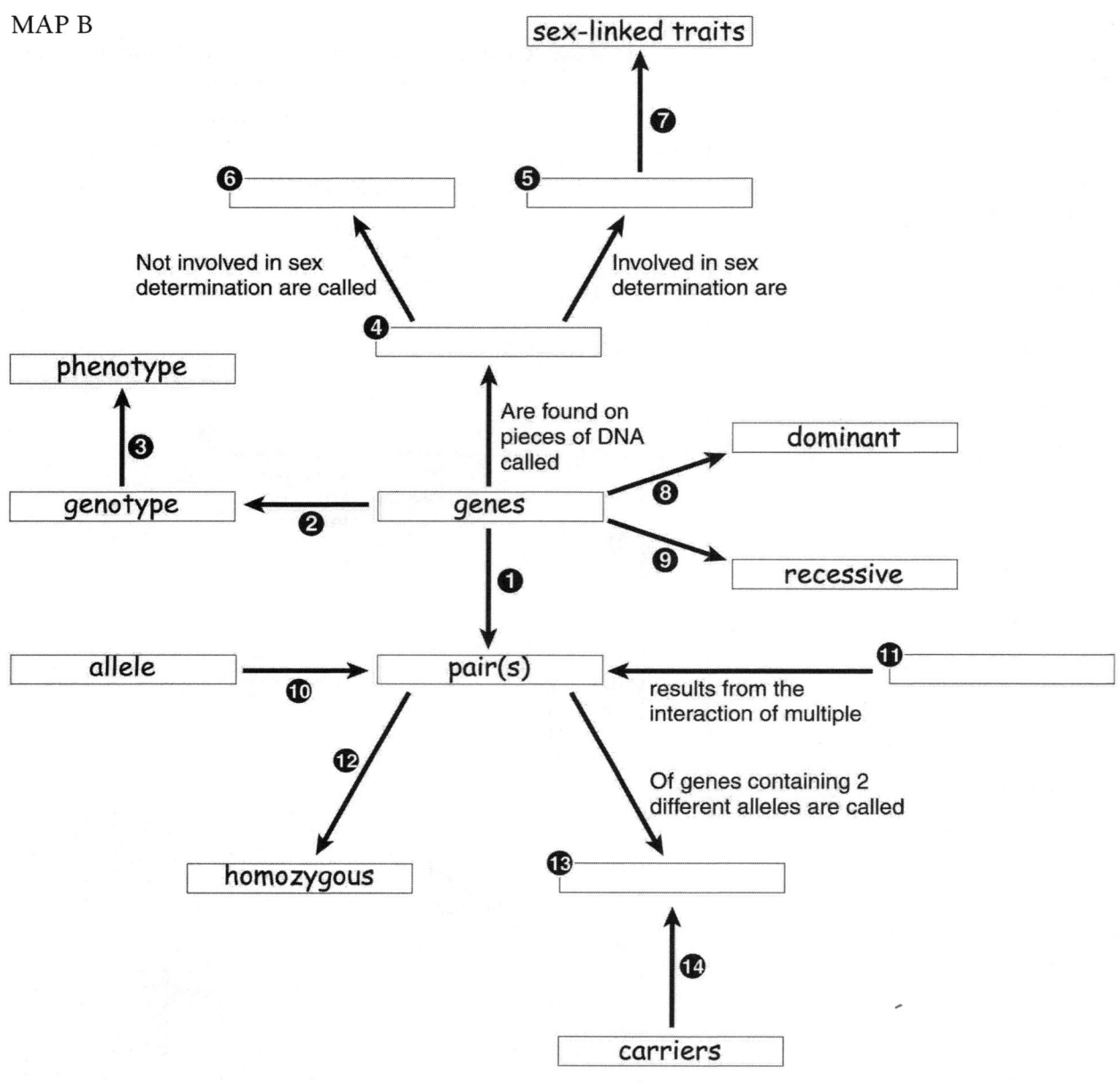

Testing Your Knowledge
Building Understanding

I. Matching Exercises

Matching only within each group, write the answers in the spaces provided.

➤ **Group A**

gestation	zygote	embryo	implantation	placenta
amniotic sac	fetus	venous sinuses	placental villi	umbilical cord

1. The fertilized egg   _____

2. The developing offspring from the third month until birth   _____

3. The structure that serves as the organ for nutrition, respiration, and excretion for the fetus   _____

4. The entire period of development in the uterus   _____

5. The portion of the placenta containing fetal capillaries   _____

6. Attachment of the fertilized egg to the lining of the uterus   _____

7. The structure that surrounds the developing offspring and serves as a protective cushion   _____

8. Channels in the placenta containing maternal blood   _____

➤ **Group B**

human placental lactogen	relaxin	human chorionic gonadotropin	vernix caseosa
oxytocin	cortisol	prostaglandins	ultrasonography
colostrum	prolactin		

1. A hormone that prepares the breasts for lactation and alters maternal metabolism   _____

2. The cheeselike material that protects the skin of the fetus   _____

3. The hormone detected by modern pregnancy tests   _____

4. The hormone that can initiate labor and stimulate milk ejection   _____

5. The pituitary hormone that stimulates milk synthesis   _____

6. The hormone that loosens the pubic symphysis and softens the cervix for parturition   _____

7. A fetal hormone that inhibits maternal progesterone and helps

   initiate labor   _____

8. A technique commonly used to monitor fetal development   _____

➤ **Group C**

carrier	autosome	sex chromosome	allele	recessive
dominant	genotype	phenotype	heterozygous	homozygous

1. The genetic makeup of an individual   _____

2. Term describing a gene that only determines the phenotype if

   homozygous   _____

3. A gene pair consisting of two dominant or two recessive

   alleles   _____

4. Term for a person who has a recessive gene but does not

   exhibit the trait   _____

5. Any chromosome except the X and Y chromosomes   _____

6. One member of a gene pair that controls a specific trait   _____

7. The characteristics that can be observed and/or measured   _____

8. Term describing a gene pair composed of two different alleles   _____

➤ **Group D**

multifactorial	sex-linked	mutation	mutagen	XX
hereditary	XY	DNA	enzyme	Punnett Square

1. The genotype of a female   _____

2. Term for a trait carried on the X chromosome   _____

3. A change in the genetic material of a cell   _____

4. Term indicating that a trait is inherited from a parent   _____

5. The substance that makes up chromosomes   _____

6. A grid used to determine all of the possible

   genotypes of the offspring of a given cross   _____

7. A substance that induces a change in DNA   _____

8. The genotype of a male   _____

II. Multiple Choice

Select the best answer and write the letter of your choice in the blank.

1. Contractions of the myometrium are stimulated by: 1. _____
   a. progesterone
   b. estrogen
   c. prolactin
   d. prostaglandin

2. The fetal circulation is designed to bypass the: 2. _____
   a. lungs
   b. placenta
   c. spleen
   d. brain

3. The second stage of labor includes: 3. _____
   a. the onset of contractions
   b. expulsion of the afterbirth
   c. passage of the fetus through the vagina
   d. expulsion of the placenta

4. Two parents with normal pigmentation can give birth to a child with
   albinism. Albinism is NOT a: 4. _____
   a. recessive disease
   b. dominant trait
   c. congenital disorder
   d. genetic disorder

5. The term *viable* is used to describe a fetus that is: 5. _____
   a. spontaneously aborted
   b. developing outside the uterus
   c. capable of living outside the uterus
   d. stillborn

6. Maternal blood is found in the: 6. _____
   a. umbilical cord
   b. placental villi
   c. venous sinuses of the placenta
   d. all of the above

7. Gender in humans is determined by: 7. _____
   a. the number of X chromosomes
   b. the sex chromosome carried by the ovum
   c. the number of autosomes
   d. the sex chromosome carried by the spermatozoon

8. Traits that are determined by more than one gene pair are termed: 8. _____
   a. sex-linked
   b. recessive
   c. multifactorial
   d. dominant

III. Completion Exercise

Write the word or phrase that correctly completes each sentence.

1. A surgical cut and repair of the perineum to prevent tearing is called a(n) _____

2. By the end of the first month of embryonic life, the beginnings of the extremities may be seen. These are four small swellings called _____

3. The mammary glands of the female provide nourishment for the newborn through the secretion of milk; this is a process called _____

4. The stage of labor during which the afterbirth is expelled from the uterus is called the _____

5. Twins that develop from the same fertilized egg are called _____

6. The normal site of fertilization is the _____

7. The clear liquid that flows from the uterus when the mother's "water breaks" is technically called _____

8. The larger sex chromosome is called the _____

9. A change in a gene or chromosome is called a(n) _____

10. The number of autosomes in the human genome is _____

11. The process of cell division that halves the chromosome number is called _____

12. An agent that induces a change in chromosome structure is called a(n) _____

Understanding Concepts

I. True or False

For each question, write "T" for true or "F" for false in the blank to the left of each number. If a statement is false, correct it by replacing the underlined term and write the correct statement in the blank below the question.

_____ 1. Ms. J is 7 weeks pregnant. Her uterus contains an embryo.

_____

_____ 2. The baby is delivered during the fourth stage of labor.

_____

_____ 3. Fraternal twins are genetically distinct.

_____

_____ 4. Blood is carried from the placenta to the fetus in the umbilical vein.

_____

_____ 5. <u>Oxytocin</u> secreted from the fetal adrenal gland may help induce labor.

_____

_____ 6. Sex-linked traits appear almost exclusively in <u>males</u>.

_____

_____ 7. The sex of the offspring is determined by the sex chromosome carried in the <u>spermato-zoon</u>.

_____

_____ 8. Carriers for a particular gene are always <u>homozygous</u> for the gene.

_____

_____ 9. A recessive trait is expressed in individuals <u>heterozygous</u> for the recessive gene.

_____

II. Practical Applications

Study each discussion. Then write the appropriate word or phrase in the space provided.

➤ Group A

1. Mr. and Ms. L had been trying to conceive for 2 years. Finally, Ms. L realized her period was late and purchased a pregnancy detection kit. These kits test for the presence of a hormone produced exclusively by embryonic tissues that helps maintain the corpus luteum. This hormone is called _____

2. The pregnancy test was positive. Based on the date of her last menstrual period, Ms. L was determined to be 6 weeks pregnant. The gestational age of Ms. L's new offspring at this time would be _____

3. During a prenatal appointment 14 weeks later, Ms. L was able to see her future offspring using a technique for visualizing soft tissues without the use of x-rays. This technique is called _____

4. Baby L was born at 39 weeks' gestation. Ms. L immediately began to breastfeed her infant. The first secretion from her breasts was not milk, but rather _____

➤ Group B

1. Mr. and Ms. J have consulted a genetic counselor. Ms. J is 8 weeks pregnant, and cystic fibrosis runs in both of their families. Cystic fibrosis is a disease in which an individual may carry the disease gene but not have cystic fibrosis. A term to describe this type of trait is _____

2. Mr. and Ms. J were screened for the presence of the cystic fibrosis gene. It was determined that both Mr. and Ms. J have the gene even though they do not have cystic fibrosis. For the cystic fibrosis trait, they are both considered to be _____

3. Ms. J wanted to know if her baby would have cystic fibrosis. Amniocentesis revealed that the fetus carried one normal allele and one cystic fibrosis allele. The fact that the alleles are different means that they can be described as _____

4. The analysis also revealed the presence of two XX chromosomes. The gender of the baby is therefore _____

➤ **Group C**

1. Mr. and Ms. B have a child with three copies of chromosome 21. This abnormality, like any change in DNA, is known as a(n) _____

2. Chromosome 21 is one of 22 pairs of chromosomes known as _____

3. The remainder of the child's chromosomes are normal. The total number of chromosomes in the child's cells is _____

4. The chromosome abnormality arose during the production of gametes. The form of cell division that occurs exclusively in germ cell precursors is called _____

III. Short Essays

1. Compare and contrast human placental lactogen (hPL) and human chorionic gonadotropin (hCG). Discuss the synthesis and action of each hormone.

_____

_____

_____

2. Name the hormones that are involved in lactation and preparing the breasts for lactation, and describe the site of synthesis and action of each hormone.

_____

_____

_____

3. Some traits in a population show a range instead of two clearly alternate forms. List some of these traits, and explain what causes this variety.

_____

_____

_____

Conceptual Thinking

1. Trace the path of a blood cell from the placenta to the fetal heart and back to the placenta. Assume that this blood cell passes through the foramen ovale.

_____

_____

_____

_____

2. Ms. J has had repeated miscarriages. Blood tests reveal a deficiency in progesterone. Could this deficiency be implicated in Ms. J's miscarriages?

_____

_____

_____

3. Are identical twins identical individuals? Defend your answer, using the terms "genotype" and "phenotype."

_____

_____

_____

Expanding Your Horizons

1. Have you ever wondered why animals can give birth alone, but humans require all sorts of technological equipment? Women rarely give birth alone, even in societies with few technological advances. The difficulties of human birth reflect some of our evolutionary adaptations. For instance, walking upright requires the pelvis to be backwards, and the large human brain size results in large fetal skulls. You can read more about "The Evolution of Birth" in Scientific American (Resource 1).

2. The movie *Gattaca* (1997) describes a futuristic world where genetic screening and engineering are the norm. Everyone has a genetic description (including lifespan) available to potential mates, and virtually everyone (except the hero) is genetically engineered. Genetic screening determines one's future on Gattaca, and genetic engineering has essentially abolished independent thought and creativity. Science fiction aside, genetic screening and engineering may soon become a technological reality in our society. What are the implications of genetic screening and engineering? Will a poor genetic outlook affect health insurance coverage and job prospects? Will society genetically engineer away creativity? Resources 2 and 3 can provide you with more information about the use and abuse of genetic testing.

Resource List

Rosenberg KR, Trevathan WR. The evolution of human birth. Sci Am 2001;285:72–77.
Hodge JG Jr. Ethical issues concerning genetic testing and screening in public health. Am J Med Genet 2004;125C:66–70.
Sermon K, Van Steirteghem A, Liebaers I. Preimplantation genetic diagnosis. Lancet 2004;363:1633–1641.Resource List